Beliefs,
Behaviors,
&Alcoholic
Beverages

Mac Marshall, Editor

ANN ARBOR

THE
UNIVERSITY
OF
MICHIGAN
PRESS

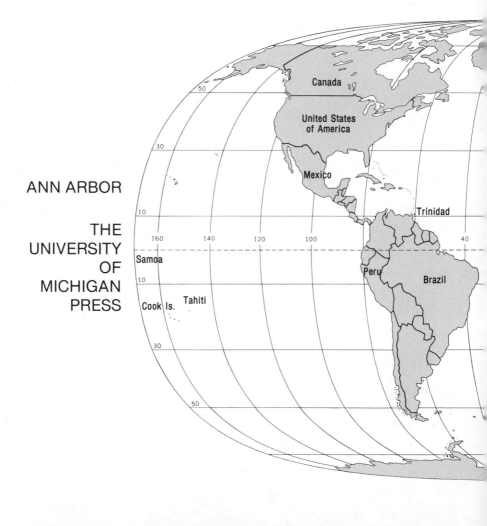

Beliefs, Behaviors, & Alcoholic Beverages

A Cross-Cultural Survey

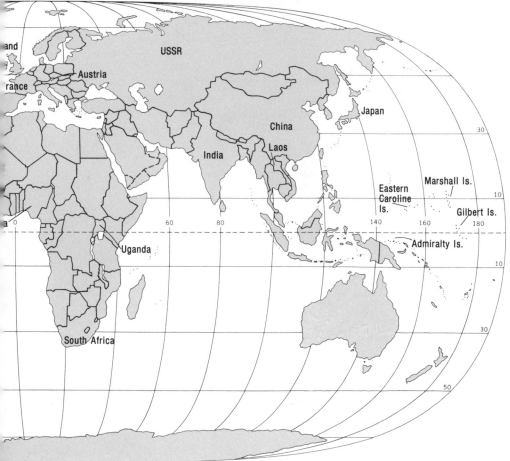

GT
2884
B44
1979

Library of Congress Cataloging in Publication Data
Main entry under title:

Beliefs, behaviors, and alcoholic beverages.

Bibliography: p.
Includes index.
1. Drinking customs—Addresses, essays, lectures.
2. Liquor problem—Addresses, essays, lectures.
3. Cross-cultural studies—Addresses, essays,
lectures. I. Marshall, Mac.
GT2884.B44   394.1'3'08   78-31552
ISBN 0-472-08580-8

Acknowledgments

Grateful acknowledgment is made to the following publishers for permission to reprint copyrighted material:

American Anthropological Association for "Beer as a Locus of Value among the West African Kofyar," by Robert McC. Netting, "Ceremonial Drinking in an Afro-Brazilian Cult," by Seth Leacock, "Forms and Pathology of Drinking in Three Polynesian Societies," by Edwin Lemert; reproduced by permission of the American Anthropological Association from *American Anthropologist*, vol. 66, no. 2, 1964. "Alcohol and the Identity Struggle: Some Effects of Economic Change on Interpersonal Relations," by Richard H. Robbins; reproduced by permission of the American Anthropological Association from *American Anthropologist*, vol. 75, no. 1, 1973. "The Role of the Drunk in a Oaxacan Village," by Philip A. Dennis; reproduced by permission of the American Anthropological Association from *American Anthropologist*, vol. 77, no. 3, 1975.

American Psychiatric Association for "Use of Alcohol and Opium by the Meo of Laos," by Joseph Westermeyer from the *American Journal of Psychiatry*, vol. 127, no. 8, 1971.

Canadian Research Center for Anthropology for "The Role of Alcohol among North American Indian Tribes as reported in *The Jesuit Relations*," by R. C. Dailey from *Anthropologica*, vol. 10, no. 1, 1968.

Department of Health, Education, and Welfare for "Alcohol in Its Cultural Context," by John J. Honigmann from *Proceedings of the First Annual Alcoholism Conference of the National Institute of Alcohol Abuse and Alcoholism*, 1973.

Docent Corporation for "Problem-Drinking and the Integration of Alcohol in Rural Buganda," by Michael C. Robbins from *Medical Anthropology*, vol. 1, no. 3, 1977.

Editors of *British Journal of Addiction* for "The Great Jewish Drink Mystery," by Mark Keller from the *British Journal of Addiction*, vol. 64, 1970, and for "Drinking Patterns and Alcoholism in the Chinese," by K. Singer from the *British Journal of Addiction*, vol. 67, 1972.

Editors of *Ethnology* for "Dynamics of Drinking in an Austrian Village," by John J. Honigmann from *Ethnology*, vol. 2, no. 2, 1963.

Editors of *Ethos* for "Drinking and Inebriate Behavior in the Admiralty Islands, Melanesia," by Theodore Schwartz and Lola Romanucci-Ross from *Ethos*, vol. 2. no. 3, 1974.

Editors of *Journal of Pacific History* for "Holy and Unholy Spirits: The Effects of Missionization on Alcohol Use in Eastern Micronesia," by Mac Marshall and Leslie B. Marshall from *Journal of Pacific History*, vol. 11, no. 3, 1976.

Editors of *Revista de Antropologia* for "Alcohol as a Contributing Factor in Social Disorganization: The South African Bantu in the Nineteenth Century," by Bertram Hutchinson from *Revista de Antropologia*, vol. 9, nos. 1 and 2, 1961.

Editors of *Slavic Review* for "Alcohol and Soviet Society," by Walter D. Connor from *Slavic Review*, vol. 30, no. 3, pp. 570–88, 1971.

B. Edsall & Co., Ltd., for "Alcoholism and the Irish," by Dermot Walsh from *The Journal of Alcoholism*, (now *British Journal on Alcohol and Alcoholism*), vol. 7, no. 2, 1972.

Insight Publishing Co., Inc., for " 'The Drunken Indian': Myths and Realities," by Joseph Westermeyer from *Psychiatric Annals*, vol. 4, no. 9, 1974.

McGill University, Centre for Developing-Area Studies for "Drinking Patterns and Alcoholism in Trinidad," by Carole Yawney from *McGill Studies in Caribbean Anthropology*, edited by Frances Henry, Occasional Paper Series no. 5, 1969.

National Clearinghouse for Alcohol Information for "Alcoholics Anonymous as a Crisis Cult," by William Madsen from *Alcohol Health and Research World*, 1974.

Rutgers University, Journal of Studies on Alcohol, Inc., for "Daru and Bhang: Cultural Factors in the Choice of Intoxicant," by G. M. Carstairs; reprinted by permission from *Quarterly Journal of Studies on Alcohol*, vol. 15, pp. 220–37, 1954. "The Epidemiology of Alcoholic Cirrhosis in Two Southwestern Indian Tribes," by S. J. Kunitz, J. E. Levy, C. L. Odoroff, and J. Bollinger; reprinted by permission from *Quarterly Journal of Studies on Alcohol*, vol. 32, pp. 706–20, 1971. "The Cultural Structure of Mexican Drinking Behavior," by W. Madsen and C. Madsen; reprinted by permission from *Quarterly Journal of Studies on Alcohol*, vol. 30, pp. 701–18, 1969. "Drinking and Attitudes toward Drinking in a Muslim Community," by J. Midgley; reprinted by permission from *Quarterly Journal of Studies on Alcohol*, vol. 32. pp. 148–58, 1971. "Sardines and Other Fried Fish: The Consumption of Alcoholic Beverages on a Micronesian Island," by J. D. Nason; reprinted by permission from *Journal of Studies on Alcohol*, vol. 36, pp. 611–25, 1975. "Changes in Japanese Drinking Patterns," by M. J. Sargent; reprinted by permission from *Quarterly Journal of Studies on Alcohol*, vol. 28, pp. 709–22, 1967. "Notes on Drinking in Japan," by B. Yamamuro; reprinted by permission from *Quarterly Journal of Studies on Alcohol*, vol. 15, pp. 491–98, 1954. Copyright by Journal of Studies on Alcohol, Inc., New Brunswick, New Jersey 08903.

Society for Applied Anthropology for "The Social Uses of Alcoholic Beverages in a Peruvian Community," by Paul L. Doughty from *Human Organization*, vol. 30, no. 2, 1971; "The 'Crisis Cult' as a Voluntary Association: An Interactional Approach to Alcoholics Anonymous," by Patricia O. Sadler from *Human Organization*, vol. 36, no. 2, 1977. Reproduced by permission of the Society for Applied Anthropology.

Transaction Periodicals Consortium for "How French Children Learn to Drink," by Barbara Gallatin Anderson. Published by permission of Transaction, Inc., from *Transaction*, vol. 5, no. 7. Copyright © 1968 by Transaction, Inc.

University of California Press for "The World's Oldest On-Going Protest Demonstration: North American Indian Drinking Patterns," by Nancy Oestreich Lurie from *Pacific Historical Review*, vol. 40, no. 3, 1971.

University of Chicago Press for "Alcohol and Culture," by David Mandelbaum from *Current Anthropology*, vol. 6, no. 3, 1965. Copyright © The University of Chicago.

Preface

During the past twenty years three collections of articles devoted wholly or in part to the cross-cultural literature on alcohol use have appeared. Each of these three books has made an important contribution to the field of alcohol studies, but each suffers from certain shortcomings that limit its usefulness for those who wish an introduction to the extensive sociocultural literature on alcoholic beverages and drunken comportment. The volumes edited by McCarthy (1959) and Pittman and Snyder (1962) have two major limitations today. First, these books are outdated in terms of the recent explosion of studies in the field of alcohol and culture (see Introduction), and second, no more than one-fourth of either book is devoted to the *cross-cultural* literature on alcohol. While Everett, Waddell, and Heath's recent volume (1976) represents a compilation of the cross-cultural literature on drinking behavior, it also suffers from two serious drawbacks: it is very expensive, and it is addressed primarily to a professional audience rather than to students and practitioners.

With this in mind, I have edited the present volume to fill a substantial gap in the literature. In a single, relatively inexpensive form, this book brings together up-to-date, readable examples from the social science literature on alcohol use and abuse around the world. Most of the articles reprinted herein have appeared since 1965, and more than half have been published since 1970. Slight editing of the original articles has been done so that the book conforms to a common cohesive style.

As a teacher I have been frustrated by the lack of good, current material in a handy format that I could assign students in my course on alcohol and culture. I am confident that others offering similar courses have also experienced this frustration. I offer this book in the hope that it will serve both student and professional for years to come as a convenient sourcebook on the subject.

MAC MARSHALL

Contents

Introduction

Mac Marshall

The cross-cultural study of alcohol presents a classic natural experiment: a single species (*Homo sapiens*), a single drug substance (ethanol), and a great diversity of behavioral outcomes. Among behavioral scientists, it is anthropologists in particular who seek explanations for human similarities and differences in natural experiments of this sort.

The few studies by physical anthropologists of alcohol use in different human populations fall within the bounds of this classic quest since no other drug substance—with the possible exception of nicotine—is ingested by so many different people around the world. Although evidence is accumulating to show that some biological differences exist among human populations, and among individuals within these populations, in reactivity to ethanol or its metabolites (e.g., Hanna 1976, 1977; Zeiner 1978), no generally accepted theory has yet emerged to explain how alcoholic beverages differentially affect "racial" or "ethnic" groups. While a better understanding of the physiological effects of ethanol on human beings seems sure to contribute to a solution of the complex psychophysiological affliction of alcoholism, the thrust of this book lies elsewhere.

There is no question today that cultural factors influence both the use and abuse of alcoholic beverages in important ways, including ways relevant to the treatment of alcohol problems. In the pages to follow we will sample the recent literature on how cultural factors define and limit the attitudes, values, and behaviors that accompany drinking. Adopting this stance by no means implies that cultural factors alone account for the revealed differences in problem and addictive drinking found around the world. Such a viewpoint does emphasize, however, that any serious attempt to understand and treat abusers of alcohol or any other drug substance cannot ignore cultural considerations.

Beverage alcohol is a nearly universal drug today and has

been so in most of the world for hundreds, even thousands, of years. Only Pacific Islanders and the indigenes of most of North America failed to discover the manufacture of alcoholic beverages on their own. In both cases Europeans introduced them to the joys and sorrows of "ardent spirits." Traditional drinks containing ethanol—the active ingredient in beverage alcohol—were made throughout Middle and Latin America in pre-Columbian times, as well as throughout Africa and Asia, and were commonplace in Europe. Because fermentation is a natural process alcoholic drinks can be produced from cereals, fruits, roots, tree sap, and a host of other media. Whatever the substance employed to manufacture beverage alcohol, however, the active ingredient remains the same; all that varies is the concentration of ethanol which depends on whether the drink is brewed (as in beer), fermented (as in wine), or distilled (as in whiskey).

Given their antiquity and geographic distribution, alcoholic beverages remain the best known and most widely used means of altering human consciousness. Ethanol's psychopharmacological properties have led humans the world over to surround alcoholic beverages with a great variety of rules and regulations bearing little consistency from culture to culture. How one should feel, how one should act, what one may say, when and where one may drink and with whom—these and other guidelines are specified in advance for the person who would consume alcoholic beverages. Despite the great diversity in rules for drinking and the behaviors that accompany it, however, certain cross-cultural generalizations that contribute in important ways to our understanding of the involved relationship between alcohol and humanity have emerged from the ethnographic literature. The articles that follow illustrate many of these generalizations which will be specified and discussed in the conclusions to this volume.

The field of anthropology has never held center stage in the interdisciplinary scientific explorations of alcohol use and abuse that have been conducted in the Western world for a century or more. A major reason for this lies not only in the fact that relatively few anthropologists have set out specifically to study alcohol use (Heath 1974b), but also because, historically, few anthropologists have been especially interested in the treatment of alcohol problems at home or abroad. Rather, as part of their larger effort to comprehend alien ways of life, anthropologists have documented the diversity of accepted, customary ways in which the world's peoples manufacture and consume these beverages. Anthropologists have been intrigued primarily by the myriad styles of *normal* drinking behavior that exist when people come under the influence of "demon rum." In keeping with the discipline's holistic approach to data anthropologists have been at pains to point out how alcohol use (and, occasionally, alcohol abuse) is woven into the very fabric of social existence. Although a majority of the sociocultural litera- ture on drinking behavior has been written by anthropologists (see Heath 1974*a* and 1976 for excellent summaries of this literature), scholars from related fields have also made important contributions to this body of knowledge. As the pages to follow demonstrate, psychologists, psychiatrists, sociologists, and historians have been especially prominent in this regard.

Anthropologists produced a smattering of publications on the manufacture and consumption of alcoholic beverages before 1940, but these topics have received a great deal more attention subsequently. This greater attention is partly a result of growth within the field of anthropology itself. It also stems, however, from publication in the early 1940s of two important works that continue to influence anthropologists interested in alcohol studies.

Bunzel's well-known paper (1940) pioneered the first major anthropological approach to alcohol and culture: keen, in-depth ethnographic reporting that seeks to explain why people in a par- ticular culture drink and comport themselves in a particular way. Bunzel's paper also represented the first "controlled comparison" between similar cultures that employed alcoholic beverages in strikingly different ways.

Horton's famous work (1943), published in an early volume of the *Quarterly Journal of Studies on Alcohol,* established the second major anthropological approach to alcohol on a solid foot- ing. Relying on the ethnographic reports of others, rather than on his own field work, and employing a sample of fifty-six different societies on which he could obtain adequate information, Horton was the first to conduct a statistical cross-cultural comparative study of alcohol use. His goal was to ascertain whether certain characteristics of the societies in his sample correlated with the differing ways their members used and reacted to alcoholic bever- ages. To this end he tested a series of hypotheses centering on the assumption that humans' major motivation to drink was to reduce anxiety brought on by either a precarious subsistence base or ac- culturation pressures.

Building on Bunzel's and Horton's contributions other an- thropologists began to explore the relationships between alcohol and culture during the 1950s. Heath (1976) asserts that the number of publications on alcohol from "an anthropological perspective" was twice as great between 1955 and 1959 as in the previous decade, and that the volume of such publications doubled again between 1960 and 1964. By the 1970s anthropologists in growing numbers were setting out to study the beliefs and behaviors surrounding the use of alcohol. This most recent development is particularly important since "a feature that sets 'alcohol studies' apart from many other topical emphases in behavioral and historical studies is that the majority of the pertinent data and observations have been serendipitous by-products of research that had very different foci of concern" (Heath 1977:4–5). Today alcohol studies in anthropology are no longer simply a result of serendipity. While observations on non-Western drinking customs continue to be made ancillary to other research concerns, alcohol and culture as a specialized subject has come to preoccupy an increasing number of scholars in the discipline. This newfound concern for alcohol may be seen in several ways.

To begin with, a substantial number of anthropological theses and dissertations completed since the mid-1960s have focused on aspects of alcohol and culture.[1] A number of major symposia[2] on alcohol use have been convened at professional meetings in recent years (e.g., Everett, Waddell, and Heath 1976; Marshall 1974a), and during the past decade the published literature on alcohol and culture has become extensive enough to spawn a variety of bibliographies and review articles designed to introduce newcomers to the field (e.g., Freund and Marshall 1977; Heath 1974a, 1976, 1977; Mail and McDonald 1977; Marshall 1974b). Finally, since 1970, the results of anthropological research projects devoted primarily or exclusively to the beliefs and behaviors associated with alcoholic beverages have begun to appear. Many of these studies offer a wealth of detailed data heretofore unavailable in the ethnographic record for non-Western societies (e.g., Levy and Kunitz 1974; Wolcott 1974; Marshall 1979).

The cross-cultural literature on alcohol use is uneven in quality and quantity. For example, the encounter of North American Indians with ethanol has been documented extensively over the years, and the very size of the literature on this subject may have contributed in part to the rise and continued existence of the "firewater myth," which suggests that Indians have a peculiar biological susceptibility to ethanol (Leland 1976). Accounts of the consumption of beverage alcohol by Pacific Islanders or Asians, on the other hand, are much more limited in number. Allowing for these discrepancies in the published record, the articles contained in this book have been selected to provide as wide a geographic coverage as possible and to provide interesting and accurate examples from the sociocultural literature on alcohol use that convey an appreciation of the range of variation in behavior and belief accompanying alcohol around the world.

In Section I, Mandelbaum and Honigmann offer succinct overviews of the diversity of topics that have been explored under the rubric "alcohol and culture." Mandelbaum discusses the relationships among individual personalities, alcohol use, and culture; the likenesses and differences in alcohol use within major world regions; changes or stability of ideas and behaviors accompanying drinking over time within a single culture and cross-culturally; and broad-scale similarities and differences in alcohol use worldwide. To this Honigmann adds the problem of intracultural diversity in reaction to alcohol, the problem of looking only at extreme or pathological use of alcohol to the exclusion of studies of normal drinking, and the varied symbolism of alcoholic beverages from culture to culture.

Section II of the book explores the meaning and use of alcoholic beverages in Mexico, Peru, Brazil, and among East Indians and blacks in Trinidad. Madsen and Madsen employ the method of controlled comparison to investigate the ways ethnicity and class interact to produce different sets of values and expectations toward drinking and drunkenness in Mexico. The authors emphasize the ways in which group drinking of pulque—a traditionally produced alcoholic beverage—has become a major symbol of the Indian way of life in Tecospan. Drinking by Indians within their own community is surrounded by an aura of sacredness carried over from Aztec times. Such drinking is distinguished by a notable lack of aggression and an emphasis on peaceful cooperation. In contrast to this integrative Indian drinking, Madsen and Madsen present data for the mestizo community of Tepepan where a great deal of belligerence accompanies consumption of alcoholic beverages. This aggressivity is heightened by the introduced Hispanic value on masculine machismo, leading the authors to conclude that mestizo drinking is socially divisive.

Dennis provides another perspective on alcohol use from a different part of Mexico. He analyzes the "drunk role" in Amilpas as a social performance comparable to that of the fool or jester in Shakespearean drama. Amilpas drunks are given great license to say things unspeakable by sober persons, and Dennis points out the important place the drunk role occupies in community life. He concludes that "social drunkenness" rather than physical inebriation is what defines the drunk role—a conclusion that may be generalized to many other societies as well.

Doughty, like Madsen and Madsen, offers a discussion of present-day mestizo drinking, this time for Peru. He observes that most drinking in Hualyas is ceremonial, that there are few problem drinkers, and that there is little ambivalence about alcohol, but notes that, despite the generally positive value placed on alcoholic beverages, Western values via acculturation have begun to lead to a modest rise in alcohol problems. Class and religious differences in alcohol use are noted, along with a description of the variety of alcoholic beverages used. Doughty concludes that the ritual of drinking in this community emphasizes social solidarity.

Leacock's material on alcohol use in the Batuque cult of Brazil presents a rather different view. Noting that the cult has African origins but that it has been heavily influenced by Indian and spiritualist beliefs, Leacock suggests that cult members believe themselves possessed by spirits (*encantados*) who "drink" through or via the person possessed. Excellent data are provided on the use of rum in curing rituals and public ceremonies, and Leacock observes that rum has become a substitute for traditional Indian hallucinogens used to induce possession.

Yawney offers controlled comparison of two different ethnic groups in the plural society of Trinidad. Whereas Madsen and Madsen argue that pulque is a symbol of Indianness, Yawney maintains that rum is a symbol of Trinidadian national identity. Even so, East Indians in Trinidad are ambivalent about alcohol while blacks are not. Yawney focuses on these different attitudes and discusses how variations in child-rearing and religious beliefs lead to what she perceives to be greater problems with alcohol among East Indians.

Section III of the book samples the large literature on North American Indian drinking. Westermeyer's contribution in this section helps demolish both the stereotype of the "drunken Indian" and the "firewater myth." This is followed by Dailey's analysis of Jesuit documents from early in the contact period, in which the complexity of Indian drinking motives and styles is given a historical dimension. Dailey stresses that liquor was just one among the many aspects of introduced European culture that affected American Indians simultaneously, and that it is not always possible to assert unequivocally that alcohol *caused*, for example, tribal breakdown. Dailey makes the important suggestion that drunken comportment was patterned on beliefs that existed before liquor arrived on the scene (e.g., the dream quest) and notes some of the ways firewater was used by whites to exploit the Indians economically.

Lurie further develops Westermeyer's point that the stereotype of the drunken Indian impedes an understanding of the myriad motives and uses associated with drinking by native Americans. She hypothesizes that Indian drinking is an established means of asserting and validating Indianness. In the process of testing this hypothesis she reinforces points made by Dennis on the drunk role and by Madsen and Madsen on the symbolic importance of alcohol as an ethnic boundary marker.

An approach unlike any other in this volume is employed by Kunitz et al. The epidemiological analysis of documentary and field-work data for the Hopi and the Navajo highlights different tribal patterns and problems in alcohol abuse. Among other things, they reach the interesting conclusion that the social drinking of Navajos places them at less risk of developing cirrhosis than does the solitary drinking of the Hopi.

R. H. Robbins is concerned with the identity of the drunk among the Naskapi of Quebec, specifically the ways in which drinking bouts serve as what he calls "identity-resolving forums." During drinking bouts persons engage in public performances designed to maintain, attain, or protect desired identities or social positions. Robbins shows how drinking bouts work to rearrange the social hierarchy in a situation of rapid economic change. Echoing Dennis, Robbins claims that the social position of the actor, rather than the amount of alcohol consumed, determines the form of drinking behavior for individual Naskapi.

Section IV of the book discusses alcohol use in Polynesia, Micronesia, and Melanesia. Lemert offers an elegant controlled comparison of drinking and drunken comportment in three historically related Polynesian cultures: the Society Islands (Tahiti), the Cook Islands, and Samoa. He shows that intoxication has become reasonably well integrated with the basic values of Society Islanders in a pattern he labels "festive drinking." Largely as a consequence of missionary pressures the islanders of the southern Cooks developed a rather different mode of drinking which Lemert calls "ritual-disciplined." This style of drinking was highly controlled and regulated, and—reminiscent of Lurie's conclusion about North American Indians—became a kind of protest movement against colonial overlords (cf. Lemert 1976). Finally, Lemert argues that "secular" drinking in Western Samoa is unintegrated with basic Samoan values and directly inimical to the Samoan way of life.

The symbolic importance of intemperance and abstinence in the contact between Micronesians and outsiders during the nineteenth century provides the central theme of Marshall and Marshall's article. Here historical materials are used to document how the renunciation of alcohol became the primary symbol of conversion to Christianity in eastern Micronesia, a matter also touched upon briefly by Schwartz and Romanucci-Ross.

In a fashion similar to Madsen and Madsen, Dailey, and Lurie for other parts of the world, Nason argues that the drinking of alcoholic beverages on Etal Atoll maintains and reinforces important traditional values and attitudes. Nason gives most of his attention to the ways in which drinking bouts permit masculine risk taking in culturally approved ways and demonstrates how drunkenness provides a social release for persons undergoing stressful experiences in this tiny, isolated Micronesian community (cf. Marshall 1979).

Schwartz and Romanucci-Ross occupy the rare and enviable position of having observed the initial public use of ethanol by persons in the community where they conducted research. They meticulously document the creation of the "state and the status" of the drunk on Manus Island, Melanesia (cf. Dennis), and provide an interesting interpretation of how drunkenness fits in with pre-existing cultural beliefs.

The consumption of alcoholic beverages throughout the continent of Asia is considered in the articles in Section V. Yamamuro and Sargent offer complementary perspectives on Japanese drinking. Yamamuro sketches the important historical and religious influences that have shaped Japanese attitudes toward alcoholic beverages. Particularly important in his view are historical influences from China, Korea, and—in the post–World-War-II era—from the Americans and the British, and the religious traditions of Confucianism, Buddhism, and Shintoism. Sargent's article is a contemporary sociological analysis of the changes in the use of beverage alcohol among the Japanese. She agrees with Yamamuro that drinking was traditionally integrated in Japan, occurring largely in a ritual and ceremonial context, but that in more recent years increasing numbers of Japanese have begun to drink to reduce anxiety.

Westermeyer and Carstairs both consider the reasons for selecting one drug over another. Writing about the Meo tribesmen of Laos, Westermeyer explains why alcohol is used by greater numbers of persons in social and ceremonial settings than is opium, and why opium is employed in other ways and contexts.

Carstairs presents a controlled comparison of two different Indian castes. Members of the Rajput warrior caste are permitted to consume alcoholic beverages and seldom use cannabis. Members of the Brahman priestly caste, on the other hand, scorn alcohol use while consuming large amounts of cannabis. Carstairs suggests that reasons for these choices can be understood by reference to sacred and secular values.

The Chinese, along with members of the Jewish faith, have received frequent mention in the sociocultural literature on alcohol because of their reputed lack of problem drinking. Singer's study of the Chinese in Hong Kong demonstrates that some Chinese do indeed develop drinking problems, but he offers cogent reasons why most do not. Like Yamamuro he gives special emphasis to the influence of Confucianism and, in addition, points out that for most Chinese alcohol is considered a food to be consumed at meals, rather than a special drug (cf. Doughty, Netting, and Anderson). Finally, in the same vein as Westermeyer and Carstairs, Singer comments on the choice of intoxicants among the Chinese.

Much of the literature on African drinking is contained in books rather than in journal articles. Section VI provides examples of the latter for South, East, and West Africa. Hutchinson presents a historical treatment of the effects of acculturation on alcohol use among the Bantu peoples of southern Africa, comparable to those of Dailey on North America and Marshall and Marshall on Micronesia. He comments on the traditional importance and integrated use of "kaffir beer" which was upset by the intrusion of European society. The article provides an excellent illustration of how changing patterns of drinking may be used as a barometer of sociocultural change.

Most of the world's major religions have at one time or another advocated abstinence on the part of their practitioners. Islam is no exception, as shown in Midgley's sociological account of drinking attitudes and behavior among the Cape Malay Muslims of South Africa.

Netting provides a case study of a society where beer occupies a central focus of daily life. Kofyar drink large amounts of beer on almost a daily basis, yet drunken fights and problem drinking are largely unknown. Netting's article illustrates the ways in which the cultural values associated with drinking limit potentially disruptive behavior.

M. C. Robbins examines the hypothesis that culturally integrated alcohol use will not lead to problem drinking. Using data from Uganda, he concludes that the hypothesis receives "modest support" from his study.

Section VII brings us full circle to the use of alcoholic beverages in Europe and the United States. In the first two articles, Madsen and Sadler present differing interpretations of the "crisis cult" analogy as an explanation for the success of Alcoholics Anonymous in controlling the drinking of its American members (see also Bateson 1971).

Walsh uses historical sources to trace Irish beliefs about alcoholic beverages and concludes that the association of alcohol with the heroic tradition in which drinking and drunkenness are glorified may partially explain the well-known Irish propensity for problem drinking.

Keller discusses the ways in which history and religion have affected changing patterns of Jewish drinking over the centuries. His account of the role of religious variables may be compared profitably with the findings of Yamamuro, Carstairs, and Singer.

In the next two articles, the place of drinking in the daily social round of an Austrian village and a French village is explored by Honigmann and Anderson, respectively. Honigmann stresses the association between alcohol and gaiety and sociability within a ceremonial context, showing how Austrian drinking forms part of a larger cultural configuration. Anderson discusses French beliefs about wine, that it symbolizes health and virility and is believed to have important nutritive value. From this she goes on to show how French children, introduced to alcohol at a very young age, grow up to view wine as an essential part of every meal.

The final article in Section VII is an insightful glimpse into drinking behavior in contemporary (European) Soviet society. Connor compiles information from a great variety of sources to illustrate the use of alcoholic beverages in the Soviet Union and governmental attempts to deal with problem drinking.

All the ethnographic accounts contained in this book show the necessity of understanding the variety of normal drinking styles in any social setting before attempting to deal with abnormal (or addictive) drinking. The sociocultural literature on alcohol use has made its greatest contribution in helping us to understand that values and attitudes—including changing historical circumstances—provide the settings within which drinking takes place. To solve the complicated riddle of alcoholism will require not only biomedical and psychological studies of alcohol use, but also

sensitive and detailed studies of the great variety of drinking beliefs and behaviors within and across cultural boundaries. Only
when all these approaches are melded together will the complete
picture of the human encounter with alcohol begin to come into
focus.

Notes

1. An extensive review conducted by the author shows that more
than thirty theses and dissertations concerning alcohol and culture were
completed at colleges and universities in the United States between 1965
and 1977. A majority of these were finished during the 1970s.

2. Appropriately, the word "symposium" literally means "a drinking together."

I. Overview of Alcohol Studies and Anthropology

Alcohol and Culture

David G. Mandelbaum

There are a great many substances that men have learned to ingest in order to get special bodily sensations. Of them all, alcohol is culturally the most important by far. It was anciently the most widespread in use, the most widely valued as a ritual and societal artifact, the most deeply embedded in diverse cultures. Tribal peoples of all major parts of the world (save Oceania and most of North America) knew alcoholic drink; it was of considerable interest in the principal civilizations, in most of them from their early beginnings onward. In some languages, as in English, the very term "drink" takes on the connotation of drinking alcoholic liquids.

Where alcohol is known, patterns for its use and for abstention are prescribed, usually in fine detail. There have been very few, if any, societies whose people knew the use of alcohol and yet paid little attention to it. Alcohol may be tabooed; it is not ignored.

In many societies, drinking behavior is considered important for the whole social order, and so drinking is defined and limited in accordance with fundamental motifs of the culture. Hence it is useful to ask what the form and meanings of drink in a particular group tell us about their entire culture and society. In a complex modern society, made up of many subgroups, the drinking patterns of each subgroup or class may reflect its special characteristics as well as the cultural frame of the whole society.

The same kind of question can be asked about the drinking patterns of an individual. Given the cultural definitions for drinking in his society, what does his characteristic drinking behavior tell us about his personality? Within most cultural prescriptions there is leeway for individual choice and manipulation. But before we can learn much about the configuration of his personality from a person's drinking activities, we must understand what choices about drinking are possible in his culture. These encompassing cultural factors are not often made clear in studies of drinking behavior and figure little in the literature on drinking pathology.

Cultural Variations in the Use of Alcohol

Cultural practices in drinking range from avid immersion to total rejection. Anthropologists know this well, but those who study the social problems of use of alcohol do not always take this fact into account. Even a brief mention of the varied social functions of alcohol and the different cultural expressions of these functions points up the central importance of viewing the act of drinking as part of a larger cultural configuration. Alcohol is a cultural artifact; the form and meanings of drinking alcoholic beverages are culturally defined, as are the uses of any other major artifact. The form is usually quite explicitly stipulated, including the kind of drink that can be used, the amount and rate of intake, the time and place of drinking, the accompanying ritual, the sex and age of the drinker, the roles involved in drinking, and the role behavior proper to drinking. The meanings of drinking, its relation to other aspects of the culture and society, are usually more implicit. Thus drinking in a particular society may be either a sacred or a profane act, depending on the context, and the people may not be aware of the basic principles and meanings that are actually involved. These may become apparent only after studies have been made of the contexts of drinking and the behavior of drinkers.

At the extremes of the range of cultural practice the meanings are relatively clear. For example, among the Kofyar of northern Nigeria, "people make, drink, talk, and think about beer." In the religious sphere, "the Kofyar certainly believe that man's way to god is with beer in hand" (Netting 1964:377, also in this volume: 352).

In contrast with those who consider alcohol to be essential and blessed are the people who regard it as destructive and dispensable. The Hopi and other Pueblo Indian tribes of the American Southwest felt that drinking threatened their way of life. They abhorred the use of alcohol so greatly that they successfully banned it from their settlements for many years (Parsons 1939; Benedict 1959*b*).

The range of religious usage is great. Among the Aztecs, for example, worshipers at every major religious occasion had to get dead drunk, else the gods would be displeased (J. Thompson 1940:68). In sharp contrast are those Protestant denominations which hold that alcohol is so repugnant spiritually that it is not allowed even symbolically in the communion rite (Cherrington 1924). Yet another contrast is that provided in India, where a villager may pour an alcoholic libation in the worship of one type of deity (usually of the locality), while to do so at a temple of one of the deities of the classic pantheon would desecrate the place and disgrace the worshiper.

Cultural expectations regulate the emotional consequences of drink. Drinking in one society may regularly release demonstrations of affection, as is common among Japanese men; in another it may set off aggressive hostility, as frequently occurs among Papago Indians (Joseph, Spicer, and Chesky 1949). Among Japanese, drinking is part of the fine ambience of pleasant physical sensation—when done at the proper time and place—and so is quite devoid of guilt or ambivalence. Conversely, there are other people among whom drinking is often accompanied by a flow of guilt feeling.

The act of drinking can serve as a symbolic punctuation mark differentiating one social context from another (cf. Honigmann 1963, also in this volume, Sec. VII). The cocktail prepared by the suburban housewife for her commuting husband when he returns in the evening helps separate the city and its work from the home and its relaxation. In more formal ritual, but with similar distinguishing intent, an orthodox Jew recites the habdalah blessing over wine and drinks the wine at the end of the Sabbath to mark the division between the sacred day and the rest of the week. Drinking may be quite purely symbolic, as it is in the habdalah rite and in the sacrament of communion, or it may be substantive as well as symbolic, as in the heavy drinking at Aztec religious ceremonies.

Among other symbolic uses of drinking are its diacritical functions, as when one group or class within a larger society follows drinking patterns that serve as a badge marking them off from others. Such a badge may be deliberately adopted by the members of the group or may be ascribed to them by others, but when a sectarian group forbids drinking to its devotees, the prohibition is often deliberately taken as a counterbadge to separate the elect from the forlorn.

The physiological effects attributed to alcohol vary just as greatly among different peoples. Some are ready to feel high effect from a modicum of drink. Thus it has seemed to more than one Westerner that a Japanese man feels the convivial glow almost before the first sip of sake can reach the stomach. Among Aleut Indians, drinking leads more to surly drunkenness than to mellow conviviality, but among them also a drinker becomes intoxicated after he has taken relatively small amounts of a fairly mild beverage (G. Berreman 1956). In other societies a man must absorb a large amount of alcohol before he shows that the drink has affected him. So is it also with hangovers and addiction; both are heavily influenced by cultural interpretations. A people who drink as heavily and as frequently as any group yet known, the Camba of eastern Bolivia, attribute no ill effects to their drinking other than the irritation caused to the mouth and throat by their liquor, an undiluted distillate of sugarcane that contains 89 percent ethyl alcohol.

Most Camba men participate in recurrent drinking bouts, which may last for a whole weekend. A drinker may pass out several times in the course of a bout and, upon reviving, drink himself quickly into a stupor again. Dwight Heath, the anthropologist who has studied Camba drinking, observes: "Hangovers and hallucinations are unknown among these people, as is addiction to alcohol" (1962:31). In general, addiction to alcohol seems to be quite rare outside certain societies of Western civilization. Among most peoples whose men are expected to drink heavily and frequently, a man does not do any solitary drinking nor does he have withdrawal symptoms if he cannot get alcohol. He may not like to do without it, but he does not feel gripped by an iron compulsion to get a drink in order to be able to keep alive.

The chemical and physiological properties of alcohol obviously provide a necessary base for drinking behavior; the same kinds of behavior are not socially derived from other widely used drugs, such as coffee, tea, or tobacco. But the behavioral consequences of drinking alcohol depend as much on a people's idea of what alcohol does to a person as they do on the physiological processes that take place (cf. Washburne 1961). When a man lifts a cup, it is not only the kind of drink that is in it, the amount he is likely to take, and the circumstances under which he will do the drinking that are specified in advance for him, but also whether the contents of the cup will cheer or stupefy, whether they will induce affection or aggression, guilt or unalloyed pleasure. These and many other cultural definitions attach to the drink even before it touches the lips.

Similarities across Cultures

Cultural variations in drinking practices are well documented, but there has been little notice of similarities in the use of alcohol across cultures. One such regularity is that drinking is usually considered more suitable for men than for women. It is commonly a social rather than a solitary activity but is done much more in the society of age mates and peers than with elders or in the family circle.[1] Drinking together generally symbolizes durable social solidarity—or at least amity—among those who "share a drink" (cf. Washburne 1961).

Drinking is more often considered appropriate for those who grapple with the external environment than for those whose task it is to carry on and maintain a society's internal activities. This distinction was anciently symbolized in India by the difference between the god Indra, the scourge of enemies, the thunderer, the roisterer, the heavy drinker, and Varuna, the sober guardian of order and morality (Basham 1954). In ancient Greece, the worship of Dionysius could transport the worshiper into an extraordinary, even frenzied, state; that of Apollo encouraged only social morality. The Greeks successfully combined the two by assigning certain functions and occasions to the one deity and a different jurisdiction and festivals to the other. Drinking was a prominent feature of the Dionysian rites but not at Apollonian ceremonies (Dodds 1956; Guthrie 1950).

In general, warriors and shamans are more likely to use alcohol with cultural approval than are judges and priests. A priest is generally the conserver of tradition, the guide and exemplar for his fellows in precise replication of ritual in ways that please the gods. Drinking rarely goes with the priestly performance of ritual, except in symbolic usage, as in the Mass. But a shaman has personal relations with the supernatural, must directly encounter potent forces beyond ordinary society. Drinking is not often considered as interfering with this function.

When the fate of many hinges on the action of a single person, that person is usually not permitted to drink before performing the critical activity. The high priests of the Old Testament, beginning with Aaron, were particularly forbidden to drink "wine nor strong drink" when discharging their priestly duties in the Sanctuary (Lev. 10:9). American pilots today are forbidden to drink for a number of hours before flying as well as during the flight. (French pilots have wine with their in-flight meals, but, as we have noted, that kind of alcohol is defined as food by the French.)

Yet another ban that appears in various cultures is imposed when it is considered dangerous to heighten the emotions of large numbers of people who gather at the same occasion. To give but one eloquent example, there is an inscription dating from about the year 5 B.C. near the stadium at Delphi which forbids the carrying of wine into the stadium on pain of a five-drachma fine. The classical scholar who comments on this also notes that similar signs are to be seen now at the football stadia of Harvard and Southern Methodist Universities (McKinlay 1951).

Drinking patterns give one set of answers to fundamental questions that must be answered in every culture. Drinking is inescapably relevant to attitudes toward bodily sensations. It is made relevant by most peoples to relations between man and woman, to the proper interchange between man and man, and to the nexus between man and god.

Change and Stability in
Drinking Practices among Civilizations

As a whole culture changes, so do the drinking mores of the people change. We can best see evidences of change and also of long-term stability in drinking practices over the long careers of the ancient civilizations.

In India, for example, changes in alcohol use reflected major changes in social structure. Drinking was done by all men in an early, egalitarian period. Then, as the motif of hierarchy pervaded and stratified Indian society, drinking was accommodated to this social theme. Liquor was prohibited for certain castes and permitted for others, just as other social functions were specialized according to caste. Within very recent years there has been a shift to a more egalitarian though alcoholically less permissive social code. Under the law of several state governments of the Republic of India, drinking is prohibited to all in the state.

The earliest Indian literary sources, the Vedic hymns, make frequent mention of intoxicating liquors. One ritual drink was soma, used only in sacrifices, and described as having inebriating effects, although it may not have been alcoholic, since it was pressed from the juice of a plant, mixed with milk, and drunk on the same day. Sura was certainly alcoholic. It could be prepared from molasses, or rice, or possibly honey, and certain kinds were made only for use in sacrificial ritual. But there was a good deal of drinking outside the ritual occasions, and such drinking is condemned in the Vedic literature as leading to quarrels and misleading men from the path of virtue (Prakash 1961; Renou 1954).

Later there came a change in the social meaning of strong drink in India. It was eliminated from the rituals for the high gods; it became polluting to those who sought to follow the edicts of scripture. The rise of Buddhism may have had some influence on this shift of Hindu religious practice, since early Buddhism discounted mere ritual, including the ritual use of alcohol.

But alcoholic drinks were not prohibited for all society. The code of Manu says only that the Brahmans should totally abstain. Those of other strata of society need not take any disgrace in drinking but also could not attain, for that and other reasons, a high state of religious purity (Jhā 1926). Since the time of Manu, drinking has been socially and religiously compartmentalized in India. It is totally excluded from the worship of the high, universalistic gods and from the way of life of the religiously purest people. Many Brahman groups are strictly abstinent, and even among those Brahman communities in which the men may drink liquor occasionally, they must abstain from drink when they prepare to approach the high deities.

The men of the *Kshatriya*, warrior tradition, customarily drink heartily. Since this class provided most of the rulers and executives of the state, there was no more thought of total prohibition under indigenous Indian princes than there was under the later regime of the British. Yet the Kshatriyas also acknowledge that the high gods dislike alcohol, and they abstain when they seek to be in a state of ritual purity.[2]

There is another set of deities, local godlings who preside over local illness and misfortunes, whose ritual is carried on mainly by those of the lower castes, though all in village society, high and low alike, may seek their intervention for personal aid. In the ritual for these deities, liquor is often applied, externally as libation, internally as invigorant. Thus there has long been a rigid separation of alcoholic use in Indian civilization. It was tabooed for those gods and men who were immersed in cosmic concerns. The influence of drink in that sphere was considered disruptive for the whole universe of religion and society. But in the more parochial domain, for local blessings, for village solidarity, for personal benefits, strong drink was liberally used.

Gandhi was strongly in the ascetic tradition, and, when the political party that he led took over the government of the country, the ascetic mode was respected. Many of the political leaders held the belief that an independent India had to be a pure India, and one way to advance national purity was by legal prohibition. This seemed to be quite in the sacred tradition, but in fact it was in one respect a radical departure from it. The Sanskritic tradition did not rule out alcohol for all in society but only for the most spiritually elevated. Yet the recent statutes prohibit alcoholic drink absolutely, for all who are within the territorial bounds of the state.

A modern example of the ancient specialization in drinking is given in Carstairs' study of a town of Rajasthan in western India. Alcoholic drink is still readily available there, but the Brahmans of the place do very little drinking. A good many of them openly drink an infusion of hashish (*cannabis indica*) which gives them a feeling of detachment quite compatible with the religious meditation enjoined in their scriptures. But the Rajputs of the town, as inheritors of martial tradition, spurn hashish and drink an alcoholic brew called *daru*. One Rajput explained that hashish "makes you quite useless, unable to do anything. Daru isn't like that; you may be drunk but you can still carry on" (G. M. Carstairs 1957:119; cf. G. M. Carstairs in this volume). Those of military heritage choose alcohol because it helps maintain their traditional posture; those of the priestly heritage prefer hashish because it helps them to pursue their eternal verities. The legal arm of the state may, in time, influence such internal controls; it does not alter them quickly and directly. In India, as elsewhere, drinking practices are tied into fundamental themes of a people's life. While these practices change as the conditions of that life change, legislative acts are only one part, and not always a critical part, of the total change.

In Mesopotamia wine was known at Jemdet Nasr, dating from some time before 3000 B.C. As Sumerian civilization became established around the temple, beer became an integral part of temple ritual and economy. It was the popular drink, indeed a staple of diet, throughout two millennia of the Sumerian-Akkadian tradition. Some 40 percent of all cereals grown, one estimate has it, went into brewing at one period (Forbes 1954). Not only was beer offered as part of the temple service, it was also drunk copiously in beer shops, and there the drinking was not necessarily seen as being morally benign.

The code of Hammurabi (who came to power about 1720 B.C.) laid down strict regulations for tavern keepers and tavern servants, who were mainly women. Taverns and inns are marks of civilization; they provide anonymous travelers and customers with food, drink, and shelter, not because of kinship or personal obligations, as is usually the case in tribal societies, but because the customer can pay. Taverns help maintain a complex society, and Hammurabi was concerned that they be operated properly. His code specified the price, the quality, even the credit terms for beer.

But, because taverns are places where anonymous people can gather, they could be dangerous to the regime. One danger was from conspirators and outlaws. A tavern keeper who tolerated such characters on her premises could be put to death. Even more stringent were the liquor laws for women who were dedicated to the gods. Such a woman could not keep a beer shop or frequent one. If she was convicted of doing so, she was burned to death, the direst form of capital punishment. It was imposed only for this beer crime and for mother-son incest (Lutz 1922). Prostitutes also gathered at the beer houses; since alcoholic euphoria could be had there for money, so also sexual pleasure. Though alcoholic drink in Sumer was used in worship and served as a means of consolidating society, in certain contexts its use was potentially antisocial and immoral, so the state tried to eliminate the disruptive side effects of alcohol.

In Egyptian civilization wine and beer were also staples of diet and ritual. One inscription states that a good mother provides her schoolboy son with three loaves of bread and two jars of beer every day (Lucas 1948; Lutz 1922). Heavy drinking, to the point of insensibility or illness, is frequently depicted in sketches and descriptions of banquet scenes. Egyptian taverns, like those in Mesopotamia, were supposed to be avoided by the social elite.

The ancient Egyptian writings include a number of warnings against drunkenness, among them a touching letter, perhaps from the equivalent of a student's copybook, written by a teacher to his student. The teacher writes that he hears that his former student is forsaking his studies and is wandering from tavern to tavern. He smells of beer so much that men are frightened away from him, he is like a broken oar, which cannot steer a steady course; he is like a temple without a god, like a home without bread. The teacher ends by hoping that the student will understand that wine is an abomination and that he will abjure drink (Lutz 1922). In ancient Egypt as in Sumer, alcohol was an essential element for human welfare when used in one context, a dangerously disruptive force in another. But there seems to have been little attempt by Egyptian state officials to regulate drinking in the manner of the Hammurabi code.

Both the moral and the immoral uses of alcohol are set forth in the Old Testament. Wine is specified for use as libation in the temple service (e.g., Num. 15:5–10, 28:7–8) but drunkenness is depicted as leading to shame and abomination, as in the accounts of Noah and Lot. Several passages in the Book of Proverbs warn against wine's dangers, and others mention its benefactions; one passage refers to both (31:4–7). According to one biblical scholar, the antagonistic view of alcohol is from an earlier, simpler stage of Hebrew history and the more tolerant view from a later period (Jastrow 1913).

In the New Testament wine is mentioned as a festive drink (John 2:3–10), as a medicament (Luke 10:34; 1 Tim. 5:23), and as supreme symbol (Matt. 26:27–29; Mark 14:23–25; Luke 22:17–18). But wine must be drunk in moderation. There are several disapproving references to excessive drinking (1 Tim. 3:8; Titus 2:3; Eph. 5:18). There is considerable continuity in attitudes toward drinking in Old and New Testaments, though the symbolic use of wine becomes greatly elevated in Christianity.

Continuities in style of drinking suggest clues to cultural stabilities. There is another kind of continuity that is of interest; it is the similarity in drinking practice over a large culture area, among many separate societies.

Culture Areas in Drinking Patterns

The functions of beer drinking that we have noted among the Kofyar of Nigeria in West Africa are important also among the Tiriki of Kenya in East Africa (Sangree 1962). Beer is a constant medium of social interchange for men; beer drinking is a preoccupying activity that few men reject. Drinking beer together induces physical and social mellowness in men. Very little aggressive behavior is ever shown as a result of drinking, and that little is promptly squelched. Pathological addiction rarely, if ever, occurs. The supernaturals are as fond and as interested in beer as are mortals, hence worshipers regularly offer beer for the spirits.

This is quite different from the style of drinking in many Central and South American societies; that drinking pattern allows or requires men to drink steadily into a state of stupefaction. Drinking is social, often done when there is a religious celebration, but not so much poured out for the supernaturals as poured into the celebrants, and always done at fiestas. Though drinking is frequent and heavy, no problem of addiction arises. This pattern has been remarkably consistent through time and place. It was maintained by the peoples of the ancient indigenous civilizations, the Maya, Aztec, and Inca. It is followed in contemporary societies, both Indian and mestizo, from Mexico to Chile, in highlands and lowlands (see J. Cooper 1948; Morley 1956; J. Thompson 1940; Simmons 1962; Stein 1961; Mangin 1957; Bunzel 1940; Metzger 1963; Viguera and Palerm 1954; cf. Sec. II, this volume).

This style of drinking is widespread but is not followed everywhere in Central and South America, as is indicated in the study by Sayres (1956) on three Colombian villages and by Viguera and Palerm on Tajin, a Totonac Mexican village. While the modern distribution of this pattern has yet to be traced in detail, the data suggest certain avenues of analysis.

Culture and Personality Analysis of a Drinking Pattern

To take the extreme case of the Camba of eastern Bolivia, why does a normal Camba man regularly drink himself into a stupor, and on reviving promptly want to drink himself right back into alcoholic oblivion? There are some eighty thousand Camba in all, living in a remote but fertile geographic enclave. They are mostly mestizo peasants, who have little contact either with the neighboring Indian tribes or with the centers of Bolivian national life. Camba men are among the heaviest drinkers on record for normal members of a functioning society.

Drunkenness for them is not an unfortunate by-product; it is the explicitly sought goal of drinking (Heath 1962). Alcohol is supposed to have some medicinal value as an internal parasiticide, but no other beneficent properties are attributed to it. The Camba could easily make wines or beers of lower alcoholic content, as do their Indian neighbors, or use other means to prolong a convivial state while drinking. But what they choose is a highly potent drink with very quick effect, and that effect is gross inebriation.

What explanation can we find for this behavior? It seems to require some further exploration. Camba men gulp down quantities of a drink that they dislike in order to attain a state in which they feel nothing. Certain conditions help maintain the pattern, though they do not explain it. Alcohol is cheap and easy to get; it is the main product and export of the region. The region is naturally bountiful, so the simple economy can be maintained even though the drinking absorbs much time and energy.

Heath offers a tentative interpretation based on the nature of Camba social relations. These are fragmented, tenuous, and atomistic. Marriage bonds are brittle, families notably unstable, and kinship ties meager. People shift residence a good deal, there is little cooperative enterprise, and enduring friendships are rare. Heath notes that all people in the world value association with others and the Camba choose to get such association in drinking parties rather than in other ways.

This seems true enough, but there arises the question why they choose to have such brief conviviality associations outside the aura of alcohol. Perhaps a single answer can be postulated for both questions, based on what seems to be a deep-seated personality characteristic. The Camba individual seems to be self-isolated, quite like individuals of another South American group about whom we have more personality data (Simmons 1959, 1962).

The men of Lunahuaná, a Peruvian town in the Andean foothills, also drink frequently, often into drunken oblivion. While their drinking practices differ in detail from those of the Camba, the grand pattern is quite the same. Simmons notes that the adult male Lunahuaneño may be characterized, in part, as timid, evasive, shy, indirect, at a loss for words, uncertain of his behavior when in the company of others, inordinately concerned with "correct" behavior, always preoccupied with what others may think of him, and always timorous lest there be unfavorable criticism. He sees other people as potentially dangerous and is characteristically suspicious and distrustful even of people he knows well.

These attitudes are instilled at an early age. Children are taught to keep to themselves, close to home, and are punished if they go into neighbors' houses. They are kept away from any visitors to the home for fear that they will not behave properly (Simmons 1962). Each person's social relations are "marked by a profound sense of distrust of others and a lack of confidence in his own ability to control the outcome of a given episode of interaction."

If we assume that the Camba have similar fear and distrust of others, similar doubts about their own abilities to cope with social relations and hence a constant attitude of defensive self-isolation, we can begin to see an answer to the questions raised above. It is that a Camba man wants to have two different kinds of relations with his fellows. He wants to insulate himself from them, and yet at the same time he wants some safe interaction with them. He achieves both through drink. From the normal isolation of the week, he comes to the drinking bout of the weekend. For two or three hours then, in the first stage of the drinking cycle, warmed by the liquor, he has pleasant interchange, is voluble and sociable. But since his fear is great and intrusive, he does not want protracted sociability. He needs the protection of isolation. This he gets through the narcotizing effect of alcohol. He regularly proceeds from normal self-isolation, through a brief episode of nonisolation, promptly into alcoholic isolation.

Two features of Camba social life give evidence in support of this formulation. Both are circumstances under which Camba men do not drink. One is at the annual reunion of the Veterans of the Chaco War, one of the bloodiest conflicts of the twentieth century. There is no drinking then; "the presence of a prevailing atmosphere of genuine camaraderie stemming from a past of significant shared experience, and a common characteristic pride may be sufficient basis to unite the veterans, during their reunion, in a way which allows warm and easy fellowship without dependence on alcohol to overcome initial reserve" (Heath 1962:33–34). The trust born of having endured great hardship and danger together dispels the normal distrust. Hence the participants feel no defensive need to drink, and when they do not have to, they do not drink.

The second instance is that of the relatively few Camba who belong to fundamentalist Protestant sects. Abstinence is part of the denominational doctrine, but there is another reason that helps explain why these few are able to deviate from the normal pattern of drunkenness. Heath observes that these Protestant converts have a stable primary group, which other Camba do not have. Three or four nights a week they meet for religious purposes, call each other "brother," and interact under favorable conditions in which each one is encouraged to take active part. The members of one of these Protestant churches form a tightly knit group, consolidated by both their internal interchange and their common opposition to the Catholic majority. So bolstered, a Protestant Camba does not need to preserve social isolation among other Protestants, he does not have the same need for alcoholic isolation, and he is able to uphold the nondrinking doctrine of his denomination.

Normal Camba drunkenness thus seems to arise from a fear of one's fellows and a desire not to interact much with them even when in their presence. This is quite different from the attitudes of Jews or Italians, whose childhood training teaches them to need social interchange and to fear social isolation. Among these people, convivial drinking is condoned, but isolated and isolating drinking is strongly disapproved.

Some interesting implications are suggested by this analysis. One is relevant to studies of the use of alcohol, and adds to the thesis ably presented by some students of the subject, namely, that drinking behavior is best understood as an outcome of fundamental social relations and that the nature of these relations must be known before the meaning of drinking, to the group and to the individual, can be recognized and any alcoholic debilitation efficiently treated (cf. S. Bacon 1944, 1945; Bales 1946, 1962; Pittman and Snyder 1962 passim).

The other opens up new queries in the study of South American cultures. The Camba, as mestizos, have kept only a very few, minor elements of the tribal Indian culture that their ancestors carried on. Yet in their drinking bouts, and presumably in their attitudes toward their fellows, they share fundamental ideas with the surrounding tribesmen. It is as though all the surface, manifest, superficial traits of Indian culture had been abandoned but certain of the basic, structural concepts retained. If this is so of the Camba, what then of all the other Latin-American peoples who follow drinking patterns that are similar in certain main respects? Could the widespread importance of machismo, the imperative necessity felt by men of these societies to defend and validate their manly qualities, be a general manifestation of fear and suspicion of others which seems to be at the bottom of Camba drinking practices?

Studies of the Uses of Alcohol

Both change and stability in drinking patterns have occurred within the frame of those ways in which alcohol tends to be used everywhere. If we should find a people in which women must drink more than men, in which drinking must be done alone or in the company of one's mentors and dependents, or in which the upholders of scripture (whether theological or political) are expected to drink more heavily than do others, we should know that we have encountered a society basically different from others so far known.

Drinking practices can be studied as expressions of pervasive behavioral themes. A pioneering effort in this direction is Donald Horton's study (1943) on the functions of alcohol in primitive societies. It was based on a survey of reports of drinking in fifty-six tribes. Horton concluded that the amount of alcohol used was related to anxieties created by food scarcity, acculturation, or war. That is, peoples who were habitually subject to these stresses drank heavily to reduce the anxieties that were so generated. Horton also noted that heavy drinking can create anxiety, and he said that the amount of drinking allowed in a culture is the outcome of the interplay between the anxiety-reducing and the anxiety-creating functions of alcohol.

This formulation has been found wanting as a valid explanation both in general and in particular cases. Two intensive studies of drinking, by Lemert among Northwest Coast Indians (1954) and by Mangin among Andean Indians (1957), found that drinking among these people was a means of social integration, a way of providing needed primary social relations, rather than a response to anxieties of the kind Horton mentions. And, from the case examples noted above, it is clear that the use of alcohol in a society cannot be explained simply as either a solvent or a source of anxiety. The Camba evidently have none of the major anxieties postulated by Horton. In the Indian village studied by G. M. Carstairs (1957), the Rajputs who drink have not been under any greater anxiety than the Brahmans who do not. The description of the beer-centered Kofyar culture gives no hint that Horton's three sources of anxiety have much to do either with heightening their continual thirst for beer or with quenching it. It well may be that where alcohol is culturally defined as a means of relieving anxiety, those groups and individuals who feel themselves under greater stress will drink more, but we must note that drinking is not necessarily so defined nor is tension relief necessarily sought through drink.

A more recent study by Peter B. Field, entitled "A New Cross-Cultural Study of Drunkenness," gives a critique of Horton's methods and offers a different explanation. "The general conclusion indicated by the findings to this point is: drunkenness in primitive societies is determined less by the level of fear in a society than by the absence of corporate kin groups with stability, permanence, formal structure, and well-defined functions" (1962:58). The presence of such group organization provides controls over heavy drinking that are not available to peoples who have looser, less well-defined kinship organization.

To be sure, if a society has strongly integrated kin groups whose members closely control each other's behavior, and if heavy drinking is seen as something to be kept in check, their drinking will be so controlled. But not every people considers heavy drinking as something to be controlled by kinsmen. Drunkenness is the normal goal of drinking in a good many South American societies, some of which have tight unilinear kin organization and some of which do not. Conversely, drunkenness is minimal in many African societies, some of them with strong corporate kin groups and some with quite loose kin organization. In India, there are both Rajput and Brahman groups that have all the social features (save only bride-price) postulated by Field (1962) as being positively correlated with sobriety, yet some of the Brahman groups are teetotalers and the Rajputs are generally heavy drinkers.

Edwin Lemert has proposed yet another approach, that drunkenness need not be considered as a symptom of either personal deprivation or defective social organization. "There is an alternative way of viewing drunkenness, which is to say as an institutionalized pattern operating in a relatively autonomous way and only tenuously related to other aspects of the culture" (1956:313). There probably are some societies in which, as Lemert says, drunken behavior is fenced off from other areas of behavior and is considered to be outside the context of morality; perhaps this occurred among the English gentry when there were alcoholic remittance men and drunken squires whose condition was politely ignored. But in most societies drunkenness is not disregarded; it may be deliberately sought, as with the Camba, or deliberately discouraged, as with the Kofyar. In either case it is closely related to the general pattern of drinking, and drinking, as has been noted above, is not culturally ignored. Most certainly it was not ignored among the English upper classes, whatever may have been their social techniques for dealing with drunkards.

One difficulty with these and some other theoretical contributions to the studies of alcohol is that their focus is so greatly on drunkenness and alcoholism. Their scope then becomes too restricted for them to be able to explain well even the phenomena on which they concentrate. Inebriety is not really dissociated from the general pattern and standards of drinking, even where drunkards are overlooked. Hence drunkenness cannot be understood apart from drinking in general, and drinking cannot be understood apart from the characteristic features of social relations of which it is part and which are reflected and expressed in the acts of drinking. At the American cocktail party, for example, participants not infrequently take in much alcohol rapidly. It has been suggested that if more food were eaten with the drinks or if drinks of lower alcoholic content were served, the social benefits of such occasions would be enhanced because the deleterious effects of the high intake of alcohol would be minimized (Lolli 1961). But whether food is taken or liquor of low alcoholic content is offered is in a sense irrelevant. We know that persons can get drunk on beer as well as on distilled spirits if they intend and are expected to do so; they can mix food and alcohol and still get intoxicated. Even more importantly, many cocktail parties seem to be mainly occasions during which one can interact gaily and superficially with a number of others in a way that precludes being relatively serious and intimate with any. If this is indeed the real social purpose of the occasion, rapid alcohol intake helps rather than hinders it.

Alcoholism in the sense of abnormal, addictive, pathologically compulsive intake of alcohol is not the same as drunkenness, which can be quite normal culturally, and should not be confused with the standard drinking practices of any society. In a paper entitled "Alcoholics Do Not Drink," Selden Bacon (1958) shows how very different are the typical practices of alcoholics in the United States from the usual American ways of drinking. Both drunkenness and alcoholism, and the manifold social, economic, and medical problems involved in them, will be understood better than they now are to the degree that they are seen in relation to each culture's normal ways of drinking (cf. Ullman 1958). Once we have clear conception of these patterns, we can assess the themes of personality that lead an individual to make certain choices in drinking, and we also can appraise the motifs of culture that become expressed in the kind of drinking that a people customarily does.

Notes

1. In France, and even more so in Italy, wine is assimilated into the definition of food and the delight that good food brings. Hence wine is drunk by all around the family dinner table. But other kinds of drink, cognac for example, are classified in a different way and drunk in non-family contexts (cf. Lolli et al. 1958; Stoetzel 1958).

2. Scotch whiskey is put in a special category. It is so costly that its main use is as a prestige symbol for the wealthiest, and so it is not nearly "as defiling as is country-made liquor" (Srinivas 1955:21).

Alcohol in Its Cultural Context

John J. Honigmann

Since classical times, travelers from the oikumene [the known world] crossing the frontiers of civilization have noted, among other exotic phenomena, the way native people use alcoholic beverages and respond to drunkenness. One of the earliest such observations, made by Tacitus on the failure of the Germans to show self-control in drinking, comes pretty close to the way we today charge certain ethnic groups in our civilization as being uncontrolled heavy drinkers.

Following the Age of Reconnaissance, descriptions of the use of alcohol in other cultures increased rapidly. They were penned by explorers, missionaries, and traders. Occasionally the observers were also the catalysts who provided liquor to Indians, Polynesians, and other native people, thereby setting up the drunken behavior with which readers were regaled. At about the time when most of the world's small-scale societies were being brought into political and colonial frontiers, anthropologists appeared on the scene. Sojourning on reservations or in the other native enclaves, they began to do research on the manner and conditions of alcohol use and, sometimes, abuse.

The early travelers, in concentrating on the style of drinking and attendant behavior, forged a descriptive approach to the use of alcohol. Anthropologists picked up the same approach but also sought for deeper understanding by questioning the connection of drinking with other aspects of social life. They asked about the functions served by drinking, especially the eufunctions since the dysfunctions were usually so plain to see that they were obvious to everyone, including members of the community being studied. Anthropologists also probed for causal explanations of the use of alcohol; that problem confronted them with the need to devise new strategies of research. To learn about causality, they had to be willing to augment their concentration on single communities with attention to comparative studies that simultaneously dealt with many cultures. Immersion in a particular culture for prolonged periods of field work can at best suggest causal relationships; it cannot test them. Serious research on cultural determinants of drinking behavior requires that drinking communities be compared with abstemious communities to observe significant variations in other factors that bear a theoretical relationship to drinking. Or else, within a single community, matched samples of drinkers and nondrinkers are compared to discover other differences between them that possess explanatory value. Anthropological research comparing social systems to determine the antecedents of heavy drinking and of certain kinds of drinking behavior was begun by Donald Horton (1943). It has led to what is probably the prevalent conception in the anthropology of heavy drinking, namely, that it results from cultural stress, for example, stress produced by culture contact.

Stress theory in its several guises has stood up well in research. It has been able to account quite satisfactorily for many cases in which drinking runs in patterns that are deviant from the norms of the society (though not necessarily from the norms enforced in the particular community where the drinking occurs). Nevertheless, it is not the only useful way of understanding the use of alcohol.

In a paper presented to the First Annual Alcoholism Conference of the National Institute on Alcohol Abuse and Alcoholism, Levy and Kunitz (1973) give critical attention to the methods that have generally been employed by anthropologists in carrying out research on the cultural contexts of drinking. One of their criticisms is pertinent in terms of my foregoing remarks. The authors point out that researchers, using what I call stress theory, have not always sought to measure stress independently of the drinking behavior that it is said to engender. Their paper is also valuable for calling attention to a comparatively new approach to alcohol forged by the authors, one of whom is a sociologist and the other an anthropologist. I refer to the clinical approach whose goal it is to measure chronic alcoholism by the incidence of cirrhosis and the withdrawal syndrome. Such a clinical approach is closely related to Levy's interest in the relatively new subdiscipline of medical anthropology.

Their paper illustrates the extent to which anthropological research on alcohol has been preoccupied with excessive and pathological drinking. Practically all the studies they cite are primarily concerned with socially and individually dyscrasic aspects of alcohol use. In fact, the clinical indicators are intended to discover patterns of excessive consumption in populations. Even when anthropologists and sociologists recognize variability in the extent to which an Indian community or American Indians in general use alcohol, they tend to pay little or no attention to nondrinking patterns or to customs of cautious and moderate drinking. Such styles of alcohol use are simply not germane to current interests. We do not regard such information as likely to be useful or helpful. We believe we have more to learn from what is wrong with social systems and individuals than from what goes well with them.

Regardless of the heuristic value of studying social pathology, to write only about heavy drinking and its unfavorable consequences in Indian tribes may inadvertently give the impression that all Indians drink a lot and get in trouble as a result. Because heavy use of alcohol in our culture still connotes immoral behavior, sole emphasis on heavy drinking may result in stigmatizing Indians, precisely what Levy and Kunitz warn against. Furthermore, undue emphasis on alcohol abuse among Indians contributes to the simplistic view that the Indian style of drinking is responsible for the adaptive difficulties that Indians face in many communities where they live. The latter folk model of American Indian adaptation, shared even by some Indians and Eskimo, does not fit the facts. To take one deduction from the model, it is not true that Americans of native background who drink heavily mostly tend to be social misfits.

In presenting facts to support that contention I must consider what is meant by heavy drinking. In the absence of a cross-cultural index, I think we are advised to work particularistically; that is, to measure alcohol use in the context of a single community, letting "heavy" be defined by the range of drinking in that community. It would be preferable to have the extremes of the range defined by the actual amount of alcohol or specific beverages ingested by individuals in a specific period of time, but in the work to which I will refer I have found it convenient to use amounts spent on alcoholic beverages (Honigmann and Honigmann 1970). The research was carried out in a newly built, far northern Canadian town, Inuvik, containing Eskimo, Indians, and métis, as well as a large number of nonnative civil servants and their families. Work with the native population failed to show the inverse correlation, predictable from the folk model, between total amounts spent on alcoholic beverages and steady employment. Instead the heaviest native spenders tend to be in the ranks of the steadily employed. In one analysis of data we examined the category of heaviest spenders, containing twenty-three native people, and discovered it to be made up of fourteen people (including eleven family heads) judged to be well adapted in their economic roles and to be meeting domestic responsibilities. None shows evidence of repetitive trouble with police on account of drinking. The remaining nine men, however, are poorly adapted by the same criteria though not, as the folk model might lead one to expect, necessarily as a result of their drinking.

The stereotype of Amerinds (a term useful for categorizing Eskimo as well as Indians and métis) all using alcohol heavily is likewise not borne out in Inuvik. Eskimo are more apt to be nondrinkers than either of the other two native groups, probably because of the force of the Pentecostal church in that ethnic group.

My intention is not to deny alcohol abuse among American Indians but to show how unwarranted it is to overgeneralize such phenomena. Only by heeding with equal diligence the whole spectrum of drinking behavior will we be in a better position to discover determinants of the abusive aspects of behavior that we wish to control.

Professor Waddell's paper (1973) presented to the same conference is in a traditional anthropological vein, but nonetheless insightful in demonstrating the sociability that surrounds drinking among the Papago Indians and the social bonding that drinking and drunkenness facilitate.

My comments will be directed to one especially noteworthy feature of Waddell's paper, his conclusion that drinking—or a style of drinking—communicates the social identity of those people who participate in it, demarcating them from other social groups or categories. To speak of securing or communicating identity through drinking goes beyond offering a functional interpretation of alcohol use. It uncovers the implicit meaning of the phenomenon as the actors see it and thereby ventures into the area of symbolic anthropology.

The meaning of alcohol in culture has tended to be a neglected topic, though the close kinship of meaning and motivation suggests that it is an important subject for anyone concerned with alcohol abuse. Several recent studies support the theory that how alcohol is used constitutes a social marker of Indian or other ethnic status. Nancy Oestrich Lurie (1971, also in this volume) points out that some Indians drink to demonstrate their identity as Indians and Hugh Brody (1970) thinks it possible that spree drinking among midwest Canadian Indians in skid rows "unites the Indians as Indians." It confers on the Indian a self-concept he does not necessarily find ennobling but that he chooses. Philip Spaulding (1966) reported for an enclave of northern Saskatchewan métis that disdain for sobriety symbolizes their adherence to a set of contracultural values. Such values were set up in deliberate opposition to the middle-class values of nonnatives who had moved into the community and threatened the autonomy of the métis. Research in the Arctic town of Inuvik (Honigmann and Honigmann 1970) bears out a similar pattern of cultural choice made by certain members of the native population. A style of reckless and, whenever liquor was available, heavy drinking had been learned from white men in the region during the previous seventy years of acculturation, incidentally a period of culture contact when it is unlikely that the population was deeply stressed. As that epoch drew to a close and the new administrative center of Inuvik began to recruit its native population, several hundred middle-class nonnative families also arrived to reside in the town. The influx of this largely transient population tremendously exaggerated the bifurcation already present between natives and a comparatively small number of local whites. Relationships between the two ethnic populations polarized. The two neighborhoods into which the town is divided, one heavily populated by Indians, Eskimo, and métis, and the other primarily for nonnative civil servants and their families, with their unequal housing and other facilities, visibly symbolize the vast cultural gap separating the two population blocs. Interaction between the two is extremely limited, with the result that the native people are left free to reinforce their identification with one another and to further their own distinctive way of life. One way a substantial proportion, especially men, do so is by perpetuating the reckless frontier style of drinking, which has acquired a new significance in the town, namely to mark off native group identity and to symbolize rejection of the other way of life that has blossomed in the region. Using alcohol in disregard of legal norms sets off the native culture from the dominant middle-class culture that has moved northward so conspicuously, and it also represents a means of repudiating certain values in that culture that native people find spurious and restrictive. Not everyone repudiates the mainstream cultural values to the same degree. Some families of native background in Inuvik, especially families containing one nonnative spouse, aspire strongly to emulate middle-class values and manage to do so with considerable success. We know of one family that strove to drink in middle-class fashion, adopting for a brief time the practice of a drink before dinner after the husband returned from work.

Drinking styles that become emblems of membership in particular social groups and categories are constructed or selected, not always consciously, for their symbolic meaning. The meaning of a style derives partly from the forms of behavior to which it is in opposition or, in the case of the family having an evening drink, from the style of behavior that they seek to emulate. A drinking style also acquires its meaning from the social and cultural context where it is practiced, where it is positively or negatively sanctioned, and where other institutions help to maintain it. Such a theory allows the prediction that when contexts are drastically altered in the perception of the group, drinking styles will change.

Earlier I described stress theory as useful to explain drinking behavior. The sociable consequences of drinking and the meaning assigned to alcohol or drunkenness also provide useful means of understanding alcohol in its cultural context. These various bases of understanding are not contradictory but may well complement one another in a given social situation. Each has its advantages and helps counteract shortsightedness in any one interpretation. Noting the positive consequences of drinking prevents overemphasis on the dysfunctions and gets at the behavior from the actor's point of view. Studying the meaning of drinking avoids the one-sidedness of approaching alcohol use only in terms of the norms set for it by the dominant society, norms which, although known to a component community, may not accord with its own standards and perception.

II. Alcohol Use in Mesoamerica, Latin America, and the Caribbean

The Cultural Structure of
Mexican Drinking Behavior

William Madsen and Claudia Madsen

The study of drinking behavior has been retarded by a lack of theoretical formulations applicable outside the context of Western civilization. Cross-cultural surveys (Horton 1943; Field 1962; and Bacon, Barry, and Child 1965) have focused on primitive drunkenness without weighing cultural differences in the definition of normal drinking. Although these studies do not specifically equate drunkenness with alcoholism, they leave the impression that primitive drunkenness is a form of pathological drinking caused by anxiety or defective social control.

The relative absence of alcoholism outside Western civilization has been noted in anthropological studies which stress the predominantly integrative function of drinking in primitive societies. Spindler (1964) has suggested that alcoholism as well as socially integrative drinking is a function of the cultural setting.

Following Foster's (1967b) theory of cognitive orientation, we shall attempt to explain drinking behavior as a consequence of cultural premises about reality. This paper shows how Mexican drinking behavior is structured by culturally defined assumptions about identity, community, and prestige. Our analysis is based on a comparative study of drinking in two peasant communities: the Nahuatl Indian village of San Francisco Tecospa, and the mestizo town of Tepepan near Mexico City.

We are particularly concerned with changes in drinking behavior produced by the introduction of Western values. Since the analysis of change requires time perspective, we begin with a discussion of Aztec drinking before and after the Spanish conquest.

Historical Change

The Aztecs who invaded the Valley of Mexico from the north were considered barbarians. In the process of conquering Mexico they absorbed the culture of earlier agricultural inhabitants. By the time the Spaniards arrived in the sixteenth century, the Aztecs had built a civilization whose cities, science, and art awed their conquerors.

The Aztecs used an intoxicating beverage called pulque made by fermenting the juice of the maguey plant.[1] Pulque was regarded as a divine gift from the goddess Mayahuel. To drink pulque was to honor the gods. Being holy and blessed, pulque

was not to be abused. People were expected to become intoxicated on certain holy days, but otherwise public intoxication was
forbidden and punished. The penalties ranged from public disgrace to death by stoning or beating. Drunkenness in secular contexts was rare except among the aged who were exempt from social sanctions prohibiting public intoxication. Excessive drinking
was attributed to the misfortune of being born with the fate of
becoming a drunkard.

The Spanish conquest destroyed the Aztec empire and reduced its proud citizens to servile members of a subordinate
group. Widespread drunkenness was one of the earliest and most
persistent responses to the shock of conquest (C. Gibson 1964).
The change from secular sobriety to mass drunkenness reflected
the deep distress of native society. Aztec sanctions were gone but
drinking was still associated with divinity and succor. Intoxication
became a blessed escape from the despair and confusion that followed the conquest. After the collapse of tribal rule, the community was the largest native social unit capable of survival. Drinking reinforced social bonds that united the Indian community and
set it apart from the conquerors.

Alarmed by the extent of native drunkenness, the Spaniards
made unsuccessful efforts to stop it. Spanish priests tried to divert
the Indians from the drunken road to Hell while Spanish rulers
took legal action to thwart the threat to their labor supply, already
reduced by the death toll from European diseases. Since the Spanish introduction of distilled beverages and drinking taverns had
contributed to native drunkenness, laws were enacted prohibiting
taverns and the sale of liquor to Indians. Efforts were made to halt
the manufacture of pulque which had become a major industry of
the Spanish haciendas. New laws provided severe punishment for
Indian drunkenness, beginning with a penalty of 100 lashes for a
first offense. Legislation, confiscation, and punishment all proved
ineffective (C. Gibson 1964).

Vagabondage increased simultaneously with drunkenness.
Many Indians wandered aimlessly from town to town and finally
settled in the Spanish-dominated cities where they abandoned
their Indian language and values. They acquired mestizo identity
through intermarriage with the Spaniards or by adopting city ways
and speaking Spanish.

Cultural Divisions in Modern Mexico

During the Mexican Revolution Indianism was idealized and still
is by many Mexican intellectuals. Nevertheless, most mestizos

look down on Indians as inferior beings akin to savages who are poor, childlike, superstitious, and dangerous.

The Mexican government is attempting to accelerate the acculturation of the Indian population into the mainstream of national culture. Technical experts and social scientists are trying to help Indian communities achieve progress. Hybrid seed, modern irrigation, and improved market resources have been introduced in an effort to better the material lot of the Indians. Education is designed to promote social progress that will bring the Indians closer to the mestizo way of life.

Mexican Indians are not always amenable to the process of being remolded into mestizos. While the Indians are often eager to improve their material welfare with modern innovations, they are rarely willing to abandon Indian communal values or the symbols of Indian identity. The Indian does not want to be a mestizo. He pictures the mestizo as being greedy, exploitative, and very far from God.

In the Indian mind, group drinking has become a symbol of the Indian way of life. Drinking is regarded as a ritual essential for social cohesion within the community. As pressures to de-Indianize increase, the Indians respond by placing more emphasis on the traditions that seem most Indian. The observance of these traditions involves ritualized drinking that serves to strengthen rather than weaken social bonds.

Tecospa

The Value System of an Indian Community

San Francisco Tecospa is a Nahuatl Indian village (population eight hundred) which may be described as a corporate peasant community. The village is located in the administrative subdivision of Milpa Alta, which is part of the Federal District of Mexico. From Tecospa to Mexico City is barely an hour's driving time.

Although most of the inhabitants are bilingual, Nahuatl is the language of the home and of communication among close friends. Spanish is the language of commerce used in the markets of Milpa Alta and Mexico City, and also in dealing with government officials who occasionally visit the town.

Nahuatl is the primary tongue in each of the eight Indian villages in the Milpa Alta area. Every village has a slight dialectical difference which can be identified by residents of the other villages. The Indians of each community feel that the Nahuatl spoken in their village is superior and purer than that of other villages. This ethnocentric feeling about dialect is associated with community and family loyalties.

As in colonial times, the local community is the primary point of reference by which the Indian defines his identity, his roles, and his obligations. A Tecospan thinks of himself first as a member of his community and secondly as an Indian. This order of classification is reversed only when he is dealing with non-Indians, especially mestizos. Antagonism and open hostility frequently occur between the Indian villages in the Milpa Alta area but when two Indians from different villages are confronted by a mestizo, they stand together as fellow Indians.

Within each community an Indian is first identified as a member of a family. However, familial role behavior is extended to all members of the community. The respect shown to parents must be displayed to all elders. Highest respect is due to the mayor, the prayer maker, and the curer who has been "chosen by God" to care for the ill and infirm. There is a general feeling that the welfare of all the residents of Tecospa hangs together and that anyone disgracing himself is bringing disgrace on the whole town. Tecospans should back fellow villagers in any quarrels, fights, or problems involving outsiders. If a Tecospan is wanted by the police for a crime committed outside the village, every other Tecospan must be willing to hide the fugitive or physically defend him from the police even at the risk of death.

This does not mean that Tecospans try to isolate themselves completely from the outside world. They are aware that they have much to gain from mestizo culture. Villagers are proud of the fact that they have obtained electricity and running water piped to several public taps. They have built a stone bridge across an arroyo in the dirt road that connects their town to the nearby paved road between Milpa Alta and Mexico City. Although the Tecospan is quite willing to accept material benefits from the outside world, he wants no part of the effort to change his identity, his primary loyalties, or his "spirit." Nor is he particularly interested in the events of the larger Mexican scene or the world. The exception is any addition to the large body of facts and folklore that reflect negatively on the mestizo.

Within the community equality is an important value modified only by the status that goes with age, the deference and obedience due to elected officials, and the respect owed to those who are "close to God." To outshine a fellow villager materially is regarded as a gross insult. Conspicuous consumption is a negative value. The accumulation of material wealth is condemned unless it is used for financing a religious fiesta or assuming the care of one of the saintly images in the church. The care of a saint may involve buying new clothes for the image, giving a fiesta with food and drink for all the villagers, and perhaps taking the image on a pilgrimage. Financing religious fiestas may take years of saving and leave the benefactor impoverished but it brings him honor and prestige.

In everyday life, respect is accorded to those who properly fulfill their culturally defined roles. A man must be a good farmer and a woman must be a good homemaker. The young must respect the old and all must respect God and the saints. Respect further depends on one's willingness to share with other Tecospans. No villager should lack field hands when his family is small, food when his larder is empty, or pulque when he is thirsty.

Pulque Production and Consumption

Both the production and consumption of pulque, which are closely associated with the daily ritual of Indian life, are believed to be sanctified and proper. Life is seen as an integrated totality; the Indian, the land, and its products form a meaningful whole. As one villager said, "Our fathers lie buried in the soil that produces our food and we shall join them there in time."

The fields which produce maize, beans, and squash are outlined by rows of maguey plants. When a maguey reaches maturity and begins to send up its thick flower stock, this growth is cut off at its base, leaving a cavity which daily fills with the fluid intended for the stock. The fluid, called *aguamiel,* is milked daily by sucking it into a large, perforated gourd and letting it flow into a container. Then the aguamiel is added to the pulque barrel in the home, where fermentation takes place. The fermented pulque at the bottom of the barrel and the human saliva mixed with the aguamiel initiate the process of fermentation which produces pulque. Early in life children become familiar with the process of making pulque. Boys are frequently in charge of milking the maguey plants and the pulque is in large part a product of their labor.

Pulque affects the Indian from conception through eternity. A pregnant woman often takes an extra serving of pulque for the one inside her. The suckling infant is given a sip of pulque from the cup of his mother or father. Once weaned, the child receives pulque at meals, since it is considered a nourishing food. The regular diet of Tecospans includes pulque at every meal.

The growing child learns that pulque is an integral part of

his universe and this universe should be harmonious. Overt aggression is discouraged by direction and example. Children are severely punished for fighting with a peer or disobeying an elder. Peaceful cooperation and mutual respect are highly prized and demonstrated in drinking behavior.

Parents teach their offspring that grown men are expected to display courtesy and dignity when they are drunk but women and children should never become intoxicated. Departure from the rule of nonviolence sometimes occurs outside the circle of drinking companions. A drunken man may beat his wife for real or imagined misbehavior. Wife beating is sanctioned and accepted by women because of the belief that a woman who has never been beaten cannot enter heaven.

Pulque is associated with the dead and the relationship of the dead to the living. Wakes for adults include copious servings of pulque and food. It is inappropriate to drink to the point of collapse at the wake. After a man's burial, his friends may gather at one of their homes to drink together in respect to their departed comrade. A drink is poured for his spirit while the mourners propose a series of toasts recalling the good deeds of the dead man. As drinking continues, the conversation turns to recollections of others who have died and stories of earthbound spirits. Such drinking sessions end in gross intoxication.

Souls of the departed continue to need the sustenance of pulque. A dead adult is buried with tortillas and pulque to sustain him on his trip to the next world. Upon arrival in heaven the souls start raising crops to provide themselves with food and pulque. When the souls return to earth on the Day of the Dead, pulque is always included in the banquet provided for the visiting spirits. Asked about pulque in Hell, an Indian replied, "The Devil is free to do as he likes, so certainly he drinks pulque. No one drinks selfishly by himself when others are thirsty, so the Devil must share with those souls he has won, for they are now his and belong to his pueblo."

Pulque must be given to the skulls buried in the four corners of fields near the highway to protect the crops from out-of-town robbers. If the skulls do not receive their pulque, they stop frightening off thieves and start frightening the owner of the field.

As in preconquest times pulque is considered a holy beverage. The myth of its divine donor has been transferred from Mayahuel to the Virgin of Guadalupe. The Indians refer to pulque as "the milk of our Mother," that is the Virgin. Ceremonial drinking is required for the celebration of all religious fiestas.

Indians of the Milpa Alta area can distinguish by taste the pulque produced by each village. Tecospans believe their pulque is superior to all others. Since pulque comes from the land of their community, the Indians feel that it constitutes a bond between them. To refuse a man's pulque is to reject the man, his family, the village, and the Indian world as a whole. The sharing of pulque symbolizes social and spiritual brotherhood.

The significance of pulque drinking was vividly demonstrated to us during the early part of the field work in Tecospa. William Madsen entered a neighboring village for the first time on the day of the fiesta honoring the village patron saint. Without obtaining permission, he photographed the dances in progress. A few minutes later he was backed against the church wall at machete point by a group of angry drunken men. Just then a group of Tecospa Indians appeared and calmed the hostile captors. The words spoken by the eldest Tecospan were, "Release our friend. He is not a stranger. He has drunk our pulque." It was enough. The machete disappeared and all present drank pulque together. The sharing of pulque as a symbol of friendship is a traditional way of terminating a quarrel.

Indian Drinking Behavior

Drinking occurs only in prescribed social contexts and drunkenness is largely confined to community or family fiestas. Ceremonial occasions for drinking include saints' days, baptisms, confirmations, weddings, house warmings, and wakes. The drinking group typically consists of men but it is not uncommon for their wives to drink beside them in a home environment.

Ritualized drinking begins with formal toasts and countertoasts. As the drinking progresses, the formality of the ritual tends to be relaxed but each person tries to maintain his dignity despite intoxication. This does not mean that he cannot display humor— there is much laughter within the drinking group. If a man "passes out" he is placed in a comfortable position and if he is too drunk to walk home at the end of the evening his wife or a friend will help him.

Any display of aggression or hostility toward a fellow drinker is unthinkable. One is drinking a sacred beverage on a ceremonial occasion and it is a time for sharing common identities rather than airing individual differences. People never display anger or physical violence in a drinking group made up exclusively of Tecospans. Group intoxication intensifies the feeling of community and oneness. Any expressions of anger are directed against outsiders and usually are shared by all. Even this type of animosity is rare.

Group drinking is a structured process of peaceful interaction among individuals who identify themselves as a unit functioning in a homogeneous and predictable social environment. The alternative of deviant behavior simply does not exist. The greater the mutual sharing of pulque, the greater is the feeling of unity. Such drinking, despite the degree of intoxication, is always integrative. It is never associated with guilt, anxiety, addiction, or social problems.

Nor is pulque drinking associated with unpleasant aftereffects. If discomfort occurs on the morning after, it is attributed to exhaustion or exposure to night air on the way home. Treatment consists of resting, drinking herb teas and a fair amount of pulque. The patterns of agricultural work are flexible enough so that a day missed in the fields for a valid reason is not seen as failure to fulfill one's working role.

Distilled beverages are seldom used in ritualized drinking. Until Tecospa was connected with Milpa Alta and Mexico City by bus service, the town lacked cash crops which would provide money to buy distilled beverages. After the establishment of transportation facilities, Tecospans began selling pulque and surplus crops. The cash income is used to buy manufactured goods as well as a limited quantity of beer, tequila, and grain alcohol. Young men buy beer at two small stores and drink it on the premises in the early evening. They rarely drink more than two bottles each. Sometimes the beer is taken home and mixed half-and-half with pulque.

Tequila and grain alcohol are not sold in the village but young men occasionally bring a bottle back from a market town. The bottle is consumed outdoors by a group of three to six men. They do not drink in a home, where the son would risk a paternal reprimand for wasting money on mestizo intoxicants. Those who choose to drink tequila or grain alcohol are somewhat marginal persons who have accepted certain mestizo values. At the time of our study only three men in the village showed a consistent preference for grain alcohol. They were regarded as deviants and referred to by the Spanish term *alcohólico* or a Nahuatl word meaning unreliable. The term alcohólico does not mean an alcoholic but one who consumes grain alcohol. The aggressive drunken behavior of these three men reinforced a general impression that they were abandoning the Indian way of life. It is significant that each of them had worked in larger towns for periods of more than a year and then returned to Tecospa. They will probably leave again and try to become mestizos.

Drinking distilled beverages in the village disturbs its homogeneity and threatens the Indian value of nonaggression. By a similar process Indian drinking in a heterogeneous setting may produce conflict or violence. Drunken disputes occur when Indians from different villages are drinking in the same town during a village fiesta. Indian bystanders usually manage to soothe the antagonists and avoid violence, but sometimes fights erupt between groups from different communities.

A more common occurrence is conflict between Indians and mestizos on occasions of public drinking in market towns. The Indians feel threatened by mestizo merchants who "cheat" them in town, wholesale buyers who underpay them for their crops, and forest rangers who arrest them for cutting timber in Indian-owned forests. Mestizos sometimes ridicule or insult an Indian during fairs or fiestas in Milpa Alta and Xochimilco. If the Indian is drunk enough to answer back in kind, there may be a fight. Policemen quickly appear and often arrest the drunken Indian. Indian conflict with mestizos increases the feeling of need for community solidarity against the outside world. After returning to their village, the Indians observe the traditional rite of social interaction by sharing pulque.

While Indian drinking can create friction or violence in a heterogeneous setting, ritualized drinking within the community performs an integrative function by reinforcing group solidarity and corporate identity. In this social context drunkenness is normative and highly valued behavior which supports the communal values shared by all members of the community.

The corporate structure of Tecospan drinking has parallels in many other Indian communities of Latin America. Bunzel studied drinking patterns in the Indian village of Chamula, in Chiapas, where drunkenness is valued behavior. In analyzing her findings, she writes, "Not only is drinking always social, it is always ceremonial. . . . Alcohol is considered a necessity, and as such it has no critics. Nor does anyone feel guilt or shame over having been drunk. . . . Alcohol is not socially disruptive among them, but a mechanism of social integration" (1940:372, 377–78, 387).

Similar observations were made by the Romneys in a study of a Mixtecan Indian barrio in Juxtlahuaca, Oaxaca. The prevailing pattern was to drink heavily during the fiesta and not at all between times. The ritualized drunkenness required during fiestas did not produce aggressive behavior. The Romneys analyze their data in these words:

> The manifest function of this drinking pattern as stated by the men is that it represents solidarity and acceptance within the group. They recognize that the pattern is very different from that [the mestizo pattern] in the central part of town and say that it sets the Indian off from the Mexican. They also say that it symbolizes acceptance of the Indians and of the whole cofradia organization and the round of fiestas that it entails. . . . Questioned about whether or not they desired alcohol between fiestas, the men in the barrio always responded as though this were a peculiar question, because obviously one drank only during fiesta occasions. Most of the men accepted this drinking pattern as the only natural and imaginable one possible. [1966:69–70]

In each of the Indian communities discussed above, drinking is culturally defined as a rite of corporate identification which strengthens group solidarity. It is not defined as a tension reliever, ice breaker, or jollifier for the anxiety ridden.

Mestizo Value Conflict

The integrative function of Indian drinking changes during the process of acculturation. The strength of Indianism is slowly eroding with the encroachment of modern Western civilization. Some Indian communities borrow from the dominant culture until they no longer consider themselves Indian. Loss of Indian identity can be best observed in market towns or administrative centers which are focal points of change.

Borrowing begins in the realm of material culture while the ethos remains Indian. When basic values begin to change, the community develops identity problems. Some people think of themselves as mestizos while others fight to maintain their Indian identity. Ultimately the change from Indian to mestizo culture involves transition from a corporate to a competitive society.

Tepepan

Such a transition is occurring in the mestizo town of Tepepan (population three thousand) located on the main highway between Mexico City and Xochimilco. Tepepan is part peasant and part proletarian. Most of the families own land used for subsistence agriculture, but wage labor has become an alternative means of earning a living. Young men commute by bus to Mexico City where they are employed as gardeners, mechanics, and factory hands. Women are hired as maids by wealthy urban families. The heterogeneous population includes residents who come from various parts of the Valley of Mexico and rootless individuals who move from one town to another. Spanish is the only language spoken in Tepepan. The older generation is familiar with Nahuatl but never uses the language of "uncivilized Indians."

Tepepan mestizos lack the sense of community and sociocultural identity that characterizes the Indian village. There is no feeling that members of the mestizo community should stick together and help each other nor is there any sense of group pride. On the contrary, the mestizo is wont to disparage his community as a disreputable lot of witches, murderers, and thieves. The individual seldom identifies with others outside his family. Even family identity is on the wane as the number of broken homes increases. Only in reference to Indians does the mestizo identify as a member of a superior group. The Indian way of life has become a target of ridicule and contempt for the mestizo who is trying to emulate the ways of city people.

Despite his contempt for Indians, the mestizo has a conflict about Indian values. Conflict between competitive Western goals and egalitarian Indian values produces contradictory definitions of appropriate behavior. Conspicuous consumption is valued by some members of the community and condemned by others. The man who is trying to get ahead fears the disapproval of his neighbors and harbors doubts about the propriety of his own behavior. There is no single system of rules he can follow to gain social recognition.

The religious prestige system is giving way to a secular system based on competitive display of wealth and power. There is a growing tendency to shun religious offices requiring large personal expenditures on community fiestas. Instead of contributing to the group, the modern-minded mestizo strives to outshine other members of the group. He wants a better house, better food, and better clothes than his neighbors. He covets the lucrative occupational roles of the wealthy city dweller and resents the fact that such roles are denied him because he lacks the requisite skills. Even when the mestizo fails to achieve his economic goals, he never stops dreaming that some day he will be rich. Accumulation of wealth is not an end in itself but a means for the individual to demonstrate his superiority over others.

The mestizo man seeks prestige by proving his machismo which is the art of displaying manly superiority. He achieves sexual identity by dominating others with his wits and his fists. The true man must be prepared to defend his honor even at the risk of death. In his relationships with women he must exercise absolute authority over his wife and make a conspicuous display of sexual conquests outside the home.

The concept of machismo is derived from the Spanish ideal of manliness which spread through mestizo society in colonial times but never penetrated the Indian community. Ramos (1938) suggests that machismo is used to mask a sense of inferiority which can be traced back to denigration of the mestizo by the Spanish conquerors.

Unlike the Indian, the mestizo expects aggression and hostility from others. His society encourages aggressive behavior and violence. Young boys are taught to fight when they are insulted or ridiculed by their peers. In the process of growing up, a boy learns by example that the aggressive male is the one who wins out in the struggle for superiority.

The woman's role has been traditionally defined as a corollary of male superiority. The domineering man requires a wife or mistress who plays a completely submissive role. The mestizo man still cherishes the image of female subservience, but many women operate on an entirely different premise. The mestizo wife who has accepted Western ideas about women's rights poses a threat to her husband's machismo. Conflicting definitions of sexual roles have produced conflicted marital relationships which not uncommonly end in desertion.

Mestizo Drinking Behavior

Tenuous family and community ties reflect the lack of corporate identity. The man who sees himself in danger of becoming a social isolate drinks in search of companionship and escape from anxiety. The implicit premises reflected in mestizo drinking are explained by Wolf:

> Uncertain of backing from his fellows, he is thrown back on his own resources . . . he often feels estranged from society. Wishing to escape reality, he has learned to "drown the pain of living" in alcohol or gambling, creating for himself an unreal world with unreal stakes. Despising life, he has learned to substitute the dream for unfriendly reality. He may rise suddenly on a crest of fantasy into a dream world of personal dominance only to fall back into a trough of self-denigration, filled with feelings of misfortune and insufficiency. [1959:240]

The mestizo man views drinking as an essential means of displaying his manly superiority. Abstinence is a negative status symbol indicating the lack of machismo. Beer, tequila, and pulque are consumed in bars or stores where men gather in the evening. To gain prestige in the drinking circle, a man must be able to outwit and outfight his fellow drinkers. Secular drinking situations commonly involve a game of verbal dueling won by putting down an opponent without letting him know he is the target of an indirect insult. If the insult is recognized, it must be repaid. The ethics of machismo require an insulted man to fight in defense of his honor. Drunken fights sometimes end in murder, with multilation of the victim to degrade the enemy and bring grief to his family.

Gross intoxication causes loss of prestige when it renders a man incapable of defending himself. To recover his prestige he must later hunt down his enemy and attack him. It is customary to drink for courage before such an attack. Sometimes an evening of drinking is followed by an attack on a rival outside the drinking circle.

Chronic drunkenness, like abstinence, is viewed as a sign of weakness. Although the drunkard loses prestige, he is not condemned, ridiculed, or ostracized. Alcohol addiction is defined as a misfortune which befalls those who are born with the fate of becoming drunkards. Victims of fate are not blamed for behavior which is beyond their control.

Marital conflict is increased by drunken husbands who beat their wives excessively without provocation. Most women define beating as normal male behavior when it is administered as just punishment for the neglect of household duties. However, the drunkard who abuses this privilege angers his wife and sometimes provokes her to take action. One Tepepan wife solved the problem by hiring a witch to "hex" her husband. She reported that the bewitched man continued coming home drunk but showed a remarkable personality change and stopped beating her.

Mestizo drinking is a socially divisive process in Tepepan which produces disruptive behavior and addiction. Intoxication intensifies feelings of hostility which lead to violence. Aggressive drinking behavior reflects the culturally defined assumption that every man is engaged in a do-or-die struggle to outshine his fellows. When he fails, as sooner or later he must, the mestizo becomes a nobody in his own eyes and in the eyes of society. Alcohol then enables him to recapture the fantasy of being a superior person.

This disruptive pattern of drinking behavior is also found among lower-class mestizos in Mexico City. Drinking provides escape from the degrading existence of the poor in a society where status depends on wealth. A slum dweller's premises about reality are described by a Mexico City youth:

> There is no law here, just fists and money, which is what counts most. It is the law of the jungle, the law of the strongest. . . . No one helps the ones who fall; on the contrary, if they can injure them more, they will. . . . If one is winning out, they will pull him down. . . . We live by violence, homicide, theft, and assault. We live quickly and must be constantly on guard. [O. Lewis 1961:237]

The slum dweller despises his community and wants to get out. If he cannot do so, he feels trapped in a hopeless situation where the only way he can gain prestige is by proving his machismo. What machismo means to a slum dweller is conveyed in these words:

> Mexicans admire the person "with balls" as we say. . . . The one who has guts enough to stand up against an older and stronger guy is more respected. . . . If any so-and-so comes up to me and says "Fuck your mother," I answer, "Fuck your mother a thousand times." And if he gives one step forward and I take one step back, I lose prestige. But if I go forward too, and pile on and make a fool of him, then others will treat me with respect. In a fight I would never give up or say, "Enough," even though the other was killing me. I would try to go to my death smiling. That is what we mean by being "macho." [O. Lewis 1961:38]

This concept of machismo is reflected in aggressive drinking behavior accompanied by bloody fights and brutality. To refuse a drink is to arouse antagonism or invite a fight. Drinking groups are composed exclusively of men who seek social interaction in cantinas or pulquerias. The atomistic structure of lower-class society fosters extensive drinking.

Middle- and Upper-Class Drinking

Attitudes toward drinking change in the middle and upper classes when the means for upward social mobility become available. Excessive drinking then becomes a financial drain, a hindrance to working ability, and a threat to reputation. Correct drinking behavior is viewed as a social skill which must be carefully manipulated to enhance the drinker's status. In contrast to the lower-class pattern, upper-class drinking groups frequently include women, but all-male drinking groups are still popular in upper-class Mexican society.

Drinking parties provide the individual with an opportunity to display his intelligence, sophistication, and wit in a competitive game in which each person tries to prove his superiority. Formal toasts usually regulate the rate of drinking. Guests must follow the lead of their host and may not drink faster than he does. Inconspicuous intoxication is the normal goal of drinking.

The upper classes condemn public drunkenness. The man who cannot control his drinking is detested as a fool who has the mind and morals of a peon. To some extent, upper-class sanctions against drunkenness have permeated the middle class.

Middle- and upper-class drinking is selectively integrative in promoting superficial interaction within social cliques whose membership is constantly shifting. Although drinking parties provide a limited sense of corporate identity, their primary function is to enhance the status of the upwardly mobile individual.

Conclusions

Since preconquest times, Indian drinking behavior has been structured by the assumption that drinking is a form of corporate communion among men and between men and gods. Pulque drinking is defined as a rite of sharing that signifies identification with the group and acceptance of all its members as social equals. These premises are reflected in ritualized drinking behavior devoid of violence and hostility.

Group drunkenness intensifies the feeling of community and accentuates the display of valued role behavior. The role of drunken Indian is enacted with exaggerated dignity and courtesy toward other members of the drinking group. Ritualized intoxication is a function of the integrated value system which structures drinking-role relationships in a noncompetitive society. Within the Indian community prescribed drunkenness seldom gives rise to addiction, social problems, or guilt.

The external threat of mestizo culture has increased the value of drinking as a means of asserting Indian identity. Common opposition to the mestizo outgroup is manifested by emphasizing behavior which seems most Indian. Sharing pulque is viewed as a sacred rite which sets the Indians apart from the mestizos.

Loss of community and identity opens the door to drinking problems. The change from secular sobriety to mass drunkenness after the Spanish conquest reflected native despair over the loss of tribal identity and traditional goals. Drinking and vagabondage provided escape from a meaningless existence.

The proletarian mestizo of modern Mexico also lacks the

corporate identity that constitutes a cultural prerequisite for socially integrative drinking. During the process of acculturation, there is no single system of cultural rules which the individual can follow to gain social recognition. The old religious prestige system is giving way to a secular system based on the competitive display of wealth and power. The man who seeks prestige through conspicuous consumption fears the disapproval of his neighbors and harbors doubts about the propriety of his own behavior. He is caught between two cultures in an anomic situation where there is no clear-cut definition of role relationships and no means of obtaining desired occupational roles. In many respects, the mestizo fits Marx's concept of the alienated proletarian who lacks sociocultural identity.

Mestizo drinking behavior reflects the hostility and anxiety created by value conflict, blocked goals, and competitive relationships. The person who is in danger of becoming a social isolate drinks in search of companionship and escape from anxiety. Secular drinking occurs in bars where role relationships are not integrated by cultural directive. Intoxication intensifies feelings of hostility and leads to violence when machismo is at stake. Aggressive drinking behavior stems from the assumption that a man gains prestige by dominating others with his wits and his fists. Chronic drunkenness produces loss of prestige but the drunkard is not condemned, ridiculed, or ostracized.

When the urban mestizo becomes fully acculturated, he loses his Indian values and acquires the means of achieving Western economic goals. Prolonged drinking then becomes a financial drain, a hindrance to his working ability, and a threat to his reputation.

Middle- and upper-class mestizos view drinking as a social skill used to enhance the status of the upwardly mobile. Abstinence is a negative status symbol. Drinking-role relationships are structured by strict rules about when, where, how, and with whom one must drink. Male drinking behavior reflects the upper-class premise that machismo should be proved not by brute force but by displaying intellectual superiority and sexual prowess. Conformity is maintained in exclusive social circles by ostracizing deviant drinkers.

Upper-class drinking standards are distinguished by the condemnation of public drunkenness. The drunkard is detested as a fool who has the mind and morals of a peon. Among all social classes in urban society, deviant drinking is associated with addiction, disruptive behavior, and the guilt or shame characteristic of Western alcoholism.

Note

1. A species of the agave (*Amaryllidaceous* genus), especially *Agave atrovirens;* also A. *potatorum,* A. *americana,* and A. *tequilana.*

The Role of the Drunk in a Oaxacan Village

Philip A. Dennis

> Invest me in my motley; give me leave
> To speak my mind, and I will through and through
> Cleanse the foul body of the infected world,
> If they will patiently receive my medicine.
> Shakespeare [*As You Like It,* act 2, scene 7]

In Amilpas, a village in the Valley of Oaxaca, a drunk wanders down the street, lurching from side to side and shouting insults at all he encounters. Little children run indoors, and people approaching from the other direction dodge off into side streets to avoid meeting him. Ordinary village street life ceases as he approaches and resumes after he has passed. Local residents seem to regard drunks as one of the hazards of village life, along with rabid dogs and loose oxen. There is a similar element of physical danger: if the drunk is armed, he may injure someone, and, in fact, most intravillage quarrels and homicides occur after drinking. My wife and I have vivid memories of dashing into our adobe house along with neighbors when bullets from a street drunk started zinging through the trees. We thought he was shooting at our Coleman lantern!

Drunks do present real physical danger, especially when armed with pistol or machete. However, the social danger represented by the drunk seems to be feared almost as much as the actual physical danger. The drunk does not have to observe the polite conventions which allow everyday life to go on in the village. Instead of a polite, "Good morning, how did you awaken?," he may greet a fellow citizen with an accusation of stealing from the village treasury, failing to repay an old loan, making someone ill (witchcraft), or some other kind of misbehavior. The visiting anthropologist quickly learns that drunks are likely to accuse him of nefarious purposes: being an evangelist, selling data to an enemy village, using villagers for his own gain. Like his informants, he learns to avoid drunks and situations where drunks are congregated. The drunk is likely to say things that were better left unsaid, to voice suspicions that are only suspicions, and by their nature are incapable of being either proved or disproved. He threatens to tear down the polite facade of ordinary social life in the village.

Offensive Information Exchange

The approach to social life developed by Erving Goffman is especially useful in analyzing the drunk's role. Goffman (1959) tells us that the social self is vulnerable and subject to discrediting, and that a general problem in social interaction is to control the exchange of potentially destructive information. Conventional rules of respect for the social situation are one way of doing this (Goffman 1963). The proper personal attire, facial expression, and attention to those speaking must be maintained. Nowhere are such rules of conduct more apparent than at festive meals and other social occasions in Oaxacan villages. Formal speeches are made as drinks and food are served, and an elaborate front is maintained by statements that guests are in their own homes, the group is united, in fact brothers, and that there are no animosities. Polite phrases are repeated emphasizing the safety of guests and the confidence and friendship enjoyed by all present. As Michael Kearney (1972) observes, this forced insistence on safety and friendship serves to emphasize its opposite: the old quarrels and repressed aggression which threaten to erupt, given a chance. The truth as perceived by participants is likely to be quite different from that expressed openly in the social gathering, but the rules of respect for the situation act as what we may call an "information control device." They block the exchange of potentially disruptive information and allow the interaction to continue. Hotchkiss (1967) has pointed out some of the other information control devices in Mexican villages: the adobe and cane fences which ensure domestic privacy, the evasive greetings used in casual encounters, the shopping basket carefully covered by a rebozo.

　　Taken together, all these elaborate conventions for minimizing information exchange may be extremely effective. They may be so effective, in fact, that they prevent the truth as perceived or suspected by community members from ever being expressed. Social life seems to require not only information control, but techniques for communicating in spite of the control devices that exist. Hotchkiss has shown that in Mexican villages one technique for circumventing information control devices is spying by children. Accorded special license, children can be almost any-where, and can report back to their parents the scandalous doings of other adults. I suggest that there is a repertoire of such tech-niques of "offensive information exchange," and that among them is the role of the drunk.

Social gatherings in Amilpas are not complete unless some-one plays the role of the drunk. At a banquet given in honor of a visiting dignitary, the district superintendent of public schools, there were after-dinner speeches. The village had been petition-ing for a second school building for several years, and had even offered to provide the labor and part of the materials. The superin-tendent had been little help. He was in fact regarded as a major obstacle in the path of getting the new school. When he had made his own pompous after-dinner speech, full of flowery promises, a drunk who had been listening on the periphery of the crowd lurched forward and stood at the foot of the banquet table. He called the superintendent a liar, asked why none of the previous promises had been fulfilled, and shouted that he wouldn't believe any of the new promises being made. There was embarrassment among the crowd, but also delight. The drunk had forcefully stated the village's real position, which differed considerably from the polite front being presented by the village authorities at the banquet table. It would have been suicidal for the authorities themselves to take such a hard-line position, but the drunk had the license to do so. The "message" contained in this encounter seemed to be as follows:

> We will play the game of being polite hosts to a visiting dignitary who controls a resource we need. He has failed us in the past and we have little reason to believe he will come through in the future. Although we will show him the correct courtesies, we will also state our real position in a forceful and dramatic fashion, but in such a way that we cannot be held responsible.

After the incident, informants commented that after all, the drunk had only been telling the truth. Put in Goffman's terms, the drunk in this case was a member of the village's team (1959). He in fact served as its licensed and privileged spokesman, ready to chal-lenge the established social front on his team's behalf.

At banquets and other formal social occasions, the drunk has a captive audience. Relatives try to calm him down or lead him off, but usually not before he has had his say. Women, who rarely play the role of the drunk as I have described it, do have an important "nonformalized" role in this regard (see Chiñas 1973). They are quick to lead away an inebriated male relative, put him quietly to sleep, perhaps cajole him into leaving a situation which is becoming unpleasant. A woman plays a sort of corollary role, that of guardian of the drunk. She is expected to enforce respect for social norms, and to manage her stronger but less responsible male relatives.

When a drunk makes offensive remarks to a gathering, a common audience reaction is embarrassed silence: individuals look at their plates, and some may exchange collusive glances. The drunk's license does not confer license upon the audience. Interviewed later, many of those present may admit they secretly enjoyed his accusations and ravings, but they cannot admit this at the moment. They must maintain their own appearance of respect for the situation, in the face of the drunk's assaults. The drunk, by social definition, refuses to respect the situation, but he cannot confer a similar privilege on the others present.

Another audience response is to ignore the drunk, and to continue polite conversation in spite of his verbal assaults. This amounts to throwing up a new barrier of information control, to prevent the assimilation of the destructive information being offered. The drunk's response—stubbornness and petulance—is really an insistence on saying what he is supposed to say in spite of the information control barriers he faces. The drunk can be seen as intent on fulfilling his mission as agent of information exchange. His is not an easy task: he must circumvent adobe walls, evade well-meaning relatives, and silence those who would ignore him. He insists on speaking partly out of the conviction that what he has to say should be heard. Perhaps in no other way will people learn that Pedro Fulano is a thief, and this is the sort of thing that should be known.

In less formal situations the drunk may have to find his own audience. Drunks are notorious for searching out social gatherings and entering uninvited to make their proclamations. Relatively little effort is made to exclude them, or to prevent them from speaking. Drunks could be easily picked up by the village police and thrown into the local jail, but this rarely happens unless there is a real threat to physical safety. After all, the drunk does provide entertainment, which is always a problem in the village setting. Conversation and gossip are partial solutions, but watching the drunk is even better. Michael Kearney's observation (1972) that in another Oaxacan village drunkenness is a way of transcending the dismal realities of everyday life, can be applied more specifically to the drunk's role. It represents one individual's release from oppressive, everyday social norms, in a performance which benefits others as well. Observers may not feel free to laugh openly, but there is little doubt they often enjoy the drunk's behavior.

There is of course a great deal of difference in the ability of individuals to play the role. In Amilpas, Demetrio the poet is a specialist. Once drunk, he speaks in rhyming couplets, stringing couplets together into barbed and witty speeches. He is often asked to speak on social occasions, to the smiles of adults and the giggles of children. The expectation when Demetrio staggers to his feet is that some scandalous and delightful piece of gossip, new or old, will be offered. At a banquet of the *cofradía* in which I served, he delivered impromptu a series of stinging couplets about myself and about the fat and greedy village priest, who had refused to attend the affair. Demetrio in effect serves as a local gossip columnist, regularly reporting goings-on about town. In a setting where very few read for pleasure, Demetrio provides in an oral medium the kind of information found in movie magazines or other scandal sheets. It is true that gossip is a major form of entertainment in the village setting, as Hotchkiss (1967) and others have observed, but it is also true that some people are better at it than others. Demetrio, once inebriated, is a skilled public gossip. After the *cofradía* banquet, apologies were offered, apparently on the suspicion that Demetrio had gone too far and that the possible offense was unjustified. Demetrio pushes the role of drunk as social commentator to its limit, but villagers recognize that he becomes sidetracked by petty gossip, invents cutting remarks for their own sake, and often misses the really trenchant social commentary to be made. He illustrates an entertaining but sometimes foolish and pointlessly offensive aspect of the drunk's role.

In the street, stumbling along, forcing passersby to turn into side lanes to avoid him, the drunk can be seen as a messenger in search of an audience, a bearer of social truths too painful to listen to openly. In such a situation, escape is the only legitimate way of dealing with the drunk's insults. Women, who spend more time than men in the courtyards and streets where they are exposed to drunks, seem to cooperate among themselves to avoid their attentions.

> ... women avoid any possibility of interaction with a drunken man by signaling one another of the approach of a borracho on the public streets, by ducking into one another's doorways and tienditas, and by many other avoidance techniques. ... I several times found myself beckoned into the solar of a woman I had never seen before because a weaving, stumbling figure was approaching, perhaps still half a block away. [Chiñas 1973:104–5]

On informal occasions when an obnoxious drunk is present, the standard escape is to slip away quietly when no one is looking. The drunk would interpret a public announcement of leave-taking as a desire to avoid his company, an insult. He would insist that one stay on and continue drinking with him, so to avoid such unpleasantness one simply leaves unnoticed when the opportunity arises. This is not regarded as impolite; it is simply prudent.

The physical danger in such a situation is partly in one's own reaction. If one is sober and one's accuser is drunk, it would be regarded as grossly unfair to strike him. An informant commented that "striking a drunk would be like striking a child. The authorities would throw you in jail and ask, 'Were you more drunk than the drunk, to react the way you did?' " The drunk is viewed as physically incapacitated, but socially liberated. He cannot be held responsible for what he says, since he is drunk, and he need not fear reprisal from a sober victim. Speaking of Chamula, a highland Maya village in Chiapas, Bunzel comments:

> Toward a drunken man everyone assumes a protective and conciliatory attitude. He is not considered responsible. If he is belligerent no one tries to cross him or argue with him. No one, unless he too were drunk, would assume a belligerent or condemnatory attitude. [1940:378]

When more than one man is drunk, of course, the situation is different. To accept an invitation to drink with someone already inebriated is to allow oneself to respond to any insults that may arise. This fact helps explain the reluctance to accept a drunk's invitation to join him; it is potentially dangerous, since once "socially drunk," one can respond in kind. As long as one is sober one must simply avoid the drunk's insults, or laugh them off as nonsense, but once drunk oneself, the aggression one feels can be legitimately expressed.

Romney and Romney (1966) interpret fiesta drinking in a Mixtec village as a form of mutual aggression, in which social pressure from the group forces each man to drink beyond his capacity. The drinking procedure provides the main evidence for the "group-drinking-as-mutual-aggression" hypothesis: each man must finish his shot glass of liquor during each round of drinks served. The drinking procedure is identical in Amilpas, but it is important to note that here aggression is expressed not only through drinking itself, but also through the words and actions of the drunk. I suggest that the Amilpas drunk in a social gathering expresses not only his own pent-up aggression, but also the generalized aggressions of the group, which may be focused in turn upon a visiting dignitary, the village president, the anthropologist, or some ordinary member of the group. Formal drinking situations could easily deteriorate into an aggressive free-for-all were it not for the role of the drunk. Instead, the drunk seems to take on himself the burden of expressing aggression, castigating in turn various members of the group under cover of extreme intoxication, to the discomfort of those insulted and the general delight of everyone else.

Related Antiroles

Goffman (1963) suggests that individuals who are visibly intoxicated are exhibiting "out-of-role" behavior, and that like those engaged in frivolous sports or dressed in costume, they are open to jokes and other familiar advances, on the grounds that they are not playing serious roles. One does not have to be careful about communicating with an out-of-role individual, since he has demonstrated that he is profane and not to be taken seriously. In Amilpas, however, the drunk is not out-of-role at all. He occupies a definite role, one which is defined as sharply critical of the everyday roles being played around him. In this sense the drunk's is an "antirole," which, within its own carefully defined rules of behavior, reverses normal role expectations.

Regarded this way, the drunk's is clearly only one of many similar roles. In Amilpas, *susto*, or "fright illness," allows some of the same kinds of behavior (Uzzell 1974). Individuals who have suffered severe fright may be understandably cantankerous and disagreeable, as a result of their illness. However, relatives must continue to interact with them and to show care and concern for them. Their behavior is not really their fault, nor is it characteristic of their personality, since they are suffering from *susto*. Illness here provides an analogous social explanation for deviant behavior, and creates a similar sort of antirole. The difference is that the *susto* victim's license provides little opportunity for offensive information exchange.

The drunk's role also reminds one of the "rituals of rebellion" described by Gluckman (1963) and others, in which individuals publicly assert their hostility: subjects castigate their king, women revile men, and so on. Gluckman's interpretation of such rituals is paradoxical. They actually reaffirm the rightness of normal roles, and demonstrate the strength of the system to withstand periodic reversals of behavior. In a similar way, the threat to social life posed by the Oaxacan drunk is a very contained one. Normal social life does go on, and no one seriously questions the appropriateness of the norms he flouts, least of all the drunk himself, once he is sober. Oaxacan drunks, like Gluckman's rebellious Swazi warriors, are not revolutionaries. They have no interest in changing the social system, only in dramatically calling attention to the conflicts and hostility it creates. The clear implication in both cases is that the open expression of conflict helps resolve it, or at least ameliorate it.

In the Swazi ceremony, the ritual context clearly demarcates the legitimate arena for rebellion. For the Oaxacan drunk, apparent inebriation serves the same function; because he is intoxicated, his behavior in public can be ignored. From the drunk's own point of view, inebriation provides a legitimate excuse. On the following day he can, if necessary, beg forgiveness on the grounds that he was drunk and didn't realize what he was saying. In Amilpas, as in the Peruvian community described by Simmons (1960), there seems to be little guilt attached to intoxication, and no hesitation in referring to it later.

The antirole which provides the best comparison is that of the fool or court jester of Renaissance times. The Roman practice of keeping mentally retarded individuals for amusement evolved in medieval times into the specially licensed role of court jester (Goldsmith 1963). By the Renaissance, the fool's role was well established, and it is familiar to us from the literature of the time. In Shakespeare's plays, the fool is easily recognized by his distinctive costume: a suit of motley (usually green and yellow stripes); a fool's cap; and a bauble or imitation scepter, sometimes tipped with a fool's head in miniature (Goldsmith 1963). On an Amilpas street, the drunk's stumbling gait and slurred speech provide an analogous means of identification, and indicate a similar license in the role being played.

Because of his supposed insanity or feeblemindedness, the dramatic fool has special license to act as an agent of offensive information exchange. Lear's Fool, probably the best known, continually reminds the king of the extent of his folly. Lear has mistaken insincere praise for true love, and has given away his kingdom. The Fool taunts Lear with having grown old before growing wise, and comments that "there's not a nose among twenty but can smell him that's stinking" (act 2, scene 4). The king's only recourse is to disregard such remarks; after all, they only come from a fool. Like the drunk, the fool has license to tell the truth, but he has no way of making others behave in terms of it. He is essentially a commentator, freed from normal restraints by reason of insanity, but incapable of seriously influencing the action of the play. The irony of the dramatic fool, of course, is that often he is not a fool at all, but a voice of common sense and truthfulness, who ruthlessly points out the defects of the other characters. Lear's Fool is not unreasonable when he suggests that in terms of foolishness, he and the king would do well to change places. Presumed insanity, like presumed inebriation, allows a painful accuracy.

Alcohol and Drunken Behavior

Amilpeños, like people in many other societies, believe that inebriation is the immediate cause of the drunk's behavior. However, it seems likely that alcohol intake itself has no "disinhibiting" effect. MacAndrew and Edgerton (1969) argue convincingly that it is what society defines as permissive behavior after drinking that determines the behavior that occurs. The "time-out" from social norms which so often characterizes drunken comportment is, they argue, a social phenomenon and not a direct consequence of alcohol intake. Time-out occasions occur in many societies without benefit of alcohol, and conversely, inebriation is not always associated with time-out. MacAndrew and Edgerton's cross-cultural examination of drunken behavior uncovers radical differences, all of which cannot be attributed logically to the same physiological cause. Alcohol cannot be at the same time a sexual stimulant and a sexual depressant, a stimulus to aggression and a pacifying agent. Instead, alcohol, when it is used as a means of defining a time-out from social norms, seems to be chosen because it affects the sensorimotor system, and is thus highly "monitorable" by both the drinker and his audience. Because of the changes it produces in body control, alcohol intake can be used as a visible and perceptible symbol of altered expectations in comportment (MacAndrew and Edgerton 1969).

　　It seems likely that all antiroles require some outside, monitorable reason for the behavior involved. In MacAndrew and Edgerton's terms, "time-out" does not occur without some explicit reason being offered. Illness in the case of the *susto* victim, madness for the fool, inebriation for the drunk, the ritual context for the rebellious Swazi warrior: each provides a convenient social explanation for what would otherwise be deviant behavior. The very idea of deviancy is related to the lack of a clear social rationale for inappropriate behavior. Where such a rationale exists, we do not speak of deviancy, but of institutionalized behavior in some form of antirole. The Oaxacan drunk is no more a deviant than the

Swazi warrior, since each behaves in terms of the expected effects of some outside agency. Intoxication becomes a simple folk explanation for the drunk's behavior, although for his own explanation the anthropologist must look to more complex social and psychological processes.

In Amilpas, the assumption is that alcohol itself is disinhibiting. Drunks, it is believed, will naturally speak their minds, and in general they fulfill this expectation. The loss of self-restraint when intoxicated is considered as much a physiological reaction as loss of motor control. In fact, the one becomes indicative of the other. Stumbling and slurring one's speech indicate drunkenness and loss of self-control, and therefore confer social license, no matter how "real" they may be.

This being the case, it becomes apparent that "social drunkenness" really defines the drunk's role, and not physiological inebriation. Amilpas drunks are often suspected of not really being as drunk as they seem, in order to perform otherwise unacceptable acts with impunity. For example, an Amilpas drunk who accosted a passing woman from Soyaltepec, grabbed her basket of freshly prepared tortillas, and threw them on the ground, was accused by the Soyalpeños of not really being drunk. He pretended to be drunk, they said, to vent his aggression on a helpless woman from a traditionally hostile village.

Of course, drunks in Amilpas are often very drunk indeed. A successful saint's day or other celebration leaves the courtyard scattered with sleeping bodies, and an occasional passed-out drunk is a common sight. Being so drunk that one cannot speak in an articulate manner may actually prevent one from playing the role of the drunk effectively. Inebriated beyond a certain point, the drunk's attempts at criticism or satire often become ridiculous, to the amusement of his intended targets. Physiological inebriation to the point of losing self-control turns the drunk from acerbic social commentator to object of scorn. Passed-out, lying in the street in the rain, or stumbling and falling into a clump of cactus, the drunk becomes a visible demonstration of human frailty. He illustrates what is regarded as an all-too-human tendency to indulge oneself to excess.

The stumbling, inarticulate drunk is pitiful, but in a more subtle way, he reminds those who see him that social rules are instituted for a function. Lying in the street, he provides a vivid example of what happens to those who push their socially sanctioned license for deviance to the limit. Like Freudian sexuality, Goffmanesque destructive social information must be expressed one way or another. Devices for offensive information exchange are inevitable, given the nature of social life, but they also involve penalties for the individuals who make use of them. The drunk who shoulders the burden of expressing destructive information is seen to suffer for having done so. Sometimes irresponsibly truthful, sometimes entertaining, the drunk often ends up as an object of pity and scorn. The elaborate code of politeness which rules everyday life may be oppressive, but the unconscious drunk demonstrates to his onlookers that the alternative is worse.

In sum, native theory regarding the drunk is that he is not responsible for what he does and should be ignored or avoided, since alcohol produces changes in behavior. In reality, apparent inebriation serves to define a crucial role in village life: the licensed drunk pierces the elaborate information control devices of the community and provides the barefaced facts and opinions which normally go unspoken. Like the fool in a Shakespearean play, the Oaxacan drunk is accorded the special privilege of speaking the truth.

The Social Uses of Alcoholic Beverages in a Peruvian Community

Paul L. Doughty

Studies of alcohol consumption in various cultural contexts have shown many different responses to alcohol on both individual and social levels, and that the use of alcoholic beverages may vary in degree, amount, and function among different cultures. In many societies alcohol usage is so thoroughly integrated into the dietary and social norms that it is taken for granted and its effects anticipated and suitably controlled. Where the use of intoxicating beverages is expected and commonplace, their special qualities are consciously utilized as a device to structure and promote social intercourse and to facilitate the achievement of cultural ideals. Examination of the specific uses of alcohol, therefore, will provide some insight into the character of the social process and its milieu. This paper describes some of the drinking customs and associated behavior in one Peruvian highland community, and will demonstrate its recognized as well as covert functions. Since the Peruvian setting has been well described elsewhere, only the most salient points need be mentioned here. The traditional Indo-Mestizo society of highland Peru provides us with abundant materials for the subject at hand because of regional differences and important social structural elements.

The highland areas of the country have been characterized by a very rigid system of social stratification, dominated by the Spanish-speaking mestizo townsmen. The rural, Quechua-speaking Indian peasantry (the lower class in most areas) has begun to achieve some social mobility chiefly through migration and the acquisition of minimal skills. The Indians residing in the Andean highlands have long comprised a socially isolated, deprived, and subordinate sector of the Peruvian population. The principal features of Indian culture today are survivals of pre-Colombian and Spanish colonial society, nurtured in a closed universe that bespeaks limitations and which offers few alternatives. In this context, Mangin notes that drinking in the manoral society of Vicos, Ancash, is largely ceremonial. As such, it has come to form an integral part of the social roles open to the Indians; in the cultural sense, drinking "fits" (1957). Mangin, speaking of Quechua-speaking Vicosinos in 1952 and 1953, observed that there was little or no ambivalence related to drinking, nor were there any problem drinkers or alcoholics in the closed community. It should be noted, however, that the pattern observed in Vicos over fifteen years ago by Mangin appears to be changing at the present time. There are now at least three or four Vicosinos with an alcohol problem to the extent that drinking interferes with their loosely scheduled work patterns and interrupts their family relationships.

A second example from Peru is described by Simmons (1959, 1960). The people of Lunahuaná, a Spanish-speaking, mestizo community on the Southern coast of Peru, have been producers of wine and brandy for many generations. As with the Indians of Vicos, the use of alcoholic beverages is integrated into the social life of the community, and there are many parallels between Vicos and Lunahuaná drinking patterns despite the cultural differences between the communities. In both places, the solitary drinker is considered a deviant, drinking is associated with virtually all ceremonial events such as rites of passage, and it is essentially a male activity. Simmons noted that heavy drinking accompanied the grape harvest in Lunahuaná. At this time teenagers learned, under some duress from their parents, to conform to community drinking norms. Drinkers attempted to make their companions drunk. Nevertheless, drinking seemed to provide an important means of reducing anxiety and aggression. Despite the apparent integration of drinking in Lunahuaná culture and the fact that alcohol consumption is taken for granted by virtually everyone over sixteen years of age (just as in Vicos), Simmons found that there was ambivalence in Lunahuaná with regard to the learning of the drinking patterns. The culture of Lunahuaná appears to present some special problems deriving from the fact that the community itself is a producer of alcoholic beverages on a commercial scale. Drinking is closely associated with the grape harvest, and, symbolically, the young men are indoctrinated into the group drinking patterns at this time. The people of Lunahuaná are, therefore, doubly involved with alcohol, more so than the average community in Peru.

The District of Huaylas

The mestizo community of Huaylas, Ancash, located in the Callejón de Huaylas in the north highlands provides a contrasting cultural situation. A political district and compact social entity, Huaylas has a population of fifty-five hundred, of which approximately twelve hundred live in the town of Huaylas. Located in a small, irrigated valley nine to ten thousand feet above sea level, the district is essentially rural in character. Almost everyone engages in small farming and stock raising whether he is a townsman or not. In addition, there are many artisans (shoemakers, carpenters, tilemakers, weavers, etc.) in the district. Huaylinos like to think of themselves as self-sufficient and self-reliant although they are closely involved with outside events and dependent upon them to a large degree. The people are largely bilingual and, by highland standards, well educated; this permits Huaylinos to participate actively in the political and economic life of the region and the nation.

Because there is neither great wealth nor grinding poverty in the district, its social character is somewhat more open than in those areas which are dominated by large haciendas, such as the region around Vicos. There is no discrete Indian population to provide sharp contrast with the mestizos as occurs in the rest of the region (cf. Holmberg et al. 1965). One finds an incipient class system based upon a combination of social, cultural, educational, economic, and political factors. Some opportunity for social mobility exists in the district.

Strong relationships with Peruvians outside the valley have long been established and Huaylinos are highly mobile geographically as well as socially (Doughty 1963). The emigration rate is very high, and over the past twenty-five years about three thousand Huaylinos left the district to live in the coastal areas, particularly Lima and Chimbote. This pattern is typical of mestizo communities in the department of Ancash as well as in much of the central and northern highland regions.

The use of alcohol in daily life by Huaylinos is frequent and follows patterns similar to those that have been described for other Peruvian communities. There are, however, a few basic features that should be kept in mind as we consider some of the details of drinking as they customarily occur in social life in general, and particularly as they form part of interpersonal relationship patterns.

Drinking Patterns in Huaylas

First, drinking is a social act and is part of virtually every social gathering. Solitary drinkers are considered deviant and at best are looked upon as unfortunate individuals, or at worst, as unfriendly or "cold" (*seco*). Secondly, the act of drinking is a ritual unvarying in form. The ritual always involves a toast, "health" (*salud*), which is spoken by the drinker and repeated by his companions. If all members of the group have glasses, they drink simultaneously. Otherwise, the drinker, upon finishing his glass, empties the residue on the ground or floor with a quick snap of his wrist and passes the bottle on to the next person, whom he toasts, and the process is repeated. This toasting ritual is a kind of social contract; once a party to it, everyone is expected to fulfill his obligation to the rest—that is, accompany them in drink. The contract can and does embrace persons of differing social classes and so constitutes a patterned, comfortable means by which communication may take place despite status differences.

A third generalization concerning drinking patterns in Huaylas is that it is expected that men will drink more than women—a trait which has a wide distribution, as Mandelbaum has noted (1965, also in this volume). Because of this, it is considered masculine to become inebriated occasionally. The fourth and final point is that drinking is considered a natural part of life. Abstinence is at best considered unusual and a nondrinker may be thought unfriendly or antisocial, as in the case of the solitary drinker. Consequently, virtually all adults drink alcoholic beverages.

There is a wide range of commercial beverages imported in Huaylas. The following imports for 1958 (the last year for which I could obtain complete records) are mentioned in order of importance by quantity: beer, cane alcohol, wine of various types, pisco, cognac, vermouth, and anisette, followed by a variety of more exotic drinks such as rum, champagne, and a cocktail called "Stronger." The Huaylas population over twenty years of age (which appears to be the age at which Huaylinos begin to consume measurable quantities of alcoholic beverages) in 1960 numbered twenty-six hundred fifty persons—a figure close to what the 1958 population must have been. Based on these figures, the average consumption of commercial alcoholic beverages in Huaylas amounted to approximately eleven liters per person per year. The sharp drop in consumption between 1956 and 1958 (table 1) was due to the termination of work on the hydroelectric plant at nearby Huallanca and the cessation of high salaries which many earned. It also reflects a decline in population, for many persons moved to the coast after the construction ended.

TABLE 1.   Types and Quantities of Alcoholic Beverages Consumed in the District of Huaylas, Ancash, 1956–58

	Quantity in Liters	
Beverages	1956	1958
Beer	19,552	13,007
Cane alcohol	19,598	10,956
Wines	3,527	1,602
Pisco	3,015	1,193
Cognac	1,731	822
Vermouth	1,761	719
Anisette	1,274	241
Other	1,480	717
Total Liters	51,938	29,257

Source: Banco de la Nación (Caja de Depósitos y Consignaciones), Huaylas, Ancash.

These figures do not, of course, include the large amounts of chicha (maize beer) consumed annually by the average Huaylino. This quantity, in liters, I estimate to be at least equal to that of beer. Chicha is brewed in the home by virtually all Andean peoples of all social classes. Chicha in Huaylas is made of dried yellow maize which, having been moistened and allowed to sprout is called jora. The jora is ground, added to water, and boiled. It is then allowed to ferment with the help of brown sugar which is added to taste. The alcoholic content of Huaylas *chicha* is low—not much over 3 percent usually. The nonalcoholic *chicha morada* is made from purple maize in a slightly different manner to avoid fermentation. Both types are customarily served at room temperature, although hot *chicha de jora* is sometimes served as a kind of punch. Recipes for *chicha de jora* vary widely and each household takes great pride in the uniqueness of its product. There is no government control over production and distribution, nor is a tax levied upon *chicha* when produced for home use. Some *chicha* is dispensed at a few *chicherías* where, of course, its sale is theoretically subject to taxation. Unfortunately, there are no available records (as there are for "commercial beverages") of how much *chicha* is produced or consumed.

Many of these beverages, which are thought to have unique properties, may be consumed at a particular time or for a special reason. *Chicha*, for example, is thought to be a food of considerable nutritive value as well as a superior thirst quencher. Persons of both sexes and virtually all age groups (except the very young) drink *chicha* either at home with meals or in the fields as refreshment during work. Most consider it a food.

Pisco, like *chicha*, is regarded as the national drink. It is taken at any time or occasion and is often used as an aperitif or may be consumed after a meal, "to settle things in the stomach." Wines, when available, are generally consumed at mealtimes. Certain other beverages or combinations of them are considered to have medicinal or health-giving properties. Thus, anisette when taken in small quantities is believed to drive out the cold, as is "captain" (*capitán*), a drink made from vermouth and *pisco*. Vermouth is also sometimes taken with tea for this purpose or to calm the pains of a stomachache.

Cane alcohol (variously called *washco, caña, cañazo,* or in jest, "whiskey *huaylino*") is consumed either straight or mixed (*templado*) with soft drinks or water. When mixed with soft drinks it is called "alcohol with a point" (*con punta*) and is thought to cause more rapid intoxication. A small glass of equal parts of alcohol and lime juice is referred to as a "little hot one" (*calientito*) and is considered a powerful cold remedy. Beer, although expensive and prestigious, if consumed when too cold—rather than at normal room temperature (about 60 degrees Fahrenheit)—is thought to induce pains in the throat, particularly if one is not feeling well. This applies equally to soft drinks.

There is no aversion to the mixing of drinks, nor indeed to the time of the day that one imbibes. At a formal meal, a guest may well be asked to partake of all the following beverages: before the meal, a small glass or two of *pisco;* during the meal, red wine, white wine, a soft drink, and several glasses of *chicha;* after the meal, one may settle his stomach with an additional shot of *pisco* and, if the host can afford it, beer. This menu of drinks is typical of family gatherings and celebrations where meals are served the guests.

The guinea pig (*cuy*), which was originally domesticated for food in the Andes, still provides the final and most important dish of any special meal. Sometimes, particularly for birthday celebrations, additional *pisco* is consumed if one is challenged to drink a *copita* containing the tiny bone of the guinea pig's inner ear. Because of its small size, the bone, called the "little fox" (*zorrito*), may remain in the glass requiring the drinker to try again until he is successful in swallowing the bone. This was the only drinking "game" encountered in Huaylas and then only infrequently.

Attitude and Conduct While Drinking

To some extent Huaylinos behave while drunk much as the Vicosinos described by Mangin (1957). According to him, behavior while intoxicated was, for the most part, simply an exaggeration of a person's normal behavior; he did not find that people changed in personality when under the influence of alcohol. This seems only partially true in Huaylas, for there appear to be a number of exceptions, quite likely due to the greater number of social roles open to Huaylinos as well as increased levels of social rivalry and aspirations. When sober, Huaylinos tend to be assertive and independent, rather "open," and given to conversation. Aggressive behavior increases with alcoholic stimulation and people insist upon having their way. In fact, they say of themselves, "*Somos muy exigentes*" ("We are very demanding"). When drinking, they become quite loquacious and bold in their dealings with companions, particularly with those of a higher social class, at times giving vent to opinions hitherto unspoken. Others are often challenged to agree or disagree with a statement by responding to the short and vociferous question, "What do you say, yes or no?"

At this stage, an invitation to drink is virtually impossible to refuse or escape without serious incident. On several occasions, for example, I met the mayor of Huaylas slipping quietly through back streets on his way to the municipal office. His explanation of this devious route was that if he went by way of Commerce Street, the "boys" in the various stores would not let him pass without sharing a round or two, thus costing him an hour or so at each place. When aggressive Huaylinos drink, they tend to become more aggressive, or valiant (*guapo*) as they express it. Some persons indicated that they sometimes drink in order to gain this additional "bravery" (*bravura*) before attempting some difficult task such as facing a discomforting social situation. Even when not under the influence of alcohol, physical contact between men is frequent and entirely normal (in contrast to the United States). An arm about the shoulder of a companion is a common stance. When drinking, Huaylinos draw closer together physically, and it is not uncommon to see persons talking to each other, standing virtually "nose to nose," arms about each others' shoulders.

With persons under the influence of alcohol, the noise level rises sharply. If there is music, there will inevitably be dancing (usually *huaynos*) whether women are present or not. There is no physical contact between partners dancing the *huayno* (a common type of Andean music), and the drunken men invent fancifully exaggerated steps, performing with much individuality and fanfare. Finally, when the level of intoxication known as being "happy" (*alegre*) is reached, one may expect considerable shouting, laughter, and occasional whoops (called *guajes:* hahahaiiii) of earsplitting volume.

The tolerance for drunks in many Latin American societies is in general quite generous. In popular songs toasts are often raised in praise of beauty or of one's place of birth and drunkenness is expected when one's sweetheart leaves him for another. By the same token the "big night on the town" is upheld in the popular mind as a recreational ideal. "*¡Qué viva la jarana!*" ("Long live the spree!") is the shout of approval one often hears in the early morning. Public behavior which might be severely and negatively sanctioned in the United States is passed off as quite normal and within the limits of propriety in a place such as Huaylas. Drunks, in fact, are usually ignored or eased out of the way if they have intruded into one's affairs. Because drinking is a social act, drunkenness is almost by definition public.

However, limits are imposed in Huaylas, either by the members of the National Civil Guard (police) stationed there or by the public officials. Truly obnoxious drunks—such as those who have been fighting, provoking conflicts, or who have not been able to make their way home—if caught or "collected" receive sentences of "twenty-four inside" (i.e., twenty-four hours in jail). If there is work to be done in the jail or in the public square, drunks are used when they become sufficiently sober to work. In

1960, according to the Huaylas police records, 11 percent of the arrests of men were for public intoxication (eighteen cases), while 4 percent of the women arrested (two cases) were taken into custody for this reason. For the most part, however, drunks are simply escorted home by relatives, godsibs, friends, or by their wives.

Few Huaylinos are total abstainers, although there are many who seldom drink or who rarely become intoxicated. Women are often served smaller portions or may be permitted to drink only a part of that which they are served. Generally, however, because it is inhospitable to return a partially filled glass, some feign drinking, and when the host is not looking surreptitiously empty their glass or cup behind a chair and onto the absorbent earthen or brick floor. Persons not wishing to drink generally plead ill health. Especially favored are references to kidney and liver ailments, throat soreness, or an illness which might be aggravated by the "cold" properties of the beverage. The theme which underlies this kind of comportment (and which can also be seen in relation to other kinds of behavior) is that it is better to procrastinate or prevaricate than to offend. Excuses for abstaining are therefore accepted with reluctance and skepticism unless the illness is proven. Such an excuse as "driving and drinking don't mix" is not yet appreciated as a valid reason for a driver to abstain. Nondrinkers maintain their abstemious posture only at considerable social cost. The few Protestants living in Huaylas were "permitted" to drink soft drinks, but were strongly ridiculed and were often the butt of jokes. Several Protestants eventually proved to be "backsliders" in this regard when the social pressure became too great.

Aside from the general age and sex differences in drinking patterns already mentioned, there are readily observable differences in drinking behavior according to socioeconomic class. The Huaylas upper class, which is largely urban in residence pattern, consumes the major share of the beer sold in the district. The upper class also drinks a high percentage of such other commercial beverages as wine, vermouth, cognac, *pisco*, anisette, and champagne. Cane alcohol, as a rule, is not generally consumed by members of this class, although they drink it when served. The same cannot be said of *chicha: chicha* is prepared in every household and is consumed by everyone (even "nondrinkers" on occasion) where served or available.

Members of the local upper class participate in a constant round of social events such as dances, birthday parties, baptismal parties, and other festivities, all of which call for the use of alcoholic beverages. Among the men of the upper class, recreational drinking requiring no special social rationale to motivate it is very common. It is a safe estimate that half of the upper-class men in Huaylas purchase beer or some other commercial beverage at least three or four times a week and especially on weekends.

The chief difference in drinking patterns between the Huaylas middle and upper classes is that the middle class consumes much more cane alcohol and much less beer. Their consumption of *chicha* is also probably greater. They have less leisure time and are less likely to spend it in recreational drinking, although this does occur. Middle-class women are more likely to become drunk during festivals than are their upper-class counterparts.

The lower class reflects this pattern in a more pronounced manner. The members of this group consume almost no beer at all (unless invited to do so), instead drinking rather large amounts of cane alcohol, *chicha,* and *pisco.* The low consumption of beer is apparently attributable to its expensiveness. At the time of study, a one-liter bottle of beer cost between 30 and 40 percent (five *soles*) of the day laborer's average daily wage. Alcohol and *chicha,* however, could be purchased in less expensive, smaller units for which it can be said that buyers received a greater return on their investments. The lower class did almost no casual recreational drinking; its consumption of alcoholic beverages occurred principally at festive events.

Place and Time of Drink

Most drinking occurs either in the home or in a public place (such as a store or a bar) in the company of one's relatives and friends. In the town of Huaylas itself, there were at the time of study five establishments which could be legitimately classified as bars, catering indiscriminately to the public (although the bar at the billiard room had a largely upper- and middle-class clientele). Most of the alcohol consumed in Huaylas is imbibed midst the friendly setting of the eighty or more stores found throughout the district. Most such commercial establishments are a combination of general store and bar. They are the principal informal gathering places for men, and it is the rare storekeeper who does not keep a few glasses and a bottle or two about for his friends.

The situational contexts of drinking in Huaylas are varied. The first is the occasion of a religious or secular festival, the celebration of rites of passage, or a party to entertain distinguished guests. A second circumstance in which alcoholic beverages are consumed is during leisure time. The frequency of such occasions varies according to one's economic condition, as indicated previously. For some of the upper class this may even be a daily event, although for most it is weekly. Games such as billiards, checkers, chess, cards, or *sapo* (a typical Peruvian mestizo game in which contestants try to pitch brass discs into the mouth of a brass toad mounted on a table) are invariably accompanied by drinks, often paid for by the losers as part of a wager.

Huaylinos also drink for what may be termed emotional or psychological reasons. Persons who feel lonely, bored, or who are in search of consolation and sympathy search for companions who may be already drinking in stores. As a consequence, one can anticipate listening to long accounts of personal problems from time to time. There are a fairly large number of persons whose drinking was more than just an escape. I knew at least eleven people (all men) whose drinking had ceased to be a cathartic device and had reached a point where it manifestly added to their difficulties. If not already alcoholics, their proclivities in this regard were recognized and commented upon by others. There may well, of course, have been more. I knew approximately five hundred fifty persons by name in the district; the problem drinkers constituted 2 percent of this group.

The fourth situation in which drinking is likely to occur is during the performance of hard manual labor or on trips to the *puna* regions (areas above the tree line). On such occasions a drink is thought to refresh the individual and to help him to carry on his tasks either by warming him up, "animating him," rewarding him, or by bolstering his resolve. Alcoholic beverages thus function, in theory, to focus one's attention on the task to be completed. The most common beverages consumed are *chicha, pisco,* and cane alcohol.

Where persons from outside the family are involved in agricultural work, either on an exchange or festive labor basis, more drinking is done than if the family alone or hired laborers are involved. House building—as with other group work situations— is often a festive occasion made merrier by the consumption of large quantities of *chicha,* cane alcohol, or *pisco.* The festive labor party, called *rantín* or *minga,* works in bursts of activity between the moments when one's spirits are being reanimated. By late afternoon, the stage which Huaylinos refer to as "happy" has often been reached. If the builder can afford it, music is supplied by a man who plays *huaynos* on a large drum and flute combination (the *caja* and *roncadora*). The day's activities thus gradually evolve into a general household festival by the day's end. It should be noted that such festive and exchange labor has declined in popularity in Huaylas and has been replaced to a large degree by wage labor.

The important distinction between festive exchange labor and communal civic work should be noted. The former takes place largely in the social context of the extended family or neighbors, whereas the latter involves the entire community on work of general public interest. "Voluntary" civic work is an important feature of Peruvian Andean community life, sharply distinguishing these peasant communities in general from Banfield's "amoral familists" of southern Italy (1958).

Civic work parties, called *repúblicas*, are a common feature of Huaylas life as in many other Andean peasant communities. Organized by the barrios, the district irrigation council, or the school-parents association, Huaylinos engage in many hours of voluntary civic work to further projects of community concern. The levels of individual involvement in district affairs as well as community accomplishment in Huaylas is considerable. Largely as a result of their voluntary public labor, Huaylinos could boast (in 1964) that their district was probably the leading rural area in the country in terms of their access to and use of domestic electricity. Thirteen schools, a network of vehicular roads, a large irrigation system, a well-kept plaza and church, a three thousand-volume public library, and other such facilities are also the results of community efforts. At the present time, the district of Huaylas ranks among the most progressive in the highlands in terms of the public facilities available to its inhabitants.

The *república*, or public work project, is the key to this record. Each barrio maintains a list of ablebodied workers (*republicanos*) who are called out by their elected barrio leaders to work at least ten or twelve times during the course of a year. Twenty to 50 percent of the men turn out on these occasions, and those who do not choose to work are asked to make a contribution in kind or in money. Donations usually consist of a bottle of alcohol or as much as a seven-gallon barrel of *chicha*.

The projects undertaken by the *republicanos* vary in difficulty and urgency, and the rhythm of work is geared to the situation. Huaylinos may work a ten-hour day on some occasions or, in less demanding situations, as little as four or five hours during the course of an entire day. But no matter what the circumstance, the festive spirit of the work party is inevitably maintained by joking, music, and seemingly liberal amounts of drink. It is thought that alcoholic beverages are required in order to keep spirits high and the work progressing. Nevertheless, barrio leaders ration the amount consumed by the workers so that "they will not drink too much and get hurt." Alcoholic beverages are purported to make the workers more valiant (*guapo*) in the face of difficulties.

During the rural electrification project which was carried out by Huaylas' *republicanos* in 1960, the eighty men from Yacup barrio did one day's work fortified by at least eight bottles of cane alcohol and *pisco* and eight seven-gallon barrels of *chicha*. This was approximately three quarts of alcoholic beverage per man, an amount considerably above the average for such occasions. More normal would be a ratio of one quart of cane alcohol or *pisco* for every seven men and a pint of *chicha* each. As seen in table 2, refreshments amounted to 6 percent of the contributions made in the course of the electrification project.

TABLE 2.   Value of Contributions Made during Fifty-one Days of Community Work on the Electrification Project, Huaylas, Ancash, 1960–61

Unit	Value in Soles	Percentage of Total Contribution
2,550 man-days worked at s/15.00 per day	s/38,250.00	77
Materials donated	8,880.00	17
Refreshments	3,020.00	6
Total	s/50,150.00	100

Note: s/26.80 = U.S. $1.00

The quantity of alcohol consumed during work is therefore not as great as it might seem at first glance. During the work analyzed in table 2, only s/1.18 (U.S. $.044) per worker was contributed for beverages, enough to buy one half-pint of beer or three ounces of cane alcohol. These estimates should be considered minimal, however, because of the probable failure to record all contributions, particularly *chicha*. Consequently, extensive drinking during public work projects is more apparent than real and the symbolic or imaginary functions are more important than the actual physiological ones. The occasion which forced the workers from one barrio to leave the eucalyptus post they were carrying at the roadside because they were too drunk to continue was not typical.

Barrels of *chicha* are normally packed on donkeys while the bottles of *pisco* or cane alcohol are safeguarded in the hip pockets of the barrio leaders or in a sack carried by a man specifically charged with the task of holding this communal treasure. *Chicha* is often served from the barrel in a tin can or gourd drinking bowl; beverages such as *pisco* or cane alcohol are consumed directly from the bottle or from a "shot" glass. On some occasions, lacking a shot glass, a vessel is fashioned from the small barrel-shaped fruit of the prickly pear cactus (called *tuna* in Peru).

Behavior on a public works project is typically masculine in the Huaylas style. There is considerable boasting about the prowess of one's barrio in getting the job accomplished and there is a feeling of competition among the barrios. Raucous shouts (*guajes*) resound through the mountain air and toward the end of the day, *vivas* ("Viva Huaylas," "viva el barrio de Shuyo," etc.) may be heard echoing from the hills. On their way home, upon completion of the day's work, the workers parade through town to the accompaniment of the *caja* and *roncadora*. They stop at several of the many bars or stores for additional liquid refreshment, often the storekeeper's contribution to the day's activities. It is also customary for those who have worked to visit the district mayor's house to be treated to some beer or *chicha*. A *república* may thus end with as much as two or three hours of festivities, lasting well into the evening. Those who do not wish to participate quietly go their ways.

As at any social gathering where drinking is relatively heavy, one does not formally take his leave, but rather slips quietly away unnoticed by the rest. To take formal leave of the host or fellow guests on such occasions inevitably leads to the insistence that one stay, making a graceful departure extremely difficult if not impossible.

The Function of Drinking

As Eric Wolf has noted, such communities require a "ceremonial fund" of traditional behavior patterns and the necessary resources to implement them in order to support and maintain the social requisites of peasant life. "The ceremonial funds of Indian villages of Mexico and Peru, for example, are very large . . . for there a man must expend a great deal of effort and goods in the sponsorship of ceremonials that serve to underline and exemplify the solidarity of the community" (1966:7). The nature of personal relationships in Huaylas is basically gemeinschaft in character. To be sure, there is no one in the district who knows everyone else. Nevertheless, Huaylinos tend to identify with each other and with the district as a whole, in spite of the many factional arguments and squabbles which wax and wane. In terms of wealth there are neither the very rich nor the very poor, and despite class differences, there is an air of egalitarianism which conflicts with the traditional hierarchical values and attitudes governing interpersonal relations generally throughout Peru.

In Huaylas, the ritual of drinking is a kind of special contract between two or more people, which legitimizes social relations. As such, it is a most important part of the "ceremonial fund." The ritual emphasizes social solidarity in Huaylas because it is applied inclusively and is standard at all social levels or between them. Social status notwithstanding, anyone is free to invite the other person to a drink and expect acceptance. With the invitation goes the obligation to accept. Finally, to drink with a person is to recognize his dignity as an individual and, through the ritual, to interact with him on the basis of respect and relative equality. Failure to reciprocate properly, such as in purchasing one's share of beverage in his turn (*mandar su tanda*), is a distinctly uncomfortable situation and a violation of the "rules." Such an event can provoke hostile relationships. The deliberate escalation of such "demand" drinking is itself hostile in intent, and the "contract" may be broken by one of the parties if the financial or social compromise is too great. Since one gains some prestige by treating others, one must be careful that his social debts do not outstrip his pocketbook.

The stamp of legitimacy given by the act of drinking together in a ritualistic manner of course is, and has been, important in many societies. Thus, one may say, "I'll drink to that," in closing a business deal in the United States. In Zinacantan, Mexico, Cancian reports that "acceptance of the gifts signals acceptance of the request, and the bargain is usually sealed with at least some of the drink that has been given (1965:48)." And in similar circumstances in Hualcan, Peru, ceremonial drinking accompanies the change of personnel in the traditional religious hierarchy (Stein 1961).

In Huaylas, the civic work system is one of the ways in which persons of varying social positions are brought into direct contact with each other. The drink, considered an indispensable element on such occasions for psychological and/or physiological reasons, serves the highly useful latent function of providing the means by which social barriers to harmonious interpersonal relations are minimized or set aside. The consumption of alcoholic beverages promotes the common fraternal, masculine, and festive aspect of the *repúblicas*. Public work may thus become an enjoyable experience, full of that good fellowship which is regarded as a reward for participation.

The negative aspects of drinking in relation to work are recognized by Huaylinos. Festive labor is expensive. Individual and group drinking certainly does not improve technical efficiency and may in fact lead to sloppy workmanship or to less work being accomplished. It is obviously costly to indulge the workers' appetites in terms of the actual expense of the drinks, the time lost in consuming them, and the time required to terminate the task after the consumption. There can be no doubt that drinking in purely economic terms is dysfunctional. Yet it cannot for this reason be dismissed. Although Erasmus has noted that when the uneconomic aspects of festive labor arrangements are perceived, and "frequency interpretations" are made, such systems apparently die out because people put "two and two together"; nevertheless, he cites the case of some Cuzco Indians who, despite the "cost accounting" of their system by Erasmus, chose to remain with their traditional ways of work (1961:144–56). The "ceremonial fund" was still a too-much-needed part of their village life.

In Huaylas, civic work projects are vital to solving district problems, and must be undertaken with popular agreement and cooperation. Thus, the cost of providing refreshments for work occasions may be seen as worthwhile, since it promotes social solidarity and group cooperation and sustains a major community resource: its unified system of voluntary public labor. Most of the work performed by the *republicanos* is semiskilled at best and thus suffers little in quality due to the acts of nonsober workers.

Yet the question should be asked whether the pleasurable cultural detail of social drinking will prove a handicap to Huaylinos as they attempt to adjust to the new socioeconomic conditions emerging in their country. It is abundantly clear that Huaylinos have been involved in these developments. The construction of the large hydroelectric complex within the district a number of years ago provided opportunities for well-paid employment and for the acquisition of new skills. The system and conditions of work were more rigid than those normally followed by the largely self-employed Huaylinos. Despite such differences, however, Huaylinos became the core of the labor force on the construction project and in fact earned a reputation for being the hardest workers. As a result, however, of the increased income enjoyed by

Huaylinos employed on this project, there was a spectacular rise in the consumption of beer and other drinks within the district (cf. Bradfield 1963). (Note the differences in table 1 between 1956, when the construction project was under way, and 1958.) Instead of simply buying one bottle of beer, the nouveau riche of Huaylas would buy each of their companions a whole case. Some of the workers could not stand such prosperity and in fact lost their jobs because they indulged their drinking habits too much.

Conclusion

Despite its integration into social life, the seeds of ambivalence with regard to drinking are being sown in Huaylas. Women participate only superficially in drinking contexts and often decry the fact that the men get drunk and miss a day's work. The parish priest denounces heavy drinking from the pulpit and the primary school teachers recite to their classes the doctrine that liquor is evil. A number of indicators—young men of Huaylas do not find themselves under pressure to drink (unlike the youth of Lunahuaná); drunks are frequently jailed; there are a number of problem drinkers in Huaylas—suggest that the more urban, more modern pressures of Peruvian society are reaching this highland district. Although drinking in Huaylas is certainly integrated into the culture, it has much less specificity as a role attribute than in Vicos, Hualcán, or apparently Lunahuaná, a result of Huaylas' greater socioeconomic complexity (cf. S. Bacon 1945).

Drinking customs still underscore and provide important ritual support for the personalistic relationships which characterize Huaylas society. The maintenance of these relationships requires time, and drinking not only provides this time but structures the manner in which it is spent. It provides a mechanism through which mutual respect may be shared and exchanged on an equal footing, and consummation of the drinking act legitimizes the relationship. Deliberate failure to complete the ritual "contract" in the prescribed fashion is insulting and has a destructive effect. Drinking has functioned in harmony with the total cultural configuration and has been a positive element encouraging patterns of solidarity. As such, the drinking of alcoholic beverages was an important, though minor, facet of work—particularly group labor situations— where there was need for all to participate in an equal manner. Until the community becomes further specialized, more directly concerned with the tighter regimentation of time observable in the urban-industrial society of the coast, and until paid construction teams replace the community labor which now meets large-scale public needs, one may predict that these patterns will continue to be a small but vital element in the culture.

Ceremonial Drinking in an Afro-Brazilian Cult
Seth Leacock

The present study concerns the use of alcohol by the members of an urban religious cult in northern Brazil. A striking feature of the ideology of this cult is the fiction that it is not the members who drink during the ceremonies, but the deities who possess them. As might be inferred from this belief, there is considerable ambivalence within the cult about drinking, due both to pressures from the larger society and to an awareness that excessive drinking is sometimes disruptive. The purpose of the present paper is to consider the role of drinking in cult activities, and to suggest some of the reasons why drinking continues as a prominent feature of the ceremonies. This will involve the consideration of the functions which drinking serves, not only in cult integration, but especially in possession.

The Batuque

The religious group to be considered is one of the so-called Afro-Brazilian cults, and is located in the city of Belém. This cult, the Batuque,[1] is similar in many respects to the other African-derived cults which are found in other parts of Brazil and in other areas of the New World, and the basic ideas and rituals seem clearly to have been brought to the New World by African slaves. The principal ceremony is a public performance during which the members of the cult dance to the rhythms of drums, sing songs designed to call down the gods, and enter trance states which are interpreted as possession by the deities. The Batuque, however, has been greatly modified by the addition of ideas of American Indian and spiritualist origin, and many of the members of the Belém cults are completely unaware that their religion is of African origin. The members are also extremely variable as far as their physical characteristics are concerned, and only a minority are clearly descendants of slaves.

It is not just in the presence of new deities, however, or in the broadened membership that the Batuque is different from the Afro-Brazilian cults which are described in the literature. One of the most striking differences is the extent to which the Batuque is individualistic when compared with the Candomblé of Bahia, for example. The typical Batuque cult center is very loosely organized, initiation is not of great importance, and the behavior of the deities when manifested in cult members is little standardized. It would be a mistake, however, to assume that because the Batuque is different from the cults described in the literature, it is therefore unusual. Since most of the scholars who have studied these cults have been interested in African survivals, they have tended to ignore cults like the Batuque, which have relatively few African traits. There are many hints in the literature, however, which suggest that such cults are both numerous and popular. It can confidently be predicted that when more is known about the *caboclo* cults in Bahia, and the "Yoruban-derived" cults in São Luis, the Batuque will prove to be representative of a type of much modified Afro-Brazilian cult which is widespread in coastal Brazil.

There is considerable evidence that drinking during ceremonies is a common practice in many of these modified cults. In São Luis, in São Paulo, and in a number of other cities as well, ceremonial drinking is known to occur, but has not been described in detail (Ferreira de Camargo 1961; Bastide 1960). Drinking is usually associated with deities which are not of African origin, and seems not to occur in any of the more conservative cults, such as the Dahomean center in São Luis or the Yoruban centers in Bahia, where the deities are exclusively African (Eduardo 1948; Bastide 1958). Drinking would not be expected in these cults in any case, since it would not be in keeping with the relatively austere and dignified atmosphere of the ceremonies.

Only a few of the deities which are of importance in the Batuque are clearly African. Many more of the deities are of American Indian origin, including several spirits associated with animals. The majority of the deities, however, have Portuguese names and seem to be figures out of Brazilian folklore and history. Collectively, all of these deities are called *encantados*, a term which literally means "enchanted ones," but which in use simply refers to any of the supernatural beings which are believed to descend during ceremonies and possess the participants. Most of the members of the Batuque are practicing Catholics, and they make a sharp distinction between the encantados and the Christian supernaturals, which are considered to be much more remote.

On occasion, however, possession is attributed to a saint, usually either Cosmas or Damian, twin saints who are very popular in Brazil.

According to cult beliefs, the encantados have much the same motivations and desires as people. There is a variety of reasons why an encantado might wish to descend and enter the body of a cult member, including the simple desire to have a good time. All encantados are believed to like to dance and sing, and many of them like to smoke cigars and to drink a variety of alcoholic beverages. It is in the context of these beliefs that drinking takes place. The act itself has few if any sacred connotations, and does not seem to be symbolic of anything else, except perhaps the obligation which a person has to fulfill the wishes of his encantado. It is also necessary to make offerings to the encantados, and these offerings are usually either food or liquor, and often both.

The relationship between a cult member and the encantado which possesses him is of course a reciprocal one. In return for being able to dance, sing, and perhaps drink, the deity does many favors for his devotee, such as looking out for his economic well-being, prescribing remedies for his sick relatives and friends, and predicting the future. If the encantado proves to be popular enough, it is sometimes possible for the cult member to engage in relatively lucrative curing practices, or ultimately to open a cult center of his own.

The most common alcoholic beverage used both for offerings and for drinking is the Brazilian white rum, *cachaça*, which is probably about eighty proof. It is less expensive than either beer or wine, and is sometimes considered too common for special offerings. In many cases, however, it is prescribed, as in offerings to Exu, a spirit with mostly evil aspects who is believed to be very prone to disrupt ceremonies. A gourd bowl filled with cachaça is placed in Exu's shrine before each public performance, and often on a regular weekly basis, to insure that he does not interfere with cult activities. Most of the encantados have a predilection for a particular alcoholic beverage, at least as far as offerings are concerned. The Curupiras prefer cachaça, as do Pedro Angaço and his son Legua-Bogi. Wine is the offering of choice for the Inhaçan Oxossi and Jurema, while beer should be offered to Xango and Rompe-Mata. Gourd bowls or glasses of the proper beverage are left for the encantado either in front of or often below the altar found in every chapel. Unlike offerings of food, which are communally eaten by the cult members, liquid offerings are either left to evaporate or are eventually poured out and are never drunk.

Ceremonial Drinking

The drinking of alcoholic beverages occurs in two contexts—curing rituals and public ceremonies. Every cult leader is also a curer, and many hold a curing session once a week. In most respects, curing as it is practiced in the cult centers is identical with *pagelança,* the shamanistic curing found throughout the Amazon Basin, both in rural and urban settings. Based on ideas borrowed largely from Tupí-speaking tribes, pagelança includes possession by a series of supernatural beings, the use of a gourd rattle and the long red tail feathers of the macaw, the smoking of a cigar or a special cigarette, and the blowing of smoke and the supposed extraction of disease objects through sucking (Galvão 1955:134). An early innovation by Brazilian practitioners was the substitution of cachaça for the narcotics often used by the Indians to induce possession. Batuque curers also drink cachaça, but it should be stressed that they drink only after being possessed and never before.

It is generally believed by cult members that the use of cachaça is indispensable during curing sessions, and no criticism of this practice was heard. Drinking is thought to "give force" to the proceedings. The one cult leader who claimed that she never used cachaça in curing explained that she had been specially prepared to work in this way, but that all other curers drank a great deal. A curing session begins with a brief period of singing and shaking the rattle, after which the cult leader is typically possessed by a steady stream of encantados, none staying over two or three minutes. Most of these encantados demand cachaça, and the curer drinks almost continuously for the hour or so that the session continues. He also smokes cigars, cigarettes, or pipes, according to the preference of the encantado, and if a child encantado should descend may be given a soft drink. From time to time patients come forward for treatment and are whisked with the macaw feathers, saturated with smoke, and sometimes sucked as a prelude to being shown some object supposedly causing the trouble. Curing is always a solo performance, with only the curer being possessed and drinking.

Drinking is general during the public ceremonies which are held every two weeks or so according to a regular annual calendar. Dancing begins about nine in the evening and continues until the next morning—sometimes until dawn. At a typical cult center, perhaps fifteen women and five men, the "mediums," wearing colorful costumes, take the floor at the beginning of the ceremony, and at a signal from the leader begin dancing and singing. The leader is usually possessed first, but there is no particular order in which other dancers are possessed, and no attempt is made to call the encantados in a rigidly prescribed order. However, some encantados do have a great deal more prestige than others, and it is these more important deities which are called first. During the course of the evening almost all of the dancers are possessed at least once, and most are possessed several times. Often members of the audience are possessed and are usually allowed to join the dancing unless they are obviously drunk or known troublemakers.

Since drinking is supposedly done by the encantado rather than by the medium who receives him, the amount of drinking which occurs will depend on which encantados descend. The more prestigeful deities which make their appearance during the early part of the evening usually stay only ten or fifteen minutes, and ordinarily do not drink. It is believed that they have too many important things to do to spend very much time in one cult center. They descend, sing their appropriate "doctrines," dance, greet other dancers, then either go away immediately or retire to the adjoining chapel to sit down briefly and converse with anyone wishing to present some problem for their consideration. After the consultation, the medium returns to the dance floor, sings a standardized farewell song, then lurches over backward and becomes normal.

Most cult members receive at least one of these important and serious encantados, who serves as his "owner" and guardian. But, in addition, most members receive at least one lighthearted deity who, it is believed, comes to possess the medium in order to have a good time. These playful encantados stay for longer periods, usually several hours, or in exceptional cases, several days. They usually begin arriving after the more important encantados have come and gone, and as the evening progresses, more and more dancers are possessed by their fun-loving deity. Since most of these deities like to drink, it is at this time that most of the drinking occurs. By three or four o'clock in the morning most of the dancers are in very high spirits, and the atmosphere of the ceremony is gay and lighthearted. In general, however, a certain decorum is always expected on the dance floor, where high spirits are usually expressed in vigorous dancing, and much of the silly horseplay which also may occur takes place off the dance floor.

Several aspects of the ideology connected with drinking during ceremonies need to be stressed. As has been indicated, the belief is that it is the encantado which does the drinking and not the medium. Cult members insist that they never have a hangover or feel any aftereffects, regardless of how much the encantado possessing them may drink. Some women maintain that they themselves never drink or smoke, even in their secular lives, but that their encantado may do both during ceremonies. Alcohol is never used to induce possession, either by the leader or by the other participants. In fact, drinking on the day of a ceremony is specifically prohibited, and if a medium does drink before the ceremony begins, the other mediums will state confidently that he is not likely to be possessed. If possession does occur, it is believed that the encantado will be angry. "Mariana does not want her children to drink before she arrives," said one cult member, and went on to tell how her brother had been drowned by this encantado because he often drank before she possessed him. Such a punishment is considered to be extreme, of course, and would be applied only to a chronic offender. Another kind of punishment for the same offense is to be forced to kneel in front of the drums and beat the hands on the floor or on a special stone. This occurs while the medium is possessed by the encantado whose ire has been aroused. Sometimes the deity simply causes the medium to fall on the floor and bruise himself.

Another characteristic of the drinking which goes on during ceremonies is that it is highly individualistic. Dancers who are possessed by encantados which like to drink periodically leave the floor in search of liquor. They usually go first to the house of the cult leader, which adjoins the dancing area, since it is here that most of the drinking takes place. If the cult center is supplying the liquor, which occurs only when some benefactor has made an unusually large contribution for some special occasion, drinks are usually doled out by the cult leader or one of his assistants, and the supply is often kept under lock and key. Ordinarily, however, the leader feels no obligation to supply drinks for the encantados, even though the dancers often complain loudly when there is nothing to drink. Many dancers come prepared and hide a bottle somewhere just in case one of their encantados who likes to drink should appear. They usually do not share this liquor with anyone else but are sometimes heard to complain that someone has been drinking from their bottle.

The amount and kind of liquor which is consumed vary greatly. The behavior of the encantados is not standardized, and one person possessed by José Tupinambá, for example, may act very differently than someone else possessed by the same deity. As far as drinking is concerned, this means that in one person a particular deity may drink cachaça, in another may drink wine, and in a third may not drink at all. Legua-Bogi in Pedro boasted that he was the heaviest drinker in the neighborhood and could put away five liters of cachaça in an evening. In Ana, a famous cult leader who rarely drank, Legua-Bogi, often stayed for hours but took only soft drinks. In general, drinking is seen as a personal matter between a person and his encantado. If a medium does not drink at all while possessed, and some do not, this is considered to be his own business and a situation which has been agreed to by his encantado.

There is a more active concern, especially on the part of the cult leader, when a cult member drinks to excess. Ordinarily during a ceremony there are few signs of intoxication, but occasionally a dancer will act befuddled, or become aggressive, or give other indications of being quite drunk. This kind of behavior is of special interest to the cult leader because he is very sensitive to public ridicule and tries to avoid any kind of scandal. He is quite aware that although both the Catholic church and the community at large have a fairly lenient attitude toward secular drinking, there is general condemnation of drinking in a religious context. Even within the cult there is a marked ambivalence to drinking, which comes out most clearly in criticisms of other cult centers. Not only cult leaders, but members as well, commonly attack other cult centers declaring that too much drinking goes on. "One cannot tell if it is the encantado or the cachaça speaking," was a common comment. As might be expected, no one is able to define how much is too much. The only point upon which everyone will agree is that if an encantado wants to drink he must be allowed to do so.

Because drinking is done in such an unsystematic fashion, and also because there is a definite effort to keep its extent hidden from public view, it proved impossible to determine how much liquor was ordinarily consumed during a ceremony. There are several considerations which would suggest that the amount is not very large. In the first place, there are rarely any overt signs of intoxication. It is true that when possessed by an encantado which likes to "play" (which usually includes drinking), a man or woman acts gay, sometimes silly, always very friendly—in short, in a manner which would be expected if he or she were pleasantly high on alcohol. However, this kind of behavior does not necessarily indicate that the medium is actually intoxicated. Repeated observations in situations where no liquor was available indicate that a medium acts in very much the same way whether he has had anything to drink or not, if a playful encantado is on hand. If a great deal of drinking occurred, one would expect that the dancers would pass from a state of exhilaration to the later stages of intoxication, where aggressive behavior or signs of depression would appear. As has been indicated, this does not often happen. Another factor of importance in estimating the amount of liquor consumed is simply the cost, which in terms of the income of many of the dancers is relatively prohibitive.

Another group of participants who drink during the ceremonies is the drummers. The music for the dancing comes primarily from three or four single-headed drums beaten with the hands. Ordinarily the drumming never stops during the entire ceremony, and beating a drum at a very rapid tempo for six or eight hours, even with breaks every forty-five minutes or so, is hard work. Although drummers have various motives other than liquor to keep them going, it is recognized that drinking is a major inducement, and ceremonies are simply not planned if provision cannot be made for cachaça for the drummers. One cult center which was known to be stingy with drinks always had a shortage of men to beat the drums. Drummers are rarely possessed, but many of them know the songs and join lustily in the singing. They ideally maintain a relatively impassive demeanor and rarely show any signs of intoxication.

It has already been noted that on occasion participants in ceremonies do drink a great deal and show it usually by becoming aggressive and unpleasant. There is no formal way of handling people in this condition, and they are ordinarily simply ignored. No reprimand is possible, of course, since this would be disrespectful to the encantado. More extreme behavior sometimes takes place within the cult center after public performance has ended. Dancers sometimes remove their clothing and have to be forcibly restrained from leaving the building, or sometimes they destroy their dancing costumes. This kind of behavior may be interpreted as being simply the work of particularly perverse encantados, of which there are a fair number, but in exceptional cases it may be alleged that the medium was not really possessed, but was merely drunk. This is the most serious charge of all and is probably never made against a fellow cult member. Only visitors who are especially obnoxious, or strangers, are ever accused of pretending to be possessed.

Cult Beliefs and Problem Drinkers

Some of the members of the cult who are heavy drinkers seem to use cult beliefs to rationalize their drinking. One man was famous for his four- and five-day drinking sprees, during which he would visit other cult members (all female) and parade around their houses nude. Since he was supposedly possessed by a female encantado named Jarina, his antics were usually considered quite amusing, but many cult members felt a genuine pity for the man because it was commonly assumed that Jarina was punishing him for various past delicts by forcing him to engage in these demeaning displays.

On the other hand, membership in the cults has helped some individuals to control their drinking problems. The best example is a cult leader named Carlos, age thirty-two, who in his early twenties was already drinking every day and going on frequent binges. Although he had never been active in the Batuque, or been possessed, he had attended numerous public ceremonies, so he was not too startled one day at a drunken party when he was told, after passing out and regaining consciousness, that he had been possessed in the interim by an encantado who called herself Mariana. Carlos was most impressed by the fact that he had no hangover, and largely ignored the visitation until he was possessed again two months later, again at a party and again after drinking himself into unconsciousness. This time he was ill for two weeks, and when he recovered began attending a cult center in order to be "prepared" to receive Mariana properly. At first, according to Carlos's account, Mariana drank a great deal when she possessed him, but he gave up drinking completely when he was not possessed. Gradually Mariana drank less and less, until today she does not drink at all. Carlos now receives a number of other encantados who do drink, but they drink only beer, and in relatively small amounts. Although Carlos obviously did not join the Batuque, or become a cult leader, just to control his drinking, he insists that this is one important result of his participation. He is quite aware that he did have a problem, and he attributes its solution to the guidance of the encantado, Mariana.

Another case may be cited to indicate some of the complications which may arise in the interaction between conscious and unconscious attempts to solve a drinking problem. Clara, age fifty-one, has been dancing in the Batuque all her life, since her mother and two uncles were cult leaders. For many years, in spite of a propensity to drink too much in her secular life, Clara was able to control her consumption of liquor because her encantado Japetequara (who does not drink) "looked after her." This supervision took the form of possession whenever Clara was about to drink too much, or punishment after she had drunk to excess. Some nine years ago, Clara's desire for alcohol seemed to have gotten the better of her when she began to receive a new encantado, Mariana, who drank everything in sight—on one occasion even some gasoline. The difficulty was that since it was not Clara who was doing the drinking, but the encantado, Japetequara could no longer intervene (each encantado is a free agent). In this impasse, Clara decided that the only thing to do was to perform a rite which would prevent Mariana from ever possessing her again. Before she could complete this rite, however, Mariana possessed her and agreed that she would no longer drink cachaça but only wine and beer. Clara now usually receives Japetequara at the beginning of a ceremony, when she acts very serious and dignified, and spends the rest of the evening as Mariana, an extremely pleasant, friendly, and gay encantado whom everyone likes and for whom a bottle of special wine is usually available.

The Functions of Drinking in the Batuque

The two functions most commonly attributed to the use of alcohol are the integration of society and the reduction of anxiety (Heath 1958; Horton 1943; Pittman and Snyder 1962). Drinking can be seen to serve both of these functions in the Batuque, but this kind of analysis would seem to provide a decidedly incomplete explanation of the role of drinking in cult ceremonies.

The use of alcohol has some effect on the integration of the cult. The men and women who dance together, become possessed together, and drink at roughly the same time (if not together), undoubtedly are more friendly and outgoing with one another after a few drinks than before. Alcohol seems to have the usual result as far as facilitating social intercourse is concerned. On the other hand, most dancers in a trance state seem to act much the same whether they drink or not, and alcohol is not in any sense necessary either for the high spirits which are manifested or the atmosphere of friendliness which prevails. The ties that bind in the Batuque would seem to include shared beliefs about the encantados and shared experiences in which possession is the central activity. Since alcohol is not used to induce possession, is not drunk as a part of a communal rite, and is not even consumed by all those present, its integrating effects would seem to be relatively slight.

One test of the importance of drinking as an integrating factor would be to consider a cult center where no drinking occurs. Such centers are very rare in Belém, but in one of the centers studied, the cult leader was opposed to drinking, and relatively little drinking occurred. It must be admitted at once that this cult center was the least united and had the least camaraderie of the three centers which were intensively studied. The basic pattern seemed to be a group of men and women with close ties with the leader but few with each other. However, it would be difficult to assign any of these characteristics to the lack of drinking. Much more important was the fact that the cult leader was so famous that people came to her from all over Belém and were not recruited from the immediate neighborhood, as was the case in the other centers. For this and other reasons the members rarely came together except for ceremonies. Interaction during the ceremonies was held to a minimum by the cult leader, who completely dominated proceedings and always stopped the dancing early when she became tired (she was in her sixties). Under these circumstances it is not difficult to understand why the cult members did not form a very close-knit group. It is unlikely that more drinking would have changed the situation in any way.

The relationship between drinking and anxiety is much more complex and difficult to define. There is no question that many cult members lead very difficult lives, have a great many fears, especially about their health and economic matters, and frequently have family troubles of one kind or another. It can be effectively argued that participation in the cult allays some of these fears, since the beliefs about the encantados are specifically designed to give the cult member assurance that he is being looked after by immediate, powerful supernatural beings. But it is not clear how these beliefs might be enhanced or made more effective by a few drinks taken after the medium is already possessed, unless the alcohol makes the trance state more impressive or convincing. The primary reduction of anxiety would seem to come in possession and the reinforcement which possession gives to beliefs about the encantados. The role of alcohol would appear to be minor, at least for a majority of the participants. If merely escaping from one's problems for a few hours can be considered a way to reduce anxiety, then drinking would help so far as it supplemented the trance state.

It would seem preferable to list the recreational aspects of the Batuque separate from the anxiety-reducing ones, since it will surely be granted that some individuals may be able to enjoy the ceremony in a positive way rather than merely by getting rid of tensions of various kinds. The appeal to the senses of the colorful costumes, the drums, the singing and dancing, is quite striking. Added to these features, for the participants, are the atmosphere of good fellowship and the sense of being the stars in a performance sometimes witnessed by several hundred people. That drinking could enhance the enjoyment of all of these aspects of the ceremony is obvious.

In addition to serving such general functions in cult activity, drinking also seems to have an important role in possession. As manifested in the members of the Batuque, trance states seem to be a considerable strain, both physically and mentally. A person who is supposedly possessed is much more active than otherwise, and every movement and attitude is exaggerated. Abundant perspiration indicates how much physical exertion occurs. But there is another kind of strain as well. A person in trance is supposed to be the encantado, and he must say things which are appropriate to a supernatural. He must solve problems about which he knows nothing; he must predict the future. His utterances should be impressive and much more fluent than ordinary speech. It has been argued that playing a god provides much personal satisfaction (Mischel and Mischel 1958), but it is clear that for a poorly educated and unimaginative man or woman such a role can be very difficult. What could be more welcome in such a situation, to reduce inhibitions and to give at least a self-impression of fluency and mastery, than a few stiff drinks? For the cult leader, who has more experience, the role of encantado is somewhat easier, but the fact that he drinks more than anyone else can be partially explained by the fact that he is possessed by more encantados and for longer periods than any of his followers.

The foregoing considerations would apply primarily to possession by an important and serious encantado. As was noted earlier, such deities ordinarily do not stay around long enough to drink, but on special occasions they stay for longer periods and do drink, especially when received by a cult leader. When the encantado is of a more playful nature, it is ordinarily not expected to dispense wisdom or prophesy, and need only be gay, effervescent, and friendly. In playing this role, which is quite similar to that of a person who is pleasantly high, what condition could be more ideal than to be, in fact, pleasantly high?

It also seems reasonable to suppose that alcohol would be useful in sustaining a medium during a long trance experience. Although all cult members vehemently maintain that they have complete amnesia for the time they are possessed, it is clear that some mediums remember practically everything that happens. It is often easy to trick a medium into reporting events and conversations in such detail that there is no question about her complete recall. It seems likely that when a person enters a trance state he is completely dissociated, but that after a fairly brief period he begins to be in some degree conscious of what is occurring. Perhaps drinking helps to preserve the illusion that one is at the most only semiconscious, or reduces uncertainties as to whether one is really possessed at all. Or the major effect of drinking may be simply to sustain the medium during three or four hours of relatively frenzied activity.

It should be stressed that in the foregoing paragraphs there are a number of assumptions about possession which are highly speculative. The basic assumption is that an individual in a trance state will react to alcohol in much the same way that he would if he were normal. This assumption is based solely on impressions derived from observing and interacting with large numbers of people in trance states who drank various amounts of liquor.

Thus far the discussion has centered on the functions which drinking serves in ceremonial activity. As was indicated earlier, however, there is a further connection between drinking and the cult, in that cult beliefs influence patterns of secular drinking. As the case histories presented illustrate, beliefs about the encantados and drinking are quite flexible, and individuals with drinking problems can apparently manipulate these beliefs to resolve a variety of conflicts. If an individual cannot control his drinking, he can deny all responsibility for his behavior by attributing his binges to possession by an encantado. On the other hand, some individuals can apparently control their drinking by transferring some superego functions to an encantado, even though the behavior of the deity is largely undefined by cult belief and may be modified at will by the person involved. The psychological dynamics involved in these ways of coping with drinking problems are outside the scope of this paper, but some of the factors involved can be inferred from the case histories presented.

Note

1. Members do not call the cult "Batuque," but refer to it as either "Nagô," "Mina," or "Umbanda," depending on minor variations in belief and ritual. Since these latter terms are used in the literature with various connotations, the term "Batuque" has been chosen as a general name for the Belém cults in order to avoid confusion. Strictly speaking, the term "batuque" is usually used to refer to the public ceremony.

Drinking Patterns and Alcoholism in Trinidad

Carole Yawney

The research upon which this report is based represents an attempt to examine the relationship between certain cultural variables and drinking patterns in Trinidad. For this purpose gross intoxication and alcoholism are considered forms of drinking behavior. Alcoholism is defined as the degree to which drinking interferes with an individual's real or apparent functioning as a member of his society. The study of the cultural network within which the individual drinker operates enables one to arrive at a definition of social pathology. There are two categories of cultural variables to be considered here. The one consists of those values, norms, and attitudes which directly define the drinking situation. The other refers to those socioeconomic factors which determine the range of variation within or the adaptation to the drinking situation; such factors (e.g., the availability of alcohol, the means to purchase it, family obligations, and work habits) also influence the pattern of pathological drinking.

Within a particular culture many aspects of these variables—however integrated they appear to be—are in fact in conflict with each other. The degree of real or perceived conflict varies from individual to individual and from society to society. The inability to integrate this conflict results in certain behavior problems, the incidence of which again varies on both individual and societal levels.

An analysis of such a culturally heterogeneous population as that of Trinidad is useful to illustrate the application of this theoretical framework. However, the plural nature of Trinidad society introduces a second perspective. Not only can a study of drinking patterns and alcoholism among East Indians and Negroes in Trinidad exemplify the role of cultural variables in relation to such behavior, but the results of research into drinking as an institution have implications for theories about models of plural societies in the Caribbean. The data presented in this essay support this contention that, at least with reference to drinking, Trinidad is a plural society. There are distinct patterns of alcohol use in each cultural group, and these patterns are not shared by Negroes and East Indians of the same socioeconomic class.

For reasons of efficiency only male drinking patterns were studied in the two cultural groups. The areas selected were those considered most representative of the social context from which the majority of known alcoholics come. The field time of eighteen weeks (May to September 1967) was divided between the rural East Indian village of Williamsville and an urban Negro area, Port-of-Spain. Rural Negroes (e.g., fishermen) and urban East Indians (e.g., businessmen) were excluded from the sample.[1] Coincidentally, the Negro population of Trinidad as a whole is primarily urban while the East Indian population is predominantly rural.

The Ecology of Drinking

It is necessary to understand the structural aspects of the drinking environment common to all Trinidadians within which cultural variation in drinking behavior occurs. By structural features are meant those fixed variables which influence the drinking situation and over which the average Trinidadian has no control. Included are such factors as access to retail outlets, legal restrictions on the sale and consumption of alcoholic beverages, and the image of alcoholic beverages presented by the communications media. The latter is considered a legitimate structural feature because advertising is manipulated by a select few who have a definite stake in the viability of Trinidad's "drinking culture." This term refers to the fact that, in the apparent absence of any restrictions on the sale and use of alcoholic beverages, Trinidadians can and do indulge themselves in a leisurely fashion. The agronomical conditions in many Caribbean islands favor a high yield of sugarcane, a by-product of which is rum. Most islands produce inexpensive local rums for home consumption and many varieties for exportation. All Trinidadians consider rum to be a product of national importance (regardless of cultural associations). Indeed, it might be said that rum is a symbol of national identity.

As in viticultural countries, there are a number of outlets through which the public has access to alcohol. There are no state-controlled retail stores. Instead what is found most commonly throughout Trinidad is the "rumshop." In the rural areas and in some of the outlying urban areas, rumshops sell food, ground provisions, toilet articles, etc. Here the rumshop is essentially a combination of the North American "corner store" and the "neighborhood tavern." In the rumshops, there are no legal restrictions on the amount of liquor that can be served to any one individual at one time. The drinking appears to be very casual because what is being enforced is the social sanction, not the "ounce sanction." Control is exercised by the group with whom one drinks. Women are rarely present; I did not observe any woman drinking in a rumshop during my entire period in the field. In addition, there are the inns or licensed restaurants and American-style cocktail lounges or bars. Such places differ considerably from the rumshop both in practice and in atmosphere. Since, apart from the licensed restaurants, these establishments are not frequented by the individuals who are the concern of this study, I do not deal with them in any detail.

The prevailing attitude toward alcohol use appears to be one of general permissiveness. This is of course reinforced by the advertising media. They have consciously reinforced the image of Trinidadians as a gay and carefree, fun-loving and rum-drinking people, predominantly Negro. In Trinidad, although both East Indians and Creoles are exposed to the same structural features, their adaptation to them is considerably different.

Patterns of Alcohol Use

East Indians

East Indian drinking is at once integrative and disruptive. It furthers social integration in an environment where it is difficult for the individual to achieve a sense of solidarity but at the expense of other relationships. In general, East Indian drinking is characterized by:

1. a high degree of ambivalence
2. inconsistent socialization into the use of alcohol
3. utilitarian attitudes toward alcohol use
4. irregular pressure to drink and situational variance of drinking norms
5. sanctions against excessive drinking

The predominant mood is one of ambivalence. As a result of a number of conflicting aspects of East Indian life, one finds ambivalent attitudes toward the use of alcohol, and ambivalence in the actual use of alcohol itself. The majority of the East Indians in Trinidad belong—at least nominally—to one of three religious denominations: Hindu, Muslim, or Presbyterian. All three faiths disapprove of the use of alcohol. This position is counteracted by a historical tradition of some depth and by existing social customs which strongly reinforce the use of alcoholic beverages. The use of alcohol is associated with the work situation in the field, the male peer group in the rumshop at any time, male groups in the home after work or on special occasions, and medicinal purposes in general.

Not only is the East Indian exposed to contradictions between religious dogma and actual behavior, but he is confused by inconsistencies between parental admonitions and parental practice. (It should be stressed that these conflicts are described here from the viewpoint of a person thirty-five to forty years of age or older. It is important to understand the social background from which the present alcoholic comes.) The East Indian community is characterized by a high degree of both interfamilial and intrafamilial conflict. The former presents many problems with respect to local government and political organization. However, it is the latter which is our concern here. Within the family (defined not only as a home, but as a kin group, although the two may be coextensive) one finds both intergenerational and intersexual conflict. Thus, repeated instances of conflict occur over the division of power and authority in the home, the upbringing of children, adultery, sexuality, male and female roles, etc.

Every alcoholic in my sample (total n = sixty-two) reported his involvement in at least one such relationship, this being in 90 percent of the cases conflict between his mother, his wife, and himself. Only 60 percent reported conflict between themselves and their fathers. On the other hand, of the twenty-seven families of nonalcoholics with whom I had direct contact, nineteen provided one or more examples of such behavior. Of the eight families which gave no direct indication of such problems, five were Muslim (including the extended family of a Muslim priest); the husband and wife of one were schoolteachers, but Hindu; and the husband of another was a very successful shopkeeper while his wife was a teacher (again Hindu). This would seem to suggest more success in integrating potentially conflicting behavior patterns on the part of Muslims or more acculturated Hindus.

My concern is with aspects of this conflict which have a direct bearing on the socialization of the child into the use of alcohol. It is the structural stability of the East Indian family, and attendant responsibilities and obligations, that force individuals into very tight and conflicting relationships and roles. The structural stability of the family is achieved through the control the parents exercise over the young. Some marriages are arranged by the parents; education is terminated if a fieldhand is needed; the residence of the newlywed couple is prescribed by parental requirements; the services of the in-marrying spouse are freely drawn upon. A system operates which encourages dependency of the young upon the adults and discourages initiative. The young people must rely upon their parents for a spouse, a home, and a job. Residence in the early years of marriage is established in the family compound if not in the same house as the parents. When neolocal residence is finally established, it is customarily in the same village as one and/or both sets of parents. The ease with which one of the partners can weaken his family ties varies greatly from individual to individual just as family demands vary. The competition for allegiance is fierce.

A three-generational family living in close quarters or at least as neighbors is not uncommon. Problems center on the in-marrying spouse. He (or she) not only has ties and obligations to his own family, but must forge new relationships with his spouse and with members of his spouse's family. There are often conflicting demands placed upon this individual, not only from his consanguineal family, but from different members within his new family. The mother and wife compete with each other for the son's time; the son and his mother compete for the daughter's services; the son and his wife argue with their parents about the upbringing of the children; the husband who is the authority figure to his wife and children is forced to defer to his parents; the son and his brothers compete with each other to gain shares in the inheritance of the land; the father tries to control the economic activities of his son. I must repeat, however, that it was the mother-son, husband-wife conflict that seemed most significant for the alcoholics at least. The highest incidence of adultery and promiscuity came from them. This introduces the second dimension, the intersexual conflict, which is of course exacerbated by the intergenerational stress. The husband and wife, in general, are very possessive of each other's time, especially the former of the latter. Thus the wife's allegiance to her family and even to the children is resented. Such problems reflect upon the issues of everyday life.

Intergenerational conflict is evident with respect to the use of alcohol. The children are never permitted to drink *with* their parents. This means that the drinking of alcoholic beverages in the home by father and son as "symbol equals" (i.e., men) is forbidden, although it is a common practice among all parents who do drink at home to give their children a "shot for the worms" whenever a bottle is opened. However, whether the father is an alcoholic, a heavy drinker, or an abstainer, the East Indian son should never drink with him or in his presence even after marriage. This value is particularly frustrating for those men who are married, raising their own families, successfully employed, and in many cases supporting their parents to some extent, for it means that the son is never fully recognized as an adult male by his parents. Yet in the eyes of his peer group he has become a man. To a child this male role model may never seem to be resolved, for there are many other indications of subordination besides drinking behavior. There is a respect relationship between the older and younger generations in East Indian culture, but one that is based on constraint, not affection.

In East Indian society the high degree of intrafamilial conflict and tension places the onus on the peer group to provide certain meaningful relationships. Pharmacologically, alcohol is a depressant; it reduces tension and minimizes conflict. Therefore, whatever potential sources of interpersonal conflict there may be between peers are suppressed in favor of group unity, however temporary or fallacious. The norm which generally describes male drinking in Williamsville is that one either drinks according to the conventions of one's peer group, or one abstains entirely. An individual cannot alternate between the two positions. To refuse to drink with one's friends at any time elicits accusations of stinginess or snobbishness; to do so consistently warrants rejection and ostracism by the group. Peer groups vary in intensity of drinking. However, the peer group most crucial to an individual's socialization (i.e., that composed of youths in their late teens and early twenties) is also the one that values most highly "drinking hard like a man."

The normative orientation is superficially convivial but basically utilitarian. First, those individuals who cannot control their drinking or who become drunk repeatedly and who indulge in aggressive acts while drinking are rejected. The attitude of the community toward drunks is more humorously cruel than humorously pathetic. Second, a wide variety of physiological reasons is given for drinking. There is positive value attached to the physiological effects of alcohol, regardless of whether or not they are interpreted as mainly stimulating or mainly tranquilizing.

Negroes

In the predominantly Negro Creole culture of Trinidad drinking is pervasive and integrated into other behavior patterns. In general it simply serves to integrate further an existing social unit which may include women on certain occasions. This is not to imply that *all* Negroes in Trinidad drink alcoholic beverages. There are definite sexual differences in patterns of consumption, but distinctions based on socioeconomic class and religious affiliation are more relevant to the concerns of this study. Middle-class individuals with upwardly mobile aspirations (and on occasion certain lower-class persons) do not tolerate drinking. This is consistent with their views regarding other aspects of behavior. For example, common law unions are disapproved and strong emphasis is placed upon regular church attendance but both norms are frequently violated. Nevertheless, such men do often drink on social occasions, but moderately. In other words, any ambivalence toward drinking on the part of the Negro is expressed by members of the middle class who are seeking higher socioeconomic status.

The drinking patterns typical of urban Negroes (both unskilled and skilled laborers) who frequent rumshops and inns are characterized by:

1. lack of ambivalence both in attitude and practice
2. consistent socialization in the use of alcohol
3. convivial goals in drinking
4. high social pressure to drink
5. permissive attitudes towards drunkenness

Specifically, the use of alcohol among male Negroes is associated with public social gatherings; meetings; religious functions; business and political transactions; weekends as a time for relaxation, "liming," and drinking; and home celebrations on special occasions.

The predominant attitude toward drinking is one of tolerance. This does not mean that abstainers or occasional social drinkers are unknown. It suggests rather that the drinking norms are prescriptive, not proscriptive as among East Indians. In the first place, the religious associations to which the Negroes belong are not characteristically puritan. The majority are members of the Roman Catholic and Anglican faiths. Even among followers of the more fundamentalist sects, there is no *real* concern with the drinking of alcoholic beverages by men, provided that one is able to control one's behavior.

Second, the socialization of the child into the use of alcohol is not exposed to contradictory behavior on the part of adults with reference to drinking. This is closely related to the character of the family group which socializes the individual. The Negro family in the Caribbean is traditionally matrifocal in nature. Although today many couples legalize their marriage if possible, common law unions are frequent. Moreover, whether one is legally married or not, the maternal kin are usually ego's closest affective relations. The child is exposed to a minimum of intergenerational conflict, and adult roles with respect to power, authority in the home, sexuality, and the raising of children are consistent. On the other hand, there are respect relationships between the generations, but these are based upon affection, not constraint. Unlike East Indian culture, there is an equal degree of respect on the part of both the adult male and his parents, particularly the mother. The adult male Negro is not forced into an ambivalent role. Thus, despite a high frequency of male absenteeism, whenever the child is exposed to a model of adult male behavior, it is at least a positive one.

The adult Negro male is not constantly placed in a position of conflict between his parents and his spouse. Demands for self-reliance and achievement are placed upon the individual from childhood. The adult is encouraged to be economically and socially independent. This is indicated by patterns of neolocal residence, common law unions, occupational mobility, etc. Moreover, there is less overt controversy about child rearing in Creole culture. The child's most affective ties are with the mother and the mother's kin. Likewise, they represent the authority figures. (This relationship, however, can be overbearing: 21 percent of the Negro alcoholics were *only* sons [total n = forty-eight], as opposed to 5 percent of the Hindus.) Therefore, even if the child is not exposed to a strong male role model (however periodically), the personality characteristics which are reinforced by the socialization process are consistent with the general image of the male in Creole culture and Trinidad society.

With reference to alcohol use, the adult male role seems to be logically consistent. Briefly it is this. If the father drinks, the child is taught the use of alcohol in the home; if the father abstains, the child is not socialized into the use of alcoholic beverages in the home. Again, the child is not subject to contradictory behavior on the part of the adult, whether father or father-figure. (In many instances, although the child rarely sees his genitor, he may recognize a series of father-figures such as maternal uncles or grandfathers.) There are no seemingly illogical prescriptions against drinking in company with the father, in contrast to East Indian culture. This is the case even where the father is a heavy drinker.

Another factor to be considered in this discussion of prescriptive drinking behavior is the general freedom of sexual expression in Negro culture. This is *not* to be interpreted as a reference to promiscuity but as a statement of independence. Interpersonal relationships are free of family control. There is no sexual repression as found in East Indian culture where, even after marriage, sexual behavior is controlled to a certain extent by the demands made by the parents and by the lack of privacy. Many East Indian informants commented that this was a constant source of tension. Moreover, many added that they often drank to summon up the courage to visit a prostitute. Among Negroes, on the other hand, drinking is commonly associated with nonmarital sexual behavior. It differs from East Indian behavior in that the consenting pair often drink together. Drinking is associated with having a good time, enjoying one's friends, and the company of women. Among East Indians drinking with women in public is prohibited.

The normative orientation in Negro drinking is distinctly convivial. Although deep intoxication is not sought, many aim to "feel sweet" and stay that way. This we may refer to as "plateau drinking." The choice of beverage may be brand rums, whiskeys, or mixed drinks. There is a considerable amount of prestige attached to imported liquors. Puncheon rum is rarely consumed in the cities. Drinking with one's friends occurs most frequently on the weekends. The drinking group may be either a male peer group or a mixed friendship group; the occasion more often than not is a fete held in a private home or an inn where food is served and music is available. It is quite permissible for men and women to drink together in certain public drinking places. This would exclude rumshops which are reserved for male peer group drinking.

The decision to drink with one's peers is based on choice, not necessity. In addition to an affective family environment, an individual in a Negro community may participate in a number of associations, clubs, or religious groups which may provide other meaningful relationships. This is unlike the East Indian community where interfamilial conflict restricts the number of social relationships possible. The norm in Negro peer group drinking is again convivial. Control over excessive drinking is exercised by the group itself. The attitude toward drunkenness is one of gentle concern, not ridicule. Intoxication can be viewed permissively on the condition that the individual does not behave in an overtly aggressive manner.

The one activity into which drinking does not extend itself is the work cycle. This can be partly attributed to the fact that the work situation in which the Negro finds himself is not structurally, let alone physically, amenable to the use of alcohol. The majority of Negroes are not involved in agricultural pursuits such as cane production which can readily accommodate the use of alcohol on certain occasions. The structure of the urban work situation, whether employment is found as laborer, skilled workman, or clerk, is considerably more controlled. The oil refineries, the rum distilleries, the shops, the offices, all closely supervise their workers. One factor of course is safety; the other is salary. Employers regard drinking on the job as unproductive from both viewpoints. Apart from these restrictions, however, it is quite legitimate and even appropriate to conduct one's financial and political affairs in an amiable atmosphere. It is not uncommon to discuss business over a bottle of whiskey. The attitudes enabling one to do so are different from those of the East Indian. It would be rare indeed to find East Indians discussing business affairs among themselves and drinking at the same time. The structure may be subverted, of course. The large number of rumshops in and around Port-of-Spain enable one to drink between work periods if desired.

Among urban Negroes, attitudes toward drinking and drinking behavior itself seem to be more integrated into the ecological structure of drinking than their East Indian counterparts. This is due partly to Creole life-styles in general and partly to the dominancy of Creole culture in Trinidad.

Drinking as a Pathology

The variables examined above not only affect the incidence of alcoholism, but influence the pattern of alcoholic behavior and the individual's response to treatment as well. The discussion to follow will be limited to East Indian alcoholics of Hindu origin and Negro alcoholics.

The average age of the Hindus (n = fifty-one) in the study sample was 40.5 years (range 21 to 58 years); treatment was first sought at an average age of 36.7 years. The Negro sample (n = forty-eight) was a little older, the average being 42.7 years; treatment was first sought on the average at 40.1 years. All but two of the Hindu informants in my sample were married, although 10 percent were in a common-law union. The range of marriage relationships among the Negro alcoholics was considerably more varied. The Negro respondents in general had a higher level of education. Although all the East Indians were residents of rural areas, only 61 percent were directly involved in agriculture as cane laborers or cane farmers. It is clear that the majority of the East Indians were rural and unskilled laborers. The Negroes on the other hand were urban and skilled workers. Such results are also a reflection of the nature of the sample.

All the Hindu respondents were raised in a structurally

stable family environment. The type of family background among Negroes was considerably more varied than that of the East Indian informants and much less structurally stable. The majority of both Hindu and Negro alcoholics in the sample fell into the extreme categories of birth order: "oldest," "youngest," or "only." The major difference between the two groups is that 42 percent of the Hindu alcoholics are either the eldest son or eldest child, compared to 22 percent of the Negroes. The majority of the East Indian (Hindu) respondents had started working in the field or at home for their parents between thirteen and fifteen years of age. Thus, the education of the sons was often curtailed rather early by economic necessity. In 95 percent of the cases, Hindu marriages were arranged for the son when he was nineteen or twenty years of age, to a bride who was four or five years younger. The majority of the Negro respondents started working on their own at an average age of sixteen years. Employment either involved on-the-job training or took advantage of a skill they had learned. In all cases it was an independent choice, unlike the East Indian respondents whose economic history was closely related to that of their parents. The marital arrangements of the Negro alcoholics varied considerably as noted above.

The data indicate that the East Indian alcoholics in general came from a background of greater alcohol use than their Negro counterparts. Fewer East Indian parents abstained and more were regarded as alcoholic (or heavy) drinkers. Although there was more frequent drinking on the part of the East Indian parents, none of the respondents as children were allowed to drink with them. In fact, the circumstances of the first drink and subsequent ones (before the individual started drinking on his own) were highly contradictory. Although over half of the respondents had been consistently exposed to models of heavy drinking or alcoholism, the use of alcohol was prohibited them except for medicinal purposes. On the other hand, first drinking on one's own was commonly associated with the first drunk. The Negro parents were considerably more consistent about allowing their children to drink. Those parents who did drink socialized the children into the use of alcohol gently. All the Negro alcoholics began to drink regularly when they started to work. The Negro alcoholics experienced their first drunk on the average of five to six years later in their drinking career.

Clearly there are a number of differences between the East Indian (Hindu) and the Negro alcoholic: in socioeconomic location, family background, life-history circumstances, socialization into alcohol use, and patterns of pathological drinking. The East Indians on the average seek treatment at an earlier age than the Negroes, and have more years of sobriety behind them when interviewed. Ninety percent of the East Indians are legally married, as opposed to 32 percent of the Negroes. On the other hand, 74 percent of the Negroes are employed in occupations demanding more training in general. The majority (95 percent) of the East Indians come from rural cane-farming families, while the parents of the Negro respondents are more urbanized and involved in industry. In addition, the East Indian alcoholics come from stable family backgrounds, and tend to be oldest or youngest sons, while the Negro alcoholics generally come from some variant of a matrifocal family and tend to be only sons.

As for pathological drinking, the East Indian tends to become psychologically dependent upon alcohol at an earlier age. Consequently he seeks treatment sooner, although there seems to be considerably more social and economic pressure upon the East Indian than upon the Negro, which would contribute to this. The severest drinking patterns in both groups are found among the commonest laborers. Apart from the Negro laborers, the majority of the Negro alcoholics are "weekend" drinkers who tend to be drawn into more serious problem drinking through social situations.

Considerably fewer Negroes than East Indians report interference with work habits. The main feature that both East Indian and Negro alcoholics have in common is that sooner or later at some point in their drinking history, biological control comes to predominate. Despite the shared medical diagnosis of alcoholism, cultural differences are also reflected in the approach to treatment by the two groups.

The Treatment of Alcoholism

In addition to private counseling and private medical treatment, there are major sources of help for the alcoholic in Trinidad: the Alcoholism Treatment Center, a state-financed ward in St. Ann's Hospital, Port-of-Spain; and Alcoholics Anonymous (AA), a nonprofit voluntary association of nondrinking alcoholics.

The AA in Trinidad can be described as a network of social relationships which parallels already existing sociopolitical systems on both local and national levels. The social nature of alcoholism is reflected by the differences in approach to AA between East Indians and Negroes, despite a shared medical diagnosis of the disease. There are of course "ecological" conditions present in Trinidad which make this differential response more apparent.

The small size of Trinidad enables members to visit other groups frequently and to come to know those in many groups. This threatens anonymity and contributes to the personalization of AA. Most of the AA groups are located in residential areas. Thus, other AA members consist of former friends and relatives. Many of the members come into contact with each other outside of the AA context in the normal course of daily life. The non-AA activities of members are highly visible and become rapidly known to each other through the AA network. Again, this contributes to a high degree of personalization, which is undesirable. This is especially so in the rural East Indian groups where interpersonal conflicts often come to light. Drinkers and drunkards are highly visible to the community and to AA members. This contributes to a high degree of evangelizing or campaigning on the part of AA members. Again, this seems to be more common among East Indians than Negroes.

Power struggles are not uncommon. Unfortunately, this has the ultimate effect of destroying AA unity on a national level. One of the problems, for example, has been the political cleavage between the northern and southern groups. There are accusations made constantly that each is attempting to form political alliances, while the AA is supposedly a nonpolitical organization.

The religiosity and suggestibility of Trinidadians again make the development of charismatic leadership highly possible. It is very easy for strong personality-types to dominate AA groups and entire areas. These former deviants are given access to a system which allows them to reach national levels of control. This is especially the case with the East Indians, who have always had difficulty in forming a political organ on a national level.

The advantage of AA and its effectiveness are readily apparent to other community members; this contributes to a rapid increase in status for its members, and makes membership in the AA particularly desirable. Because of the emphasis in AA placed upon the reading of the "Big Book" and other kinds of literature, many formerly poorly educated or illiterate people have learned to read, improve their vocabularies, and express themselves in public. The AA has had, in fact, a side effect in the education and producing of leaders. This is an advantage especially in East Indian communities which have always had difficulties in organizing themselves.

A content analysis of the testimonies recorded reveals differences between East Indian and Negro approaches to the AA. The East Indians repeatedly stress "material" gains as being the primary advantage of staying sober through the AA: their family accepted them once again; they set an example for their community; employers prefer to hire AA members; they benefit financially and can provide their wives and children with necessities, especially education.

The Negroes, on the other hand, do not let AA dominate every aspect of their life as quickly, if at all. The East Indian immerses himself in AA and accepts it wholeheartedly. Negroes tend to consider all phases of the program before making any deep commitment to it. Of course, there may not be such a high degree of family pressure upon Negroes as upon East Indians. Those Negroes who do accept AA give greater religious connotations to the program. They seem more concerned with God and spiritual fellowship. The East Indian is more rigid in his concept of AA. He strives for compulsive role playing and insists upon stricter adherence to AA ritual and practices. This is contradictory because it is precisely the East Indian who has the materialist attitude towards AA. The Negro is more inclined to adapt AA to the group and to minimize competition for the sake of solidarity.

Conclusion

Not only normal drinking behavior but any related pathologies are immeshed in culture. Certain cultural variables which affect such behavior patterns have been discussed. The comparison of the East Indian and Negro cultures has been facilitated by speaking of each as a cultural isolate. However, one must be aware of an additional perspective which cannot be examined in detail in this essay—an understanding of the effect of the presence of one cultural group on the behavior of a second group with a very different life-style.

Note

1. This also explains why the rural/urban dimension was not a significant factor in determining the two behavior patterns.

III. Alcohol Use by North American Indians

"The Drunken Indian":
Myths and Realities

Joseph Westermeyer

Perhaps no stereotype has been so long-lasting and so thoroughly ensconced in our social fabric as that of the "drunken Indian." Our federal government gave it official recognition by prohibiting the sale of beverage alcohol to Indian people for over a century. Until recently, many missionary groups required that Indian converts take a pledge of total abstinence. Many citizens—both Indian and non-Indian—have seen the "drunken Indian" as a hopeless, powerless figure who had no alternative to drunkenness with which to cope with poverty, the destruction of his culture, and the undermining of his family.

My purpose here is, first, to examine the misconceptions and associated political strategies that flow logically from the non-logical stereotype of the "drunken Indian" and, second, to review the data on the alcohol usage and alcohol-related problems of Indian people.

Common Misconceptions

MISCONCEPTION 1. *Indians cannot hold their liquor.* This stereotype presumes that Indian people who drink do so to excess and inevitably encounter problems as a result of their alcohol usage. Generally this presumed tendency is felt to be due to some inherent racial trait that results in alcohol's affecting Indians in a specific and unusual manner.

This notion has recently gained prominence as a result of studies showing differences in the vasomotor response to alcohol and in the rates at which Indians and whites metabolize alcohol. But the samples in such studies have been matched for only a few of the variables important to such investigation. In addition to marred method, the logic for such physiologic studies has been poorly worked out so far. For example, the observation that Orientals respond to alcohol in a physiologically different manner from whites has been used to explain why Orientals have less alcoholism, but the same argument for the same reasons has been used to explain why Indians (a group quite similar to Orientals in numerous hereditary characteristics) have presumably more alcoholism (P.H. Wolff 1973). And it is a long step from merely demonstrating physiological differences to explaining what role, if any, they might play in the etiology of alcoholism.

MISCONCEPTION 2. *Alcoholism rates are very high among Indians.* First, we have the problem of what comprises a case of alcoholism. In the opinion of most people, simply imbibing alcohol or behaving in an intoxicated manner is not a sufficient criterion for alcoholism. Students of this problem generally define a specific alcohol-related behavior or problem in order to quantify and then compare populations, rather than relying on simply case counting, when the diagnostic criteria are so vague and subject to individual interpretation.

Second, when considering such specific alcohol-related events, we have considerable evidence that all American Indians do not comprise a single group concerning which generalizations can be made. Considerable differences exist among tribes, even taking into account the small populations of some tribes that make reliable intertribal comparisons difficult. Also, within tribes there are subgroup differences, and within subgroups there are considerable individual differences. These differences, and the reasons for them, have been neglected in most studies so far.

Finally, when Indian rates are compared with national averages, some groups and tribes do have rates of alcohol-related problems that exceed the mean, and some have rates that are much lower. These points will be elaborated in the next section.

MISCONCEPTION 3. *Alcoholism is the major problem among Indian people.* Even among Indian groups that do have high rates of alcohol-related problems, it is difficult to know whether a given problem is caused by alcohol or by various social, economic, historical, cultural, and/or political factors. Alcohol problems are often associated in a given individual with such stresses as migration from the reservation to a non-Indian community; racial and ethnic prejudice; health impairment; unemployment or marginal economic status; outside interference by non-Indian social agencies in family and community affairs; and lack of control in his own community over the education of his children, law enforcement, religious institutions, and health and welfare resources.

For any one Indian or group of Indians it is difficult to separate racial prejudice, family disintegration, or economic oppression from alcohol in the genesis of various problems. However, the danger exists that if alcoholism is focused on as the biggest problem, urgent political and economic issues may be ignored. This is especially true because much of what is done regarding alcoholism is done at the individual level, ignoring important social, cultural, and intercultural problems.

It is accurate to state that alcoholism is often associated with a variety of social problems in some Indian communities today, but the relationship between alcohol and these problems is not a clearly causal one. In other words, simply attending to individual cases of alcoholism alone may neither help the alcoholic Indian himself, nor prevent new cases of alcoholism in the community, nor resolve the problems facing Indian communities. This is not to say that alcoholism treatment programs should not be undertaken, but rather that they should not be considered an across-the-board panacea for all the difficulties faced by Indian people.

The Research on Indians and Alcohol

Over the last few decades a considerable store of knowledge has slowly accumulated regarding Indians and alcohol. Originally these observations came from anthropologists who were not particularly interested in alcohol usage or alcoholism. More recently students of chemical dependency, clinicians and behavioral scientists, have begun to provide us with an information base to replace the simplistic stereotypes of the past.

1. *Alcohol usage patterns among Indian people vary widely.* The stereotypic "Indian" drinking pattern consists of the early appearance of intoxicated behavior with small doses of alcohol; binge drinking over many hours or several days, separated by days or weeks of abstinence; group "party" drinking that may entail movement from one location to another; and continued purchase of alcohol until financial resources are exhausted. It is thought to contain a "time-out" element: that is, some Indian people, while drinking, may behave in ways that would not be acceptable to them or their cultural peers if they were not drinking.

To be sure, this stereotypic pattern has often been observed among various Indian peoples. However, it has also prevailed among non-Indian groups—frontiersmen, men living together away from a family setting (such as soldiers and lumbermen), conventioneers in a strange city, adolescents and young adults, and homeless single men without regular jobs. Thus, it is not only an "Indian" pattern (MacAndrew and Edgerton 1969).

In addition, other patterns have been reported among Indian people in both historical and contemporary times. Many Indian people use alcohol in a "white middle-class" fashion, limiting their use in amount, time, and place and behaving in a manner not greatly different from their nondrinking behavior. Also, the abstinent state is voluntarily chosen by many Indian people. To make matters even more complex, the same person may employ "Indian" drinking, "white" drinking, and/or abstinence at various times in his life, depending on social factors, his own preference, or life events (Levy and Kunitz 1973; Westermeyer 1972*b*).

Thus, the actual state of affairs appears considerably more complex than indicated by the usual stereotype. The public nature and "deviant" aspect of "Indian" drinking (at least from the non-Indian point of view) make this pattern the one most widely observed and commonly reported by non-Indian people. Since abstinence and "white" drinking among Indian people are less publicly evident and less apt to merit attention, most non-Indian people tend not to appreciate their widespread occurrence among Indians.

2. *Alcohol use can occur concomitantly with untoward events in the lives of some Indian people, but it can also be associated with beneficial effects.* Among many people alcohol usage promotes social cohesion, facilitates social interaction, and enhances feelings of well-being. By removing inhibitions (whether by psychological or by pharmacological means), the use of alcohol can aid in the giving and receiving of interpersonal warmth and support. Within a group of Indian people, "Indian" drinking may serve as an admission ticket to socialization with the group. Binge drinking can at times provide an alternative means for handling grief or stress for some Indian people.

Several investigators have suggested that "Indian" drinking may actually permit traditional Indian values and attitudes to continue. This viewpoint has evolved as it has become evident that many Indians have not abandoned traditional tribal ideals in order to be assimilated into the majority society. Living as they do in a political and economic state that is imposed and directed by non-Indian people, such persons are subject to innumerable double binds, since Indian social systems and norms often conflict with those of the majority society. Faced with such dilemmas, the Indian drinker, while "drunken," can behave irresponsibly in a way that other Indians do not approve. However, the drinker can expect that other Indians will blame the alcohol, not the drinker, for the behavior. The same "drunken" behavior serves a complementary function among non-Indians: it advertises that the drinker can still "act Indian" in a way that the majority society cannot influence. Assuming this hypothesis to be true, one can expect "Indian" drinking patterns to continue as long as the majority society (1) dominates the economic life and self-governance of Indian communities and (2) limits ways in which Indian people can maintain their own ethnic social identities.

3. *The relationship between alcohol use and certain problematic events may be more fortuitous than etiologic.* That is, certain difficulties among Indian people now associated with alcohol may not be due solely or even in part to alcohol use. For example, Navaho suicide and homicide rates have remained essentially constant since 1880. Over that time the use of alcohol by the Navaho has steadily increased, and such violent events now commonly occur along with alcohol usage (Levy and Kunitz 1969, 1973). The same is true for the White Mountain Apache (Levy and Kunitz 1969). Thus the relationship between this violence and alcohol is apparently a complex one that cannot be readily understood in simple cause-effect terms.

The same may be said about a number of other alcohol-related events, including arrest rates. Indian people are often arrested for alcohol-related behavior that they consider socially and morally acceptable but that the dominant society considers unacceptable and has deemed illegal. In such cases the arrest rates may indicate intercultural discontinuities as readily as they indicate alcohol problems (Stewart 1964).

In sum we must beware of equating a statistical correlation with a causal explanation. The social and cultural context should always be weighed heavily in alcohol studies, and the more so when people representing the majority concern themselves with the alcohol use of a minority group. Besides historical and intercultural factors, consideration must be given to socioeconomic status, political issues, religious biases, and personal preferences.

4. *Considerable differences exist among groups of Indian people regarding rates of various alcohol-related events.* Difficult problems prevent the ready assessment of these events among Indian people, including small base population rates, migration, and accurate measurement of problematic events associated with alcohol usage. Despite these obstacles, however, studies have shown differences among tribes within given tribal groups.

For example, the Navaho death rate from Laënnec's cirrhosis has been lower than the national average, while the Mountain Apache and Hopi cirrhosis rates have been higher (Levy and Kunitz 1973; Kunitz, Levy, and Everett 1970; Kunitz et al. 1971, also in this volume). The death rates from suicide (often alcohol-related) among the Shoshone-Bannock, Cheyenne, and Apache have been inordinately higher (Resnick and Dizmang 1971), while those among the Chippewa and Navaho have been relatively low (Levy and Kunitz 1971; Westermeyer and Brantner 1972). Within a given tribe, differences have also been noted; for example,

Laënnec's cirrhosis prevails more among Navaho close to alcohol supply sources than among those living in more remote locations (Kunitz, Levy, and Everett 1970).

Thus it is risky to make any general statements that are meant to apply to "all Indians." While certain general statements may apply to the entire Indian population in the United States (such as the high homicide and accidental death rates prevalent among all Indians as a racial group), one must be wary of applying these notions to specific tribes or parts of tribes.

5. *Alcoholism, in the sense of physiologic dependence on alcohol (as evidenced by the withdrawal syndrome) or in the sense of classic medical problems associated with chronic, heavy alcohol use (such as Laënnec's cirrhosis), does occur among some Indian people.* For a long time it has been common to think that some Indians are "heavy drinkers" or "drunkards" but not really alcoholics. The studies of Laënnec's cirrhosis among Navaho, Hopi, and Apache people referred to above have shattered this notion. Studies comparing Chippewa with non-Indian alcoholics who are hospitalized or in a detoxification center show that similar percentages of each group go through physiologic withdrawal from chronic, heavy alcohol use (Westermeyer 1972a). Blood studies of Chippewa people at autopsy have shown alcohol levels quite comparable (both in percentage of cases and in level of blood alcohol) with those occurring in non-Indians (Westermeyer and Brantner 1972). In short, by whatever definition one chooses, some Indian people do indeed become alcoholics.

6. *Indian people with alcohol problems can benefit from treatment for their alcoholism.* Until recently, few majority treatment programs wished to include Indian patients. Many of those that did try to do so had limited or no success. As Indian people have become active in the planning and staffing of alcoholism treatment programs, early reports suggest that the previous trends are being reversed. Indian people troubled by their alcohol usage are seeking treatment in increasing numbers within a variety of treatment modalities (Shore and Von Fumetti 1972; Westermeyer and Lange n.d.; Savard 1968). Those treatment centers planned and staffed by Indian people appear to be having more success than the previous non-Indian-oriented programs in helping the Indian with alcohol-related problems.

Conclusions

Certain general statements regarding alcohol usage can apply to some Indian people more than to non-Indians, at least sometimes.

However, any such statement tends to have so many exceptions that a useless and misleading stereotype results. With regard to both alcohol usage and alcohol-related problems, an extremely wide variation exists among Indian tribes, among subgroups within tribes, and among individual Indians. Thus statements about Indians and alcohol should specify which Indians, in what place, during what period, and under what circumstances.

Alcohol problems that exist among Indian people bear many resemblances to those common to many ethnic groups in the United States. Attention to Indian alcoholism should not mask or preclude attention to the many social problems and inequities against which Indian people now struggle. Indian-planned and Indian-led programs to counteract alcoholism appear to offer promise of alleviating this problem when it occurs.

Data now becoming available have increasingly undermined the stereotypes of yesterday. It is to be hoped that current studies will provide more useful guideposts for Indian people and social institutions than have been available so far.

The Role of Alcohol among North American Indian Tribes as Reported in *The Jesuit Relations*

R. C. Dailey

Whenever one considers the reasons for the destruction of the North American Indian it is commonplace to find alcohol cited as the principal cause. Certainly this was the opinion of the early French Jesuits who sought to convert the Indian tribes of New France. For them, alcohol was the major obstacle to the success of their mission. *The Jesuit Relations and Allied Documents* (Thwaites 1896–1901) are filled with references to liquor and its adverse effects. As the subject of Indian drinking is currently of interest to several disciplines, particularly anthropology, I felt it might be of value to assemble all the data from this important ethnohistoric source in one place. In view of this, I have analyzed in some detail what the Jesuits wrote about Indians and their use of alcohol as they witnessed it in the early historic period.

Though the idea that alcohol destroyed the Indian has been accepted since the days of the Jesuit mission, it is, on the other hand, often overlooked that liquor was not the only item of European culture that had an impact. It is, therefore, virtually impossible to isolate the effects of one European culture trait from those of another. Here, even the role of the Jesuits themselves cannot be omitted.

Initially, alcohol was introduced to the Indian through the fur trade. However, it quickly came to have far-reaching social, economic, and political implications for Indian and white alike. In evaluating its place in history the popular view has been to stress the role of liquor as the villain and to accept the fur trade as an absolute necessity. This is not unexpected since despite the threat of both secular and ecclesiastical punishments, ranging from the stocks to excommunication, nonetheless, efforts to abolish the liquor traffic were unrealistic. For one thing, without a successful fur trade the solvency of the colony could not be assured. For another, even if the French had ceased to use alcohol in their relations with Indians, there was no agreement with the Dutch or the English that they would also stop the practice. Indian allies were important in the power struggle for the control of North America. The regular distribution of alcohol was a means of maintaining Indian loyalties as well as gaining new friends.

Though the Jesuits inveighed against what they saw as a wholesale debauching of the Indian, they were unable to secure more than token support for total interdiction. Bowing to church pressure the colonial administrators in France did agree to stop the liquor traffic, and several of the governors of New France actually attempted to enforce the regulations, notably Champlain and the governor of Tadoussac, but in the long run they were ineffective. In his *Canada and its Provinces,* Shortt has nicely summed up the problem: "The real issue, therefore, which the church and the colonial government had to face was whether the Indians should have brandy and orthodoxy at the hands of the French, or rum and heresy at the hands of the Dutch and the English" (1914:468).

My concern here, however, is not to review the history of the problem further, but to examine the effects of the introduction of alcohol on the Indian. Three questions come to mind: (1) What behavior among the Indians was attributed to the effects of liquor? (2) Was this behavior new to the Indian way of life? and (3) How did the Indians view this behavior, and in particular, was it disruptive to them?

As to the first question, a few direct quotes will serve to identify the kind of behavior most frequently condemned by the

Jesuits. Liquor was blamed for most of the general disorders and physical violence among the Indians. "Every night," they wrote, "is filled with clamors, brawls, and fatal accidents, which the intoxicated cause in the cabins" (46:105).[1] Whole villages were sometimes affected: "It [drunkenness] is so common here, and causes such disorders, that it sometimes seems as if all the people of the village had become insane, so great is the license they allow themselves when they are under the influence of liquor" (51:217). These drinking parties are said to have lasted as long as the liquor supply, usually three to four days but sometimes as long as two weeks.

The "disorder" to which the Jesuits refer included fatal accidents, murders, and maimings—not even one's own friends and relatives were spared: "Last summer, four Onneiouts (Oneida) were killed by their comrades, while Drunken; yet this accident did not make the others any wiser" (51:125). "I count seven who were murdered by drunkards in two months" (62:67). "When these people are intoxicated, they become so furious that they break and smash everything in their houses; they utter horrible yells and shouts, and, like madmen, seek their enemies to stab them. At such times, even their relatives and friends are not safe from their fury, and they bite off one another's noses and ears" (67:39).

In addition to physical violence, drinking "disorders" included immorality. Young men would cause girls to get drunk in order to seduce them, or they would both drink willingly and solicit one another. Drunkenness was blamed, too, for the breaking up of families: "Disunion and dissolution of their marriage invariably result from their drunkenness, owing to the sorrow and despair of their wives when they see themselves despoiled by their drunken husbands who take everything from them to obtain liquor; and who are deprived of the proceeds of the hunting, which belong to them, but are taken from their husbands before they reach the village by their creditors" (67:39, 41). Consequently, women and children went hungry and villages were neglected. "Drink is a demon that robs them of their reason, and so inflames their passion that, after returning from the chase richly laden with beaver skins, instead of furnishing their families with provisions, clothing, and other necessary supplies, they drink away the entire proceeds in one day and are forced to pass the winter in nakedness, famine, and all sorts of deprivation" (46:103). One case was reported where a whole village was destroyed by a warring Iroquois band, because all its members were drunk and had neglected to leave even one sentinel (47:141).

Now to the second question, how much of the above behavior which so bothered the Jesuits was new to the Indians' way of life? Or to put it another way, what behavior patterns would have manifested themselves following white contact even if liquor had never been introduced? While no conclusive answer is to be expected, one might begin by examining the behavior patterns reported at the time of contact. Consider first their mode of eating, and especially the custom of consuming everything at one sitting. It becomes clear then that it was only the alcohol which was new, not the practice of consuming everything at once. Hence, the "brandy feasts" as they were called, were on the same pattern as the "eat-all feasts" described in the following quotations: "In feasts, it is the rule by general consent and custom of the race, that all the food shall be consumed. If anyone eats sparingly and urges his poor health as an excuse, he is beaten or ejected as ill-bred, just as if he were ignorant of the art of living" (1:285, 287). Similarly, in the case of liquor, "give two savages two or three bottles of brandy, they will sit down and, without eating, will drink one after the other, until they have emptied them" (6:253).

Even more important was the question of physical violence. Though the Jesuits blamed alcohol for increasing murders, and a general diminishing of the Indian population, there is no evidence to confirm this. Indeed, murders motivated by dreams or sorcery or revenge in gambling bouts may have been just as prevalent before Indians began using alcohol as they were afterwards. Hence, it seems appropriate here to consider the similarity between intoxicated behavior and that resulting from dream experiences. Moreover, since the effect or power of alcohol was not understood by the Indians, intoxication was included in the category of the supernatural. Under its influence the inebriated person was given full license to behave as he pleased, even if it meant killing a person. This was the identical treatment accorded those compelled to act out their dreams. The significance and power of these is demonstrated in the following passage: "What each boy sees in his dreams, when his reason begins to develop, is to him thereafter a deity, whether it be a dog, a bear, or a bird. They often derive their principles of life and action from dreams; as for example, if they dream that any person ought to be killed, they do not rest until they have caught the man by stealth and slain him" (1:287). This kind of murder was not restricted to their own people; the French, too, were in danger of becoming victims: "If during the night they dream they must kill a Frenchman, woe to the first one they meet alone. They attach great faith to their dreams" (4:217). On this point it would be interesting to know whether there was a decrease in the traditional methods of attaining spiritual experience after the introduction of alcohol, i.e., fasting alone for days, and whether alcohol was used as a short cut, as seems probable.

It was considered essential for the welfare of the community as well as for the individual that his dream be carried out in detail, for only then would the soul of the man be satisfied. The soul was a powerful part of the person acting independently from the rest of the body, making its wishes known through dreams: "For they think that there are in every man certain inborn desires, often unknown to themselves, upon which the happiness of individuals depends" (1:259). Actually, more than the happiness of the individual was involved: "All that they dream must be carried out: otherwise, one draws upon himself the hatred of all the dreamer's relatives, and exposes himself to feel the effects of their anger" (51:125). It was as important to discover the desires of the soul as it was to carry them out. Many of their illnesses were believed to be caused when these wishes remained unrecognized or forsaken. The only cure was to satisfy them. If the desire was not recognized, a medicine man would provide the service of drawing it out. Since dreams were the sole means of communicating with the spiritual part of the body, it is not surprising that the dream quest was so prominent. Everyone was at one time or another involved in this quest, particularly the young males. A person in the process of dreaming was considered somehow sacred, as was an intoxicated person. There must have been much similarity in the behavior of the inebriated man and the dreamer half-starved, full of expectations, and hallucinating. Both could be seen running about seemingly possessed, disturbing the village with their screams.

There was another social situation in which violence or disorderly behavior occurred. Gambling was a common recreational activity. As the stakes were high it was not unusual for a man to lose everything he owned, including his children (16:199–201). "Gambling never leads to anything good; in fact, the Savages themselves remark that it is almost the sole cause of assaults and murders" (10:81). Again this suggests that brawls and murders were not unknown before the introduction of liquor, despite the fact that the Indians were noted for their stoicism and lack of aggressive demonstrations.

There was one celebration in particular which provided a social setting wherein it was legitimate to display behavior similar to that shown in drunken brawls. "This celebration is called

Ononhouaroia, or 'upsetting of brain,' because all the youth, and even the women and children, run about as if they were mad, insisting upon obedience being paid to their Demons by making them a present of something which they proffer with an enigma, and which has been suggested to them in a dream" (23:53). To these Indians the idea of "upsetting the brain" was known and accepted. Losing control over their mental processes had no shame attached, and indeed, was a sought-after means of transcending the physical to obtain a spiritual experience. Because this experience was highly valued and admired, they would openly and proudly announce their intention to drink, shouting, "I am going to lose my head; I am going to drink of the water that takes away one's wits" (52:193).

In the early historic period when only traders were in contact with Indian communities, these forms of explosive behavior while dangerous were not disruptive. However, as white settlements were built and contact became more and more regular, the Indians soon realized that the act of "losing one's wits" had to be controlled. A common method was to tie down those of their comrades who became violent when intoxicated. In other instances potential inebriates were required to surrender their weapons: "Indeed, so sensible are they of their own infirmities when in this state that when a number of them are about to get drunk, they give up their knives and tomahawks, etc., to one of the party who is on honor to remain sober, and to prevent mischief, and who generally does behave according to this promise. If they happen to get drunk without having taken this precaution, their squaws take the earliest opportunity to deprive them of their weapons" (Weld 1800:480; this was already 1795–97). However, it is impossible to be sure to what extent such precautions were used, or to what extent these methods were influenced by the laws and penalties of the white man. A murder excused by the Indians would receive the death penalty from the whites. "An Algonquin in a drinking-bout killed with three stabs of a knife a poor soldier who was quietly working in a house at Montreal. Arrested on the spot, the Algonquin thought he would escape punishment because he was drunk and did not know what he was doing. He was condemned notwithstanding to be hanged; but as the executioner was away he was killed by a blow on the head" (68:267). Most of the reports of attempted control describe Indians who were in fairly close contact with whites, either under the influence of the Jesuits or the surveillance of the white man's law. Even though some of the restrictions were undoubtedly voluntary, they were still dependent on the cooperation of the white traders. Also, the restrictions were meant to curb extreme violence and bloodshed more than intoxication itself.

The frequently reported drinking brawls where violence occurred do not seem so unusual when compared with gambling behavior as already discussed, or with the torturing of captives. The Iroquois, for example, were noted for their fierce torture practices, though many authorities suggest that this reputation is highly exaggerated. Many of the cases where individuals were assaulted or murdered by intoxicated men actually involved Christians as was the woman in the following passage: "A drunken man who had just crippled another old woman entered her cabin. The only person who was with her at once ran away, and abandoned her to that furious man, who with a wooden pike, bruised her entire face, broke her jaw, pierced her shoulders and left her for dead on the spot" (57:171). The important difference made by alcohol was that now such hostilities were turned against their own friends and relatives, particularly if they happened to be Christian. However, it is uncertain on what scale this took place. It is possible that it did not happen very often but that when it did, it created such an impact on the minds of listeners that it became a sort of infamy that was reported several times without reference to time or place. It must be remembered that the Jesuits were writing to an audience in France, whom they were obliged to please and shock in order to get financial support. This is not to deny the violence against their own friends that was touched off by liquor, but only to question its frequency and intensity, and motive. These incidents demonstrate, among other things, that the Indians could not have completely "lost their minds" since when they drank they were sufficiently aware to carry out purposive and directed action.

These kinds of murders were not too different from those committed by Christians in Europe, who tortured and burned infidels and "witches" in the name of God. In a way, this type of behavior is a defensive reaction against forces which threaten the cohesiveness of the society. Also, this was one way that the Indians could demonstrate their aggressiveness towards whites. Symbolically it is very neat: the white man provided the means, liquor, with which the Indian could murder those who had fallen under the white man's influence. Furthermore, no guilt or blame was attached since it was the liquor that had control over the person.

As for the increase in immorality and licentiousness imputed to the effects of liquor, there is not much to say. The native's moral code, which among other things condoned premarital sex, was so removed from the Christian code that the Fathers could conceive of it only as caused by some evil force such as liquor.

I think one may conclude with some justification that alcohol did not introduce any strictly new forms of behavior. Of course, some were intensified, and as frequency was increased, daily routines were upset. The only unique behavior that could be attributed to liquor was the actual search for alcohol. This led inevitably to more contact with the white man; to dependency on him for its supply; to loss of their own goods; to the neglecting of homes, women, and children; and to indebtedness and economic penury.

Yet it would be incorrect to conclude that liquor really caused no problems that were not already present. Such would be premature since the dangers of liquor were recognized by the Indians themselves. But I believe it is necessary to recognize the similarities between drunken and socially accepted behavior with the understanding that intoxication was somehow alien, thus leading to some sporadic attempts to curb it.

This brings me to the final question: was drunken behavior causing disruption to the Indian himself? There were many who believed that liquor caused misfortunes, and that it would someday bring about their destruction. This was especially true of mission Indians but there were others too who wanted restrictions on the liquor supply and on insobriety. "Some of their captains have come to plead with the French not to sell them brandy or wine, saying that they would be the cause of the death of their people" (5:51). Another captain (Abenakis) wanted to address the deputy of the English: "Thou deputy of Pleimot and Boston, paint our words on paper and send them to those on whom thou art dependent; and say to them that all the allied Savages dwelling on the river Kenebek hate fire-water," or brandy, "as much as they hate the Hiroquois; and that if they have any more of it brought hither to sell to the Savages, the latter will believe that the English wish to exterminate them" (38:35, 37). The Indians themselves began to exercise a measure of discipline and in some cases with the help of whites, formed councils to decide on penalties for drunkenness. Offenders were even put to the chevalet or were forced to leave the village and their plot of land. Acts of murder were not everywhere excused and some murderers were executed (9:145, 203; 62:53; 63:103; 68:267).

Despite these rather severe penalties Indians continued to use alcohol on a grand scale. And while to the white man it was the liquor itself which caused the disruption, to the Indian it was the difficulties involved in obtaining it. For example, it was the long trips to trading centers, or towns like Three Rivers, that were disruptive—not only to those who went but also to those who were left behind in the villages. Even if they did not seek out the liquor, the French would travel two hundred to three hundred leagues to meet up with the Indians to entice them with brandy. Cases where liquor was brought back to the village for the purpose of feasts could not be called disruptive from the Indian's point of view if the feast involved the members in a common activity and followed a familiar pattern. Rather, the major disruption occurred when the men left the villages to go on hunting parties and returned sometimes weeks later, empty-handed, indebted, and intoxicated. Meanwhile, the women and children were left without food in the villages.

Interaction with whites was always to the disadvantage of the Indian who could not control his desire for liquor. Even when he had no money, he would run up such debts that for months to come he would receive nothing in return for his furs. As already mentioned, families starved over the winter, or they broke up because the husband could not provide for them. "These savages, loaded with debts and despoiled by their creditors, who leave them not even their guns, are frequently obliged to quit the country and go among the English, because they cannot hope to pay what they owe" (67:41). When the Indians pleaded for the restriction of liquor trade, they were at the same time pleading for the restriction of any contact with whites. Liquor came to symbolize white contact and its demoralizing effects. The assumed relationship between drunkenness and disruption was a serious one—perhaps it never occurred to the Jesuits that the white man's way of life and his business practices could have negative effects. For them, liquor became the scapegoat. Drunkenness was the catchall category that was to blame for any vices or disorder that occurred. Their own shortcomings were rationalized to be the fault of liquor, so that drunkenness was blamed even for the fact that the Indians were hard to Christianize. "But the greatest evil done here by drunkenness is, that its consequences Utterly estrange the savages from Christianity" (62:67). The Fathers lamented that if only drunkenness could be abolished, the natives could and would settle down to the Christian way of life. As the Jesuits saw it, there were two demons, drunkenness and dreams, and they could not decide which caused the greater disorder or which interfered more with the conversion of the natives. Later, even the dream quest was thought to be due to drunkenness, as it was inconceivable that someone would voluntarily involve himself in non-Christian rites unless he was somehow possessed. But the evil connected with liquor had to do at least as much with its procuring as with its intoxicating effects. It is true that while inebriated they would commit crimes against their own people which they later regretted. It is interesting, though, that the blame was attached to the white man and his liquor, not to oneself. This is evident from the following statements: "It is thou . . . and thine, who killed him; for, if thou hadst not given us brandy or wine, we would not have done it. . . . Thou art my brother, I love thee; it is not I who wounded thee, but the drink which used my arm" (5:49, 51). They were well aware of who supplied them with liquor, even against their own wishes at times, so that any disorder stemming from it could ultimately be blamed on the white man. If the Indians made any causal connection, it would probably have been between disruption and white man, not merely disruption and drunkenness.

Perhaps it is not valid to distinguish between drunkenness and contact with whites since in a way they are inseparable. On the other hand, the white man's behavior and business tactics added considerably to the consequences of Indian drunkenness. He was in control of the amount of liquor sold, the prices charged, and the credit and loans given. Indirectly, he determined whether a man would have any money left to feed his family or whether he would, in fact, go back to his family at all. It was not the case that the Indian had the power to *force* the white man to give him liquor—in fact, he was happy when the white man refused. Quite aside from the management of liquor, the white man's way of life and his values were very different, and when imposed on the Indian, helped greatly to disorient or demoralize him. This aspect of social contact and the problem of assimilation has already been the topic of many books, and concerns this paper only indirectly. In any case, it was not white man's liquor alone that caused disorder.

The question of moral blame here is a very interesting one as it helps us to understand how the Indian could ask the white man to stop supplying him with liquor at the same time as he was drinking it. How can one blame the white man if the Indian sought him out and demanded liquor at any price? On the other hand, how can one blame the Indian if the white man continued to supply even after the former had pleaded him to stop? In the eyes of the whites, the Indian was the weaker; in fact, they often thought of them as children. Anybody who understands the law of supply and demand would realize that a plea to stop the supply is not equivalent to an actual reduction in demand. It was up to the Indian to show a determination to end the demand. Unfortunately, he was not familiar with this economic law. His behavior was based instead on a moral code involving trust and honor. On this account the Indian and white man never understood each other. If anything, the Indian, to the white man, appeared untrustworthy and immoral. The Indian made his situation very clear to the white man, a tactic which to us seems naive, but to the Indian, honorable. He admitted he could not resist alcohol as long as it was available. He never thought of this as constituting a weakness. Thus he put the onus on the white man to stop the trade. Here may lie the roots of the long historical dependency of Indians on whites. If the white man complied with the code of honor, he should stop the supply. Since he did not, the Indian put all the blame on him and his liquor. He could not blame himself for his behavior while under the influence because he was not even in possession of his mind at the time, and as has been intimated, they thought when one can transcend one's body, the person is qualitatively different. Another mistake the Indian made was to trust the white man to be interested in his welfare. This may have been a touch of ethnocentrism on his part. At that time, whites were not interested in his welfare. They only wished him well enough to trap more furs, with liquor providing the principal incentive.

Why did the Indian drink? There is no single explanation, but this analysis of the *Relations* suggests the following. One of the most obvious is the novel physical sensation brought on by the physiological effects of alcohol in the body. Many Indians seem to have felt that under its influence they became exceptional people such as great orators. Secondly, there is the suggestion that some Indians used alcohol so that they would be excused for committing acts of violence they would otherwise have had to suppress. Thirdly, as whites assumed more and more control over Indian affairs, the former integrating effects of warfare and other village-wide activities were replaced by the search for and communal use of alcohol. Lastly, and most important, liquor greatly facilitated the attainment of dreams which was for the Indian his most valued experience. Through alcohol he was able to achieve a degree of ecstacy never possible in prehistoric times. But though the Indian interpreted these intense emotional outbursts as the only real form of human experience, to the early European and particularly the

Jesuits, alcohol remained, as Parkman has written, "a fiend with all crimes and miseries in his train: and, in fact, nothing earthly could better deserve the epithet infernal than an Indian town in the height of a drunken debauch. The orgies never ceased till the bottom of the barrel was reached" (1909:388).

Note

1. In text references to *The Jesuit Relations,* the first number refers to volume number; numbers following the colon refer to page number.

The World's Oldest On-Going Protest Demonstration: North American Indian Drinking Patterns

Nancy Oestreich Lurie

When I read Craig MacAndrew and Robert Edgerton's *Drunken Comportment* (1969), I felt a bit as Alfred Russell Wallace must have felt upon learning about the work of Charles Darwin. I had presented an initial version of this paper at an anthropological meeting shortly before receiving a copy of *Drunken Comportment.* The book validates beyond question some of my early speculations and documents in detail my historical generalizations. However, it concentrates on one item of "conventional wisdom" while my paper is directed at another.

The apparently self-evident common sense which MacAndrew and Edgerton systematically demolish is the widely held notion of the public and temperance societies—and even many medically and psychiatrically oriented researchers—that alcohol disinhibits and causes what they term personality "changes-for-the-worse." In case after well-documented case from all over the world, MacAndrew and Edgerton demonstrate conclusively that the unquestioned physiological effect (i.e., sensorimotor dysfunction) which accompanies the ingestion of alcohol is given different cultural interpretations by different peoples. These interpretations are manifested in different kinds of locally patterned, learned forms of drunkenness ranging from changes-for-the-worse to changes-for-the-better. The authors also point out that the widespread occurrence of drunken disinhibition and changes-for-the-worse are not evidence of any inherent quality of alcohol, as conventional wisdom assumes; alcohol has merely been diffused to many peoples across the world by the adventurers of Western society who also introduced their own cultural patterns of drunken behavior.

Accepting MacAndrew and Edgerton's findings, I would like to challenge the conventional wisdom concerning American Indian drinking that starts out with the assumption that real American Indian identity is only preserved in museums and that Indians drink because of an identity crisis. According to such thinking, Indian culture has just about phased out, if it is not entirely gone, and excessive drinking by the minority group that still persists as Indian must be due to low self-esteem, feelings of rejection, and the effects of prejudice and material deprivation vis-à-vis white, middle-class culture and society. It is only common sense, according to this argument, that Indians get drunk to escape into a glorified, romanticized past and try to regain a sense of identity as Indians, at least temporarily, because they encounter so many difficulties in assimilating into and being accepted by the dominant group and its culture. This layman's view is even shared by scholars as a recent publication of the Canadian Alcohol and Drug Addiction Research Foundation demonstrates: "drinking . . . activities are explicable as responses to acculturation anxieties and as substitutes for previously institutionalized interaction" (1966:1). Similar arguments are advanced by J. H. Hamer and Bernard J. James.

> Drinking . . . permits persons temporarily to assume desirable status positions when there has been interference with, and inadequate substitutes for, the traditional social structure. [Hamer 1965:285]

> Ojibwa culture . . . has become deculturated and . . . its minimal appropriation of new cultural traits has produced a "poor White" type of subculture. . . . The anxiety that casts it[s] shadow across the entire gamut of Ojibwa behavior is a product of both the physical deprivations that attend reservation experience . . . as well as the conflicts and uncertainties that characterize status inferiority. . . . Alcohol acts to reduce the sense of isolation and to permit the ventilation of anxieties. [James 1961:728, 735, 741]

Marshall Clinard draws the same general conclusion when he insists that "the primary problem from which 'problem drinking' has its genesis is the strain which structural barriers or prohibitions put upon the realization of success goals" (1964:202). Perhaps he is right, but it is pertinent to ask in the case of Indian drinking whether we know which success goals are being thwarted.

As Indian people struggle for a workable cultural and social pluralism, adapting contemporary American economic necessities and some of the amenities to their own systems of values, their strivings seem to be frequently misunderstood. Although at the present time Indian spokesmen are gaining a wider hearing, their insistence that they want to be *Indians* still tends either to be dismissed by "practical" whites as being as unrealistic as trying to bring back the buffalo or encouraged by "sympathetic" whites as envisioning an actual return to the kind of Indian life depicted in museums. When Indian people begin to bring off what they evidently have in mind, improvement of their material welfare on their own terms, their success is interpreted as fulfilling the highly individualistic aspirations of middle-class white society and as a stepping-stone to total absorption into it.

All of the authorities cited and many others besides advert to the stereotype, designated a negative stereotype, of the "drunken Indian." I find that their observational data support my conclusions better than their own. There are two points that are glossed over. First, there is a positive stereotype of the noble red man that is supposedly the identity which Indians seek in drunken delusions but which is actually exploited by cold-sober Indians who lecture and engage in theatrical performances. Rather than denying Indians this identity and thereby compelling them to seek it in alcohol, the larger society accepts and promotes it as evidenced by Boy Scouts and similar groups who even play this kind of stereotypic Indian. Secondly, while we have the stereotype of the "drunken Indian," we do not have the "drunken Negro" or the "drunken poor white," the latter group otherwise considered analogous to Indians by Bernard J. James (1961:733). These other minorities may not drink at all, or they may drink as much as Indians and get just as drunk, but neither their own spokesmen nor concerned outsiders see such drinking as a special problem of the minorities.

In trying to get ahead in terms of white success goals, black people particularly have suffered far more of the indignities, prejudice, rejection, and disappointments which are used to explain why Indian people drink. Black people are also stereotyped negatively but in ways distinct from the Indian stereotype—child-like, irresponsible about property, and dangerous if not "kept in their place." In the nascent and early stages of the black civil rights movement, as eventually given explicit expression by Martin Luther King, black people tried to justify their demands for fair and equal treatment by promoting an ideal image of themselves as ambitious, hardworking, and in their forebearance outdoing the white man at his own game of Christian ethics. The dominant society would not accept this stereotype. Once black nonviolence was organized, however, it communicated itself as violence and was met with violence. This was returned in kind by black people who then began getting results. It is now common knowledge that even middle-class black people believe the riots and civil disturbances did more good than harm, despite the fact that these people might deplore the need for violence and not engage in it personally. Black violence, like Indian drinking, communicates in mutually understood terms in the respective intergroup confrontations. The negative stereotype of the black, like the "drunken Indian," becomes a virtue or useful weapon to the in-group so stereotyped, at least up to the point of demanding attention and getting action. "Internalization" of the negative stereotype—that is, accepting it and even acting it out—does not, as James would have it, lead the Indian person "to conclude that he is, in fact, an 'inferior' person" (1961:732). Quite the contrary. Indian people appear to have long understood what blacks have recently discovered: the value of the negative stereotype as a form of communication and protest demonstration to register opposition and hold the line against what they do not want until they can get what they do want.

My hypothesis, then, begins with the assumption that Indian people want to persist and succeed on their own terms as Indians, while at the same time borrowing freely from the material aspects of white culture. It does not matter to the hypothesis whether this is a good thing or whether in the opinion of the non-Indian they succeed. The fact is that they have maintained this sentiment and have endured for well over a century in the face of public expectation that they would vanish and despite official policies and programs that have been directed explicitly toward phasing them out. My hypothesis is that Indian drinking is an established means of asserting and validating Indianness and will be either a managed and culturally patterned recreational activity or else not engaged in at all in direct proportion to the availability of other effective means of validating Indianness. Three other means of validating contemporary Indianness will be dealt with in some detail later on as a preliminary test of the hypothesis.

In testing the hypothesis, my research design requires that we treat Indian drinking as a cultural artifact, applying Ralph Linton's four-part analysis of artifacts—form, function, meaning, and use (1936). The "form" of Indian drinking (as opposed to other kinds of drinking Indians may also indulge in) is getting purposefully drunk to confirm the stereotype of the drunken Indian. Its function, that is, its relationship to other aspects of the culture or the culture as a whole, is maintenance of the Indian-white boundary by conveying a message: "like it or not, I am an Indian." Its meaning, the affective part, is to feel good or at least better. This is often verbalized, as many anthropologists and others can attest from personal observation, but I believe the wording is frequently misconstrued. When Indian people say they drink "to feel like an Indian" or words to that effect, I am not convinced of the conventional interpretation that they are seeking identity in drunken delusions of living in the golden past or expressing sheer bottle courage against white presumptions of superiority. Indian drinking plays upon the notion, widely shared by Indians and non-Indians, that Indians "can't hold their liquor like white men." Untenable physiologically, this belief, nevertheless, has a good deal of functional utility in communicating in mutually understood terms (MacAndrew and Edgerton 1969). Finally, the "use" of Indian drinking, the way an artifact is manipulated, employed, or applied, is to get drunk according to prescribed form with greater or lesser frequency or intensity as it is called for situationally among one's own people, other tribes, or white society. Drinking to get drunk may make a person feel good in terms of a very old shared recreational activity of the Indian community. This may not be the non-Indians' idea of good, clean fun but on close analysis it can be seen to be carefully managed without real personal or social harm (Hurt 1965). Drunkenness may also be an effort to relieve frustration when other means of asserting Indianness are not readily available. Not so well managed in these cases in regard to personal and social side effects, such drinking is still within its own cultural framework of patterned and calculated bad behavior and understood as such by other Indians and even whites in terms of the stereotype of the drunken Indian.

Before discussing alternatives to drunkenness as means of validating Indianness, I would like to comment on a number of features of Indian drinking which are pertinent to the hypothesis and gave rise to it. Despite acceptance of the stereotype even by Indian people that they cannot hold their liquor like whites, it does not take very extensive field work to observe that the irresponsible drunk on one occasion may on another occasion ingest just as much or more alcohol and maintain an appearance of sobriety. Indian people, like anyone else, have differential capacities for alcohol. What is important in any case are the specific social conditions relevant to differences in behavior. My own observations suggest that Indian people are more likely to get drunk when they feel thwarted in achieving Indian rather than white goals or when their success as Indians or simply individuals apart from Indian-white comparisons is interpreted as success in achieving status as whites.

Indian suggestibility to drunkenness has been widely observed as has the Indian community's ambivalence toward drunkenness which seems to be related to the suggestibility. Drinking and drunkenness are deplored on the one hand, while the drunk is treated tolerantly on the other. People may withdraw from the obstreperous drunk to lessen his destructive impact on others but do not hold him seriously responsible for criminal and asocial acts as if he were sober. J. O. Whittaker's observations on the Standing Rock Sioux apply quite generally: "social sanctions against the heavy drinker or alcoholic are virtually nonexistent" (1963:90). Possibly some community tolerance is due to the fact that many Indian people have similar problems and can empathize with the drunk's behavior vicariously while still being forced to recognize that the drunk is a community nuisance. The question remains, what is it the drunk is trying to accomplish that other Indian people understand and thus tolerate? I believe there is a "good" message in drunkenness no matter how "bad" the individual drunk may be. The community regrets the need for drunkenness just as the middle-class black deplores the need for violence to achieve given ends. There is also the realization that, in actualizing the stereotype or becoming habituated to its use and overlooking other alternatives to achieve given ends, undesirable side effects may offset the original idea intended by the demonstration. As Edward Dozier notes, many Indian communities have sought to reduce the problem by making liquor harder to get:

> The prohibition of liquor by tribal councils on most Indian reservations after repeal of the federal restrictive law is indicative of the Indians' own concern about abuses in drinking. [1966:73]

Similarly, North American revitalization movements, such as the religion of Handsome Lake among the Iroquois and the pan-Indian Native American church (peyote), interdict liquor while endeavoring to assert Indianness by means of such alternatives as the revival of customs and use of objects that are unmistakably derived from Indian tradition. Such religions assume that Indians are by nature different and cannot hold their liquor like whites. Where no such movement of this kind provides strong group assertions of Indians' rights to be Indians, it is difficult for the community to bring strong pressures to bear to discourage drinking, the more so because of widespread Indian reluctance to question anyone else's personal decisions. It is deemed better if temptation is simply removed as much as possible.

But even if the supply of liquor is reduced, it is not difficult for people to get drunk if they are determined to do so. The usefulness of feigned drunkenness, whether consciously or subconsciously engaged in, doubtlessly helps to explain the familiar Indian suggestibility to drunkenness. Whittaker's statements on the Standing Rock Sioux are again applicable to many Indian communities. Aggressive behavior is "virtually unknown in sober individuals" while "drunkenness, on the other hand, is frequently associated with violence" (1963:85). Statistics on Indian criminality demonstrate that Indians have a high arrest rate, that crime is almost always alcohol related, and that the crimes are largely unplanned and often terribly conspicuous offenses (Stewart 1964:61–66). While I have no argument with universalistic frustration-aggression theory, I suggest that if you are an Indian and need to work off frustrations, whatever their cause, you are doubly frustrated. Your stereotype of whites is that *they* are aggressive. As J. H. Hamer has observed, and I believe correctly, drinking gives the Indian person "an escape from anxiety about the expression of overt aggression" (1965:285). Thus, before giving vent to aggressive inclinations, you get drunk or convince yourself and others you are drunk, in order that no one mistakes you for acting like a white man. James, with whom I took issue at the outset, provides what I consider a telling incident in this connection although I think he draws entirely erroneous conclusions from it.

> A band of carousing [Ojibwa] villagers broke into a church and its tabernacle in search of wine. The aisles of the building were left littered with beer cans. While such sacrilegious outbursts shock the community, there is no clear evidence that they are triggered by hostile feelings toward the mission. They seem to be the result simply of the lust for drink. [1961:731]

The beer cans strike me as rather elaborate evidence to show that the carousers were already drunk when they broke into the church.

James and others who subscribe to the idea that Indians drink because they have a low sense of self-esteem and are seeking identity rely on phrases like those I have also collected in the course of field research: "I can't get ahead because I'm an Indian" or "I'm as good as any white man." I feel such expressions of sentiment are used selectively and misconstrued. To me, they seem of a piece with other phrases having nothing to do with anxieties over status deprivation in assimilating into white society. In the course of collecting more data on Indian drinking than I ever sought, it has struck me that the Winnebago tribesman is as likely to say, "I'm as good as any Potawatomi" as "I'm as good as any white man." Friend Potawatomi answers in kind, sometimes with a punch in the nose to make his point that he is as good as any Winnebago. Despite the young Indian nationalists' insistence that Indians should identify first as Indians and then by tribe, tribal affiliation remains the primary means of establishing identity. There is also the oft heard challenge, "I'm a bigger Indian than you are," or, put sarcastically, "You big Indian, you!" The challenge is more philosophical than physical since such phrases are simply "Englished-out" of native languages and often not understood by the non-Indian observer who, if he thinks about it at all, puts his own interpretation on what he hears. What is really meant, in effect, is "I'm more genuinely Indian than you are."

This is not to deny the existence of classic self-hate and identity crises among Indian people as among other minority groups. However, in my own experience these are most frequently found among families or individuals who are estranged from the life of their Indian communities and would like to treat their obvious Indian ancestry as their white neighbors might advert to Norway or Ireland or some other "old country" beyond which they feel they have progressed. They acknowledge their origins, even with pride and some cultural tokens, but this has little to do with the everyday business of contemporary American life or even the contemporary cultures whence their ancestors came. If such Indian people can only manage to be genteelly poor, then there is no question that they suffer low self-esteem and a sense of deprivation. They may even get drunk for these familiar reasons, thus supporting conventional wisdom and nullifying my hypothesis in such cases. However, I find they are often the very people least likely to get drunk or drink at all. Are they perhaps afraid of being mistaken for *Indians*?

Likewise, feelings of frustration and inadequacy in white society are commonly expressed by perfectly sober Indian students who are in a state of anxious ambivalence created largely by the school situation where white authority figures and peers badger them directly and indirectly to stop being Indians. They are made to feel by their own people that staying in school and succeeding as well as white students is a kind of betrayal. This is difficult to understand for well-intentioned white people, including scholars, who have never been praised, overtly or subtly, for their apparent denial, lack, or denigration of their "whiteness." Finally, I would like to turn to historical considerations and show the evolution of Indian drinking from an institutionalized "time-out" period from ordinary canons of etiquette (a function it still serves on occasion) to its gradually expanding function of communication and protest in order to maintain the Indian-white boundary.

Liquor, of course, was a novelty to all North American Indian tribes except for a very few southwestern groups. It also proved to be an exceedingly attractive novelty. Too often frontier histories suggest that the introduction of liquor to the Indians led only to wild, drunken orgies. This view is contradicted by the numerous primary sources cited by MacAndrew and Edgerton (1969) on the first encounters of many Indians with alcohol. They show that the inevitable sensorimotor dysfunctions were given widely varying interpretations, ranging from apparent delight in "instant vision" to repugnance. As liquor was "pushed" by traders and became generally available, some, perhaps many, Indians never developed a taste for it, but, for those who did, cultural patterns of drunkenness became apparent which included expansive conviviality, the letting down of customary decorum, and, in some cases, serious dignified drinking into a comatose state. In time the drunken behavior of traders and other adventurers was emulated and improved upon by Indian people, but—and this is the point I wish to emphasize—they seem to have done so for cultural reasons of their own. These reasons relate to a number of entrenched, ubiquitous Indian values and ideals which transcend tribal considerations.

Recorded in the earliest documents, the Indian values are still noted in contemporary field studies as explicit ideals which are manifested in Indian behavior (Wax and Thomas 1961; Hallowell 1955; Friedl 1956). Primary among these attributes are the beliefs that one is expected to take full responsibility for his own actions,[1] to exhibit concern for personal dignity, to take pride in resourcefulness and to adapt what is at hand in order to survive, to demonstrate openhanded generosity and gracious acceptance of proffered gifts (essentially a strong sense of reciprocity),[2] and to show "respect" for other people. Some observers interpret the last as "permissiveness," a view which I consider too simplistic; it is simply too difficult for most whites to keep their noses out of other people's business, especially if they think they are saving people from their own shortcomings. These core values may have become demanding beyond their functional utility by the time of white contact, and thus drunkenness, in the form of disinhibited changes-for-the-worse, may have been seized upon in the way that Christianity was readily accepted and adopted by the taboo-ridden Hawaiian aristocracy. The missionaries provided a socially acceptable way around cherished traits without giving them up entirely since they still served functional purposes. The Hawaiians actually had a native, fermented drink, kava, but its entrenched functions, meanings, and uses militated against using it for disinhibited reduction of tensions about taboos. Furthermore, there is nothing innate to alcohol to suggest it could or should be used for such a purpose. As the Hawaiian case illustrates, cultures do not universally deal with the need for outlets from tension with what MacAndrew and Edgerton term socially acceptable "time-out" periods of disinhibition or license. Thus, Indian drunken time-out was not an inevitable development, but it was apparently a highly expedient innovation to meet a felt need to reduce tension or perhaps replace existing methods whose nature is lost to history. Innovations are always reworked to some extent to make them fit the borrowing culture; moreover, they may be continuously adapted for functional utility as the culture undergoes change.

If all this strikes the historian as farfetched speculation, I would merely note how little attention is paid to the fact that the Indians' tobacco was as attractive to Europeans as European alcohol was to the Indians. Europeans took over smoking with only slight modifications of form and use but the religious functions and sacred meanings of smoking and tobacco itself were irrelevant and were replaced with things familiar to European thinking—the sociability and relaxed comfort of spirits in moderation, perhaps. Smoking doubtless also appealed to those who attributed sophistication to familiarity with the new things brought to Europe in the great age of discovery. Furthermore, these desires were quickly exploited by colonials seeking lucrative export crops and by home governments interested in tax revenues. The present alarming reports relating tobacco to cancer and a host of other ills have prompted Pan-Indian humorists to refer to tobacco as "the Indians' revenge"—for bringing alcohol!

Now, if Indians institutionalized patterns of drunkenness for their own internal, cultural reasons, they were encouraged by Europeans for their own, largely economic reasons. We tend to forget that there was a long period when Indian societies dealt as powerful equals with representatives of competing European groups in negotiations for trade and alliance in warfare. The Europeans needed the Indians' skills and good will as much as the Indians wanted the Europeans' trade goods. The Indians accepted and adapted vast amounts of material items from Europeans, even to completely replacing analogous native items, but they kept their own cultural, social, and political counsel as did the Europeans who were growing rich on the Indians' furs as they puffed on their pipes and haggled over prices.

The initial and continuing encounters and interactions between whites and Indians were intimately associated with alcohol. Liquor was more than a borrowed item like steel traps which became part of Indian culture. Generous distribution of liquor was soon discovered to be a good way to begin business with Indians. It augured a satisfactory contract for both parties. There was no advantage in trying to befuddle Indians in order to cheat them, at least at the beginning of contact and for a long time thereafter. The Indians could simply take their business elsewhere (A. Wallace 1970*a*). The fact that Indians responded somewhat differently to liquor than did whites in their extremes of drunkenness was not attributed to cultural differences. Both sides simply assumed that they were by nature constitutionally different from each other. Furthermore, for several centuries the very differences between Indian and white society were worth maintaining as each side managed what it excelled at and exchanged with the other. But, as trade declined, as international boundaries in North America were firmed up to prevent Indians from playing different white nations against each other, and as severe competition for land set in, the nature of Indian-white relationships changed. Indians still kept their own cultural, social, and political counsel but whites deemed them a nuisance with nothing to offer in exchange to justify their separate existence.

In the meantime, trade had worked changes within tribal cultures. Leaders were often elevated to greater power as they took on the roles of negotiators with whites and distributors of goods. The old pattern of the generous hunter-leader had been extended insofar as he had more to give away. With the decline of Indian power, drinking took on increasingly desperate proportions, remaining one of the last features of the good old days. Thus, Harold Hickerson observes of the Ojibwa:

> Brawls occurred chiefly during periods of orgiastic drunkenness in the vicinity of trading posts. Drunkenness itself was symptomatic of the decay of the old mechanisms enforcing hospitality; the distribution of liquor fell to the lot of successful trappers, perhaps at

times to shamans, and thus enabled them to assume the guise of "chiefs." Under the fur trade, provisions were only sporadically available for distribution; such items as venison and wild rice were traded in large amounts to the traders, and trade goods were consumed within small extended family units. The function of the distribution of liquor to be consumed communally within the band, then, was the assertion and maintenance of leadership. [1971:181–82]

As the mutually advantageous features of Indian-white interaction deteriorated and Indian life became increasingly impoverished, ideals of Indian behavior became ever more difficult to sustain. Additionally, there were the pressures to give up entirely ideals of Indian behavior. Getting drunk remains a very Indian thing to do when all else fails to maintain the Indian-white boundary. It will remain so until Indian groups can achieve new, mutually satisfactory relationships with whites appropriate to contemporary opportunities.

At this point, I would like to discuss three alternatives to drinking as a means of validating Indianness. My examples are drawn from over twenty years of regular association with the Wisconsin Winnebago and four extended visits during the last ten years among the Dogrib of northern Canada. The generalized descriptions of the alternatives derive as well from briefer associations with other tribes in the Midwest, Plains, and Northwest Coast and from experiences with intertribal communities in Detroit, Chicago, and Milwaukee. The alternatives are not mutually exclusive. People who employ them may also drink, but drinking seems to be managed effectively in direct relationship to the effectiveness of the other alternatives.

An important validation of Indianness is the ability to maintain a reputation as an exemplary person in terms of basic ideals already discussed: dignity, responsibility, resourcefulness, respect for others, and reciprocal generosity. This complex is expressed in providing adequately but not conspicuously by local standards for oneself and dependents—usually a far larger group than the average white breadwinner is expected to provide for—and reasonably regular participation in activities that the community defines as Indian.

Mountain Wolf Woman, a Winnebago friend whose autobiography has been published, operated almost entirely in terms of this first general criterion of Indianness (Lurie 1961). She worked hard to provide adequately for her family which included grandchildren and great grandchildren and on occasion children of distant relatives and Indian friends who had hit on hard times. She was secure in her position in the Indian community and commanded respect as an Indian among whites. She found in the peyote religion whatever comfort she needed in times of crisis, and worked off anxieties with tears or great bursts of physical activity, such as chopping wood or housecleaning. She never drank, and expressed disapproval of drinking for its social and personal destructiveness, but she was tolerant of the drunk, firmly believing Indians were physiologically different from whites in their capacity for alcohol.

A., a middle-aged, monolingual Dogrib, is a thoroughgoing "bush" Indian. He works hard at fishing, trapping, hunting, and occasional wage work to support his large family which lives well by bush Dogrib standards. He engages in community activities but only recently took on a formal leadership role. He is exceedingly dignified, almost severe, in manner. However, he will join in peaceful community brew parties. When he leaves his small village to trade he makes sure that all the groceries and other family needs are provided for before sometimes treating himself to a bottle or two of rum. He finds convivial companions to share his liquor and gets hilariously drunk with them. He does not flaunt his condition or get into trouble to be picked up by the Mounties. When A. gets drunk, he does so as an exemplary Dogrib enjoying himself. He is not trying to assert Indianness. He does not need to. His drinking seems to be a socially acceptable "time-out" period from the demands of being an exemplary Dogrib without any reference to problems with white society.

A.'s brother, B., speaks a little English and is more outgoing and jovial, but not without a certain dignity of manner. He is liked in the community and considered an essentially good, hardworking man, but quite literally crazy. His nickname among the Dogrib is "White Man," partly because he likes to show off his English. But what makes him really crazy, like a white man, is that he does not drink and is openly critical of those who do. B. is so thoroughly Indian otherwise in life-style that the nickname is an endearment and he is considered harmlessly crazy. He is not distrusted like those educated English-speakers with steady jobs who are suspected of being sellouts, at least potentially, to the white establishment.

Such a man is C. who, while sharing B.'s outspoken ethic about the evils of strong drink, drinks moderately if the situation warrants it. He will take a drink with Indian friends out of politeness and engages in sober social drinking with non-Indian friends.

He tends to be house- and possession-proud, but his emulation of white standards is really part of a general orientation toward raising the community standard of living as well as his own. He sought special training and qualified as a community worker employed by the government. From a white point of view, C. would be the ideal tribal interpreter because of his objective intelligence and sophisticated grasp of English. But he is rejected by the monolingual chief and council men in favor of two far less competent and benevolently motivated men. If not entirely exemplary, their life-style is clearly Indian and their relationship to whites, including in-laws in the case of one of them, is manipulative rather than cooperative or emulative. They indulge regularly in Indian drinking primarily in its recreational form but there are overtones of boundary maintenance in the case of one of the men. C. knows he is not trusted to react and interpret from a position of total Indianness, as defined by the Dogrib, in Indian-white confrontations. However, by dint of positive accomplishments in the community interest on the community's own terms, C. manages to keep up his credit as a Dogrib and finds personal security and satisfaction in being a successful innovator.

A second alternative to drinking to validate Indianness is Indian expertise. The acknowledged authority may command traditional lore and ceremonial prerogatives (or even quasi-traditional roles in revitalization movements) or the local church if it is considered the community's own institution. He may be an expert singer or dancer at powwows or an Indian guide to white sportsmen. The authority may be particularly well informed and consulted by Indians and whites about his tribe's history.

D. is a successful expert. A bilingual Dogrib in his sixties, he has a long reputation of capitalizing on his bush skills, general Indian resourcefulness, and bilingualism in relation to whites. In his younger days he carried mail, guided, and performed other tasks in which whites were dependent for their very survival on his exemplary Indianness which among the Dogrib includes tremendous physical endurance. During the last ten years he has regularly filled the role of anthropological and linguistic informant. He is respected in the Indian community as a responsible emissary, spokesman, and representative of their best qualities to the outside world. He also manages to live as well as C., the community worker, supporting his family by hunting, fishing, trapping, wage work, and foster-child care. His outlook is Indian and, although he is completely at ease among whites, he always deals calculatedly, albeit in a genuinely friendly manner, with an alien people. D. enjoys well-managed but properly tipsy Indian recreational drinking. His attitude is well illustrated in a recent incident when a convivial party turned into a fight during which a participant knocked out one of D.'s teeth. D. was philosophical. The fellow was drunk and did not know what he was doing and, furthermore, he was sorry enough when he sobered up to give D. five dollars by way of apology.

Another expert was the late Charles R. (Charley) Lowe Cloud, a Wisconsin Winnebago. He wrote a weekly column, "The Indian News," for the *Black River Falls Banner-Journal,* by which it achieved a national circulation among Indian cognoscenti. Although a Carlisle graduate, Charley seems to have excelled mainly in football and other sports. Since his formal education was skimpy, his broken English accounts were no put-on as sometimes alleged. A classic of journalistic brevity under his by-line once summed up the complications of his life: "Not much news this week. Indian report in jail."

Charley was frequently in jail because he was frequently drunk. The authorities would pick him up when he seemed too drunk to care for himself rather than to punish him or to imagine that they could rehabilitate him. This Charley knew and appreciated, expressing neither shame nor remorse over his bouts with the bottle. Getting drunk was something Indians did. Nor did the local Winnebago people view his drinking with anything but tolerant amusement. They were ambivalent, however, about Charley's role as newsman. They admired and quoted his outspoken criticism of the white man and approved his obvious commitment to Indian values and traditional beliefs. But they were also sometimes embarrassed by his writing insofar as it often appeared to lampoon Indians and make them appear undignified to white readers. Charley, I am sure, never realized that at times his grammar and spelling were not only funny but gave rise to unconscious double entendres. He was in dead earnest in his indignation and concern for the Indian community. It seemed to puzzle him that his efforts received a mixed reaction among the Winnebago but he was a man with a sense of calling and went on writing. I believe that his drinking was a desperate validation of Indianness among Indians and a classic example of exploitation, albeit probably unconscious, of Indian tolerance for the drinker. If what Charley wrote sincerely in the community interest turned out to be unintentionally offensive, Winnebago people would (and, in fact, did) forgive him since there was always the likelihood that he was not entirely sober when he took pencil in hand.

A third way of validating Indianness is what might be called leadership. I confine this definition to situations in which Indian people are in positions to promote community interests vis-à-vis white society, particularly in regard to government agencies. This is a difficult role because successful liaison efforts in communicating with whites are so easily interpreted as selling out the community or profiting at the community's expense. Yet, leaders are recognized as necessary if the Indian community is to prosper and survive at all. The successful leader usually manages both to get things done in the community behalf and to maintain personal exemplariness in Indian terms.

E. is a traditionalist Winnebago, intelligent and sensitive but with little formal education. As he approached middle age he took on more attributes of exemplary Indianness and, as far as I know, had no reputation as a drinker when he became an active leader. He derived great satisfaction from the learning process involved in leadership and in seeing his efforts, in concert with other tribal leaders, result in material improvement for his people without in any way compromising Winnebago values. Unfortunately, as so often happens in Indian affairs, governmental agencies supplying funds for tribal work gained control of decision making and began undercutting the work accomplished by the tribe on its own initiative. E. labored to right the situation and get power back into the Winnebagos' hands but was unable to do so. He held out longer than many of his original co-workers in the new regime but finally he too resigned his office. Another Winnebago reported to me with evident approbation that E. had quit and gotten "good and drunk." Whether he did or not, it was important that people thought he did. Suspected of being a sellout, he had redeemed himself.

F. is a mixed blood Dogrib with a history of apparent identity problems. He was a heavy drinker and might have been written off as a classic example of drinking because of a sense of status deprivation and inability to assimilate as white. He seemed to be moving in a white direction since he had taken himself off the rolls as an Indian. Canadian law has now changed, but until the early 1950s treaty Indians could not vote or buy liquor. F. may have had other motivations but the right to buy liquor often accounted for people opting out of official Indian status. A brief community development project instituted by the Canadian cooperative movement permitted F to use his white education, bilingualism, and basically sound intelligence as a leader. Although F. had long been identified by the traditional full-blood community as a member of the "no-good" faction of mixed bloods, the efforts of the co-op began providing employment and serving the real interests of the total community. Scarcely launched, the project was terminated by political considerations in Ottawa. Whites took over the community service contracts which the Indian Co-op needed in order to prosper. Predictably, only the small handcraft end of the co-op's operation was allowed to remain in Indian hands, thus reinforcing the idea that Indians can only manage things that whites can recognize as "typically" Indian in the museum artifact sense. When the bids of the Indian Co-op to handle brush clearance and other community services were rejected, although the bids were sometimes lower than those of white competitors, F., who had pretty well "dried out," went back to drinking. When last seen, he was blearily insisting he was an Indian, treaty or no treaty, and indulging in the familiar expressions that he could not get ahead because he was an Indian and that he was as good as any white man. Actually, F. is one of the few Indians whose skills could assure him a good job if he wished to compete with local whites. He would suffer no personal financial loss and have greater acceptance by the white community than he had in his role as Indian Co-op leader. It is not that he drinks because he cannot get ahead in terms of white success goals; the drinking actually interferes with his getting ahead and, to me at least, seems a desperate validation of Indianness when denied the opportunity to exercise other alternatives. F. can verbalize his anger and frustration to anyone who has the patience to hear him out. The Indian community, he believes, could have handled its own affairs in its own way, namely with a cooperative, but the white government favored greedy whites whose management assured them most of the profits.

To return to my original hypothesis, I have admittedly stuck my neck out knowing I would not have space for qualifications and extensive documentation necessary to pull it back. I have only tried to make clear that I believe most studies of Indian drinking start with a mistaken assumption that it is simply *bad*. In my opinion, as an old, patterned form of recreational behavior, it is managed and probably no more hazardous to health than karate, mountain climbing, or mushroom hunting. If Indian people decide to give up recreational drinking (as it is, its intensity and frequency of occurrence vary from tribe to tribe), I am sure it will be for cultural reasons of their own, just as I believe they developed the drinking patterns initially for their own reasons. Middle-class whites concerned about Indian welfare—missionaries, social workers, psychiatrists, and others—confuse their concern for health and well-being with their embarrassment and disgust at any behavior which to them is déclassé. Getting drunk for its own sake, like sexual promiscuity, may be fun but something "nice" people do not do, or at least do not flaunt. A persistent white, class-oriented ethnocentrism prevents recognizing the otherwise exemplary, competent, "successful" Indian for what he is—an Indian doing contemporary Indian things, whether dressing decently, driving a car, or going to college. Somehow, his undignified behavior when drunk, or if he does not get drunk himself, his unwillingness to disavow or interfere strenuously with those who do, imply that he is not quite yet "just like us." The fact that Indian drinking distresses and disturbs whites and forces them to take notice may well explain why it can so easily become a form of protest, assuming my hypothesis is correct, in Indian-white encounters and can even help restore credit where one's Indian investment in the Indian community is called into question.

But protest demonstrations by definition involve extraordinary behavior and are hard to sustain indefinitely. The tragedy is that the Indian protest has been so prolonged that in some cases it becomes a way of life with disastrous consequences for the people concerned. I do not agree with Vine Deloria, Jr.'s syllogism that young Indians were sold the notion by anthropologists that Indians live in two worlds; people who live in two worlds drink; therefore, to be real Indians they must drink. But, like Deloria, I, too, have "lost some good friends who DRANK too much" (1970:86). Some took their lives before managing to drink themselves to death. And, like Deloria, my grief evokes anger and bitterness that they died as they did and that others are likely to go the same route so long as we pursue policies that continue to deprive Indians of lands, water rights, and other natural resources or so long as we offer them the opportunity to achieve decent living standards only if they measure up to our particular philosophical standards.

The one bright ray I see at present is that Indian people are finding increasingly effective, and sober, means to express aggression and protest which are unmistakably Indian. Many Indians have turned from defensive action to offensive tactics. The last few years, for example, have witnessed the occupation of Alcatraz, the development of influential and unifying Indian publications, such as *Akwasasne Notes*, the ejection of unwanted tourists from Indian land, and the successful campaign of the National Congress of American Indians to force withdrawal of a liquor ad which humorously exploited the stereotype of the drunken Indian.

Notes

1. Taking responsibility for one's own actions does not have moral connotations in terms of guilt-shame analyses of cultural compulsions to conform. Rather, it means simply a willingness to take the consequences of one's decisions—figuring things out carefully before taking action.

2. Reciprocal generosity implies that it is bad form to refuse gifts or to demonstrate a selfish desire to avoid having to give. Frances North-end Ferguson (1968) notes that this attribute has aided the program of prescribing drugs for Navaho problem drinkers in order to reduce their craving for alcohol. It is impolite to refuse the offer of a drink but the known fact that a person will get sick if he drinks while on the medicine allows him to refuse without fear of criticism from other Indians.

The Epidemiology of Alcoholic Cirrhosis in Two Southwestern Indian Tribes

S. J. Kunitz, J. E. Levy, C. L. Odoroff, and J. Bollinger

Alcoholism has long been a scourge of American Indians. In general, explanations of excessive drinking among the Amerinds have focused on the fact that their traditional cultures have been destroyed and that they have been denied access to the goals of the general American society. In the present study we explore the different responses that two Southwestern tribes have manifested to somewhat similar external circumstances. Without denying that Amerinds have in fact been victims of the expansion of white American society, we will attempt to show that the patterns of alcoholic liver cirrhosis observed in these tribes are in part a reflection of their traditional social organization and cultural values rather than an expression of cultural disintegration. Now that various federal agencies and tribal groups are showing an increasing concern with the problem of drinking, it is of some importance to determine what differences may exist between tribes in order that treatment programs may be designed appropriately for specific groups with different cultural heritages.

The two tribes we studied have lived for several centuries side by side in northern Arizona. The Hopi tribe numbers about six thousand. Their reservation is nine hundred square miles in area and is completely surrounded by the Navaho. The Hopis are a Puebloan group living in compact village communities and traditionally practicing arid-land agricultural techniques. They have tended to eschew visionary experiences and practice a highly organized formal religion.

The Navaho population numbers between one hundred thousand and one hundred and twenty thousand. They are semi-nomadic herders who practice some agriculture. They have traditionally lived in isolated extended families. Whereas the Hopi have been known as "the peaceful people," the Navaho have historically practiced raiding, both on white settlers and on the Hopis. While adopting many of the features of the Puebloan religious structure, the Navaho have maintained alongside it features of their more vision-oriented Athapaskan past.

The White Mountain Apaches are one of the Western Apache tribes, Athapaskan like the Navaho, but having had less contact with the various Puebloan tribes. Their reservation covers about twenty-six hundred square miles in central Arizona and has a population of five thousand. Because we have only examined death certificates for this tribe and have not personally done field work there, the bulk of our discussion will concern the Navaho and the Hopi with whom our personal experience and record investigation has been more extensive.

Methods

The vast majority of the members of each tribe obtain medical treatment at United States Public Health Service hospitals and clinics which are free and relatively accessible. Even those living off the reservations in border towns or in Phoenix utilize these facilities, particularly when the illness requires long and expensive hospitalization. In such cases private and mission hospitals transfer their Indian patients to government hospitals. Thus, since Indian care tends to be centralized in one agency, a review of the hospital discharge sheets in the area offices in Phoenix and Window Rock gives fairly accurate information on the incidence and prevalence of those diseases which at some time in their course require hospital treatment. Alcoholic liver cirrhosis falls into this category.

The discharge sheets include name, address, sex, and marital status as well as primary and secondary diagnoses. All the sheets in both area offices were reviewed to obtain this information on all members of each tribe who had been diagnosed as having cirrhosis, either as a primary or subsequent diagnosis. To determine the geographic distribution of cirrhosis, only cases diagnosed as Laënnec's or alcoholic cirrhosis were utilized. To tabulate death rates, however, all cases of cirrhosis were included to make our data comparable with national reporting, which does not distinguish between types of cirrhosis. In any event, there were no Hopi cirrhosis deaths from anything but Laënnec's cirrhosis and only one Navaho death from any other type.

In our previous study of Navaho cirrhosis (Kunitz, Levy, and Everett 1969) only records from the Window Rock office were surveyed as we were interested primarily in cases on the reservation and in nearby border towns. These records were complete for the latter half of 1964, all of 1965 and 1966, and the first half of 1967. Subsequently, when we gathered similar information on the Hopi, we reviewed records of the Phoenix hospital because it is a primary referral hospital for this group. In so doing, we found a number of Hopi cirrhotics living in Phoenix. To make the Navaho data as comparable as possible, we reviewed Phoenix hospital records for 1965–66 to find any Navaho cirrhotics living in Phoenix. We found three more cases, which explains the discrepancies between Navaho cases reported in this and in our previous paper. None of the Phoenix Navahos died in the period under discussion. In addition, death certificates from New Mexico were reviewed for both Hopis and Navahos and no additional cases were found living off-reservation in that state.

For the Hopi, the problem was somewhat different. Again records from both areas were surveyed. In Phoenix, records were complete from 1956 to the present. In Window Rock, records from the second half of 1964 to the present were complete. Accordingly, only data from 1965, 1966, and 1967 were used to tabulate mortality rates for the Hopi while data from 1956 through 1967 were used to tabulate the demographic characteristics of Hopi cirrhotics.

The White Mountain Apache, like the Hopi, have their health services administered from the Phoenix area office. The death certificates were reviewed for the same period as for the Hopi. As there were only three deaths from cirrhosis (all alcoholic), we will not describe the population of this tribe nor the characteristics of the patients. Cause of death was verified from death certificates on file with the Arizona State Health Department.[1]

Distribution of Populations

Hopi

Although the total Hopi population is estimated to be about six thousand, it is not known with any reliability how the population is distributed on and off the reservation. A census was beyond our means. Because gallbladder disease (cholelithiasis and cholecystitis) is extraordinarily common among most Amerinds, including the Hopi (Sievers 1968; Reichenbach 1967; Comess, Bennett, and Burch 1967), to estimate this distribution we assumed that it affected adult Hopis regardless of their area of residence. We then reviewed the discharge sheets of all Hopis from 1956 to the present to obtain the same demographic information obtained for the cirrhotics. Next we assumed that the geographic distribution, marital status, and religion of all gallbladder patients over the age of twenty was the same as the distribution of all Hopi adults. Conceivably dietary differences between those living on and off the reservation could cause some error in this method. It is also conceivable that, since gallbladder disease tends to affect people in their forties, we would be seeing a biased sample. To assess this possibility we distinguished between those above and below age thirty. There was no difference in geographical distribution by this age classification. Although it is possible that the distribution of gallbladder cases does not reflect the population distribution, we have not found any evidence to contradict that assumption. We shall therefore herein use gallbladder cases to estimate population distribution.

Because the samples we were dealing with were relatively small, we chose not to distinguish between all the communities on and off the reservation but to cluster them under three different types: traditional reservation village, reservation wage-work community, and off-reservation community. Those living off-reservation in areas where care is obtained from facilities not administered by the Window Rock or Phoenix area offices are excluded from this survey. This limitation is unavoidable but it is believed not to be an important source of error.

Table 1 gives the distribution of pathologies by village type for gallbladder disease, cirrhosis, and epilepsy. Epilepsy is included in the tabulation to protect against the possibility that dietary factors may affect the distribution of gallbladder disease.

The distribution of the three pathologies by village type is unequal. The appropriate chi-square test is significant (chi square $=19.49$, 4 df, $p<.001$). The test comparing gallbladder disease with epilepsy (chi square $= 0.91$, 2 df, $p<.64$) indicates no significant difference between the distribution of the two diseases. We therefore used the distribution of the gallbladder cases as an estimate of the population distribution between the village types. When the gallbladder and epilepsy groups are pooled and compared to the cirrhosis group, the difference was significant (chi square = 18.27, 2 df, $p < .0001$). We shall return to the problem of cirrhosis below.

The traditional village contains about 52 percent of the tribe. As their name implies, in these villages traditional Hopi values are more firmly maintained than elsewhere, agriculture is more actively pursued, and the traditional family constellation more adequately preserved.

The reservation wage-work communities contain about 26 percent of the tribe. Here there tends to be a higher number of converts to various Christian churches, and more people work for wages in either government, tribal, or private enterprises. The traditional religious system is said to be more attenuated.

About 22 percent of the tribe live off the reservation completely. These people tend to live in nuclear families, do wage work exclusively, and are less involved in the traditional religious system.

None of these distinctions is in any way absolute. For instance, residents of traditional villages may also participate actively in the wage-work economy; reservation wage-work community residents also maintain many traditional religious values; and off-reservation dwellers frequently return to the reservation to participate in ceremonies and visit their families.

This typology reflects the traditional anthropological concern with acculturation as a determining factor in social disintegration and social pathologies. Using this theory we would predict that cirrhosis would increase as one moves along the continuum from traditional village to wage-work village to off-reservation town.

Yet another way of dividing the Hopi population is the way they most commonly distinguish among themselves: whether they are for or against the tribal council. Traditionally, each Hopi village was ruled by a theocracy. The federal government, however, in order to facilitate its dealings with the tribe as a whole, encouraged the tribe to form a democratically elected council. They were given the option to vote for or against the institution of a tribal council, but many of the traditional villages refused to vote at all, as this would have implied de facto recognition of the federal government's right to make decisions regarding their rule. Therefore, those who did vote, voted for the council. The division between council and anticouncil factions in the tribe crosscuts the division between wage work and so-called traditional ways of gaining a living. Using the prevalence of gallbladder disease as the gauge of population proportions in each faction (on-reservation only), the procouncil faction contains 63.5 percent and the anticouncil 36.5 percent of the tribe. Among the procouncil, sixty-one had gallbladder disease, nine cirrhosis; among the anticouncil, thirty-five and zero.

Navaho

Among the Navaho the problem is somewhat different. The Public Health Service has divided the reservation (including the Crownpoint checkerboard area) into eight service units, each served by a hospital or, in two instances, by a field health and outpatient clinic. The Chinle and Kayenta service units are isolated, known for their traditional communities, and in the case of Kayenta, border on an off-reservation area which lacks towns and is sparsely populated. The Shiprock, Tuba City, and Crownpoint service units have more access to off-reservation towns of some size, are served by paved roads, and have saloons at those points where the highways cross the reservation boundary. All of these areas, however, also embrace vast tracts of isolated traditional hinterlands. The Winslow and Fort Defiance service units differ from the previous three in one important respect: they are adjacent to the Santa Fe railway and US Route 66 on the south. These major routes of transportation provide a continuous line of small cities, towns, and saloons across the entire southern reservation boundary. The Gallup-Tohatchi service unit includes a portion of Route 66 with several small settlements, a paved road to the north, and, most important, it has the city of Gallup as its communication center (Kunitz, Levy, and Everett 1969). The Public Health Service has estimated the proportion of the reservation population living in each service unit; these data are the ones we have used. Unfortunately, no reliable data are available to estimate the number of Navahos living off-reservation.

It will be immediately apparent that the methods of grouping the Hopi and Navaho are not precisely comparable. In large part this is because their situations are so different geographically. Almost all on-reservation Hopi live in villages equidistant from off-reservation areas. We therefore need categories other than proximity to border towns to distinguish between them. The sociological categories of means of making a living or political alignment are therefore appropriate. For the Navaho the political issues are not clear. It is somewhat easier to categorize areas roughly by the style of life of most of the people living there. This is what we have attempted to do in our characterizations of the service units from more isolated and traditional to increasingly urban orientation. In addition, because proximity to off-reservation areas is a complicating factor when dealing with the Navaho, it must be taken into account in any typology, as we shall point out further in the next sections.

Results

Table 1 shows the distribution of cases of cirrhosis and gallbladder disease for the Hopi classified by wage-work community. The distributions of cirrhosis and gallbladder disease are significantly different: 64 percent of the cirrhosis cases are off-reservation compared with 23 percent of the gallbladder cases. However, when the distributions of cases between traditional villages and reservation wage-work villages are compared, excluding off-reservation cases, there is no difference between the two groups: 67 percent of both the cirrhosis and the gallbladder cases on-reservation are in the traditional village.

TABLE 1. Distribution of Pathologies by Village Type among the Hopi

	Gallbladder		Cirrhosis		Epilepsy	
	No.	%	No.	%	No.	%
Traditional	69	52	6	24	13	43
Reservation						
wage-work	34	26	3	12	10	33
Off reservation	30	22	16	64	7	23
Total	133		25		30	

Note: 1 vs 3, chi square = 0.91, 2 df, $p<.64$; 1 + 3 vs 2, chi square = 18.27, 2 df, $p<.0001$; total, chi square = 19.49, 4 df, $p<.001$.

When the on-reservation Hopi cases of cirrhosis are divided along procouncil and anticouncil lines, the difference between the distribution of cirrhosis and gallbladder disease approached significance: 62 percent of those with gallbladder disease (61 cases) were in the procouncil villages while 100 percent of the cirrhotics (9 cases) were in those villages ($p<.06$ by Fisher's exact test).

Table 2 shows the distribution of cirrhosis among the Navaho and the estimated population in each service unit. The number of cases of cirrhosis is less than expected in isolated areas but, moving closer to off-reservation communities, increases to higher than expected levels. The expected number of cases was com-

152   Beliefs, Behaviors, and Alcoholic Beverages

puted from the estimated population distribution in these areas. The service units are arranged roughly from isolated to increasingly urban oriented, reading downward in table 2.

TABLE 2. Geographic Distribution of Navaho Cirrhotics

Service Unit[a]	Population (in percent)[b]	Observed Cases[c]	Expected Cases	Percentage of Cases
Chinle	13.5	4	9.6	5.6
Kayenta	7.0	1	5.0	1.4
Tuba City	10.6	4	7.5	5.6
Crownpoint	8.4	5	6.0	7.0
Shiprock	20.2	9	14.3	12.7
Fort Defiance	13.9	13	9.9	18.3
Winslow	9.6	10	6.8	14.1
Gallup-Tohatchi	16.6	25	11.8	35.2

Note: Chi square = 27.7, 7 df, $p<.005$.

a. The Service Units are arranged roughly from isolated to increasingly urban-oriented, reading downward.
b. Data from United States Public Health Service, Division of Indian Health, Albuquerque Area Office. Memo: Window Rock Field Office population statistics. Albuquerque; 1964.
c. An additional 20 cases had off-reservation addresses. As there is no accurate estimate of the total number of Navahos living off reservation, they are not included in the tabulation. However, our strong impression is that this represents a higher than expected number of cases.

The average age of Hopi cirrhotic men was 42.1, and women, 37.7; Navaho men, 41.2, and women, 44.3. There were 15 Hopi men and 10 women, 55 Navaho men and 36 women; in other words, in each tribe 60 percent of the cirrhotics were men.

The marital status distribution of Hopi and Navaho cirrhotics was not significantly different from that of the rest of the population (table 3).

The Navaho data require a word of explanation. Hillery and Essene (1963) have given estimates taken from the 1960 census of marital status of a number of southwestern tribes. Unfortunately, their data include all people over the age of fourteen. This heavily weights the sample toward single people. As cirrhosis virtually never occurs in people below the age of twenty, these data were not helpful. Instead, we relied on field interviews with a random sample of 86 people over the age of twenty and used these as our basis of comparison: Navaho cirrhotics tended to be overrepresented in the single category (12.5 to 5.8 percent) and underrepresented in the married category (63.6 to 74.4 percent). When the

TABLE 3. Marital Status of Hopi Gallbladder Disease and Cirrhosis Cases, and of Navaho General Sample and Cirrhosis Cases, in Percentage

	Men		Women	
	Gallbladder	Cirrhosis	Gallbladder	Cirrhosis
Hopi[a]	(n = 28)	(n = 15)	(n = 99)	(n = 10)
Married	68	80	78	80
Single	7	13	3	0
Widowed, divorced, separated	25	7	19	20
	$X^2 = 2.4, p = .30$		$X^2 = 0.3, p = .86$	
	General Sample	Cirrhosis	General Sample	Cirrhosis
Navaho[b]	(n = 43)	(n = 50)	(n = 41)	(n = 33)
Married	84	68	68	67
Single	9	18	2	6
Widowed, divorced, separated	7	14	30	27
	$X^2 = 3.1, p = .21$		$X^2 = 0.6, p = .44$	

a. Three gallbladder cases of unknown marital status omitted.
b. Two cases from the general sample and eight cirrhotics of unknown marital status omitted.

widowed, divorced, separated, and unknown category are pooled the percentages in the cirrhotic and general sample are about the same (23.9 to 20.1 percent).

There were no significant differences in case fatality rate between sexes within the two tribes. However, there appears to be a tribal difference in case fatality rates: 19 percent in the Navahos compared to 40 percent in the Hopi ($p<.03$).[2] Ten Hopis died of cirrhosis (6 of 15 men and 4 of 10 women) during the period 1956 to 1968. In the Navaho the distribution was as follows: of 36 women cirrhotics, 10 died; of 55 men, 7 died.

The death rates from cirrhosis among the three tribes show some interesting differences. Among the Navaho the observed number of deaths was 6 in 1965 and 7 in 1966, not very different from the expected 4.9 deaths by the low population estimate (100,000) and 5.6 by the high estimate (120,000).[3] Deaths among the Hopi (2 in 1965, 2 in 1966 and 4 in 1967) and the Apache (1 each year) were the same or higher than the expected (0.3).

The death rates from all types of cirrhosis were as follows: In the U.S. general population, 12.8 per 100,000, and among all Indians, 26.7 in 1964 (U.S. Dept. of Health, Education, and Welfare 1966); among the Navaho, 6.8 two-year average, 1965–66); the

Hopi, 43.2 (three-year average, 1965–67); the Apache, 20.0 (three-year average). The age-adjusted rates (to twenty years and over) were: in the general population, 19.9; Navaho, 13.0 (high population estimate) or 17.0 (low); Hopi, 104.0; and Apache, 44.0. The rather small numbers of Hopis and Apaches make the rates somewhat imprecise, but evidently the death rate from cirrhosis in the Navaho is close to the national rate, while those of the Apache and Hopi are two to four times the national rate.

Discussion

The differences in patterns of cirrhosis between the Navahos and the Hopis require explanation. Field work, as yet unreported, indicates that while drinking is common on the Navaho reservation in the traditional and wage-work communities and on the Hopi reservation in both pro- and anticouncil villages, different patterns exist in each tribe.

Among the Navaho, it is the traditional, pastoral group that evidences the most serious drinking problems as gauged by the various scales devised by Mulford and Wilson (1966). The wage-work group seems to have fewer problems with alcohol as judged by the same scales. However, in both communities fewer people drink than in white communities in Iowa. According to Mulford's data, 26.8 percent of Iowa residents were abstainers. In the two Navaho communities, 61 percent were abstainers, of whom 22.1 percent were lifelong abstainers and 41.9 percent had given up drinking.

This indicates a different natural history of alcohol use among the Navahos and the Anglos. Navahos, especially those leading a traditional, pastoral life, and to a lesser degree those living in a reservation wage-work community, tend to drink excessively when they do drink but are much more likely than Anglos to stop drinking entirely at some point in their lives. This appears to be an all-or-nothing phenomenon. In addition, those who drink tend to be young men who drink in groups. The phenomenon of peer-group drinking has been remarked on by other observers as well (Ferguson 1968; Savard 1968) and seems to be a Navaho pattern.

We suggest that drinking in Navaho society is a normal pursuit of young men and tends to be outgrown. The drinker is not ejected from his community except in extraordinary circumstances. The higher prevalence of cirrhosis near border towns is likely to be a reflection of the easier access to alcohol and the fact that drinkers develop cirrhosis before they have a chance to outgrow their drinking. At the same time, we are not yet in a position to reject the alternative hypotheses that severe problem drinkers are in fact ejected from their communities and move off reservations or that those living in border areas are more acculturated and therefore manifest more anxiety and drink for "neurotic" rather than for "normal" reasons. However, our field work in traditional isolated groups seems to indicate that there is a great deal of what would be called "alcoholic" drinking in Anglo society, but that limited access to alcohol combined with the maturation of the individual drinkers serves to protect against the development of cirrhosis.

By maturation we refer to the fact that in two Navaho communities where we have done intensive interviewing, the proportions of those currently abstaining from alcoholic beverages were 42.5 and 43.6 percent. This contrasts with 26.8 percent abstainers reported in Iowa (Mulford and Wilson 1966). The two samples included a rural, pastoral group, and residents of a reservation wage-work community. The reasons for giving up drinking had to do primarily with the threat to health that it represented and the social turmoil that it caused. Many of those currently abstaining had been very heavy drinkers previously and some no doubt would have been diagnosed as alcoholics. Nevertheless, they stopped drinking with relative ease and without the problems commonly reported by Anglo alcoholics. These drinking patterns are the subject of continuing research, and here we will only suggest that the reasons for excessive drinking among the Navaho do not appear to be the same as those among Anglo alcoholics with whom they are often compared. In addition, the fact that drinkers are not ejected from the community and do not become isolated seems to serve as some protection.

Without denying the importance of high economic access (Graves 1967) we would suggest another possible interpretation. What in fact we may be seeing, in the Navaho at least, is a traditional pattern of beliefs and behavior which predisposes people to drink excessively when alcohol is available (it was not available aboriginally). The Navaho do not seem to regard self-control as a social value in the same sense as do the Hopi. In addition, there are some data to indicate that alcohol historically became associated with high status. Before alcohol was readily available, a rich man would often dole out liquor to his less fortunate dependents after he had obtained it at considerable expense from white bootleggers. Drinking has thus historically been a social affair among the Navaho, and this pattern has persisted with the increasing availability of alcoholic beverages. At present, drinking tends to be a highly visible public spectacle.

Among the Hopi the situation is different. The "Hopi way" has valued harmony and peace and eschewed "acting out." In addition, the traditional method of social control among the Hopi has involved a reliance on gossip, witchcraft accusations, and ultimate ejection from the community (Aberle 1967).

However, preliminary field work has led to two observations. Alcohol use is common in both pro- and anticouncil villages, and many Hopi drinkers report solitary drinking as a means of avoiding social censure. We suggest that in the case of the Hopi we are seeing at work two somewhat different mechanisms of social control. The traditional mechanism has been ejection from the community. In anticouncil villages where the theocracy still exerts power, the traditional means of controlling deviants may still work. That is, when drinking becomes serious enough to evoke a response from the theocracy, the deviant may be ejected from the village to an off-reservation town. In such circumstances, he may become isolated and freed of all constraint. His drinking may therefore proceed to the point where cirrhosis develops.

In procouncil villages where the theocracy has been replaced by the Anglo-Saxon legal structures of courts and police, the deviant is not as likely to be ejected from the community. It is for this reason, perhaps, that cirrhotics are found in off-reservation towns and procouncil villages but not in anticouncil villages. At present, field work is being carried out to determine whether the off-reservation cirrhotics do indeed come from the anticouncil villages. As yet we are not able to reject the alternate hypothesis that drinking in off-reservation areas is a result of acculturational stress. However, the fact that we cannot predict the prevalence of cirrhosis on-reservation by distinguishing between wage-work and traditional agricultural villages gives us pause before involving any of the traditional gauges of acculturation in explaining the patterns we have observed.

In addition to the differences thus far discussed, there is an indication from case-fatality ratios that cirrhosis may have a different natural history in the two tribes. Of 25 known Hopi cirrhotics, 10 died. Of 91 known Navaho cirrhotics, 17 died. Although we recognize the limitations of our data, the higher ratio of deaths to known cases in the Hopis is consistent with the above discussion that the Navaho pattern may be one of heavy drinking when young which is outgrown, presumably at a time when the cirrhosis, if it exists, is still reversible. The Hopi pattern may be one in which the drinker is ejected from the community, becomes isolated, and then continues to drink until the disease proves fatal.

There is some confirmation for our suggestion in the data from the Apache who, even more than the Navaho, have been an acting-out tribe, as their high homicide rate attests (Levy and Kunitz 1969). However, the Apache fatality rate is at least not higher than that of the Hopi. Their drinking behavior, like the Navaho, is generally described as a highly visible group spectacle (Curley 1967; Mail 1967). In addition, since 1960 alcoholic beverages have been obtainable legally on the reservation at tribal package stores so that availability is not the problem that it is for reservation Navahos and Hopis. Yet they still have lower death rates from cirrhosis than the Hopi. Accidental and violent deaths do not seem to explain the disparity, and we would suggest that in this case, too, we are seeing the persistence of an earlier mode of behavior which does not predispose to death from alcoholic cirrhosis.

A number of other possible explanations should be mentioned although we feel that those described above are probably of prime importance. Conceivably the different death rates are a reflection of nothing more than the size of the respective reservations. It may simply be easier for Hopis to reach a source of alcohol than for many Navahos living in remote reaches of the reservation.

Another possibility is that there is inherited susceptibility among the Hopi to develop cirrhosis. Klatskin has "been impressed with the inordinately high incidence of alcoholic cirrhosis in certain families." Admitting that environmental factors may account for such instances, he feels that "the possibility of an inherited susceptibility to the disease cannot be excluded" (1961:449).

Although a considerable amount has been written on patterns of inbreeding among both the Hopi and Navaho (Woolf and Grant 1962; Spuhler and Kluckhohn 1953; Allen 1965; Woolf and Dukepoo 1969); we are not yet equipped to deal with this issue. Our impression is that inherited susceptibility or resistance to cirrhosis is not of as much explanatory value as the suggestions we have outlined above (Kunitz 1970). Clearly, however, this is an area that merits further investigation.

Although it is still too early to go much beyond the speculations offered herein to explain the differences we have observed between the various tribes, enough has been said perhaps to indicate that the problem of Indian alcoholism is not the same from tribe to tribe. Now that the Public Health Service, the Office of Economic Opportunity, and various tribal councils are becoming increasingly involved in treatment programs for Indian problem drinkers, it is of some practical as well as theoretical interest to try to determine more precisely the magnitude of the problem in various tribes, the etiology in each case, and whether, in fact, a real problem exists. Certainly at this point that favorite catchall, "acculturational stress," may serve to disguise many distinctions that are important to make.

Notes

1. The diagnoses as recorded on the hospital discharge sheets most commonly were not verified by either biopsy or autopsy. This is clearly a problem that bedevils all record research of this kind. In the case of the Hopi, we interviewed all the patients or their survivors to verify the drinking history and to collect ethnographic data not reported in this paper. In all cases the histories we obtained were in agreement with those recorded on the hospital chart and were compatible with a drinking history severe enough to lead to cirrhosis.

2. Details of the statistical methods may be found in G. W. Snedecor, and W. G. Cochran, *Statistical methods*, 6th ed. (Ames, Iowa: Iowa State University Press, 1967).

3. The expected numbers of deaths from cirrhosis in the three tribes were computed by applying the age-specific rates of the United States white population to the estimated age-specific census data from the three Indian populations. The rates used were the pooled age-specific rates for men and women for cirrhosis (ICD Code 581) both with and without mention of alcoholism. The apparent difference between the Hopi and the Apache can be assessed by assuming that the rates are the same in the two groups and by using the variance test for the Poisson distribution on the three-year totals for each group: the upper 1-tailed test gives a p of .11. Navaho mortality from cirrhosis is provided for 1965 and 1966, the years for which we have complete records (Kunitz, Levy, and Everett 1969:677).

Alcohol and the Identity Struggle: Some Effects of Economic Change on Interpersonal Relations

Richard Howard Robbins

Kenelm Burridge (1969) has recently drawn attention to the role of economic change in promoting various types of millenarian activities. He proposes that the introduction of a money economy into a society will bring about a questioning of the nature and distribution of power, and that this questioning will effect an effort to change the means by which persons may secure prestige, this effort manifesting itself in millenarian activities. However, there are other activities of a less spectacular sort that appear to result from the same circumstances. Codere (1950), for example, notes that following the introduction of wage labor among the Kwakiutl there was an increase in potlatch activity. Salisbury (1962) observes an increase in ceremonial exchanges among the Siane following the introduction of indentured labor, and Middleton (1960) remarks that following the introduction of migrant labor among the Lugbara there was an increase in witchcraft accusations. In each of these instances, the introduction of a wage-money economy produced, not an increase in millenarian activities, as Burridge proposes, but an increase in those institutionalized and ritualized activities that serve to express and resolve interpersonal conflict. The aim of this paper is to explore this phenomenon focusing initially on the drinking behavior characteristic of Naskapi Indian males in Schefferville, Quebec. More specifically, this article investigates the following hypothesis: When economic change alters persons' means of access to status-conferring goods or activities, or increases the availability of such goods or activities, there will be an increase in frequency of interpersonal conflict, and an increase in occurrence of those cultural processes which serve to resolve this conflict. A secondary hypothesis holds that Naskapi drinking interactions serve as a locus of interpersonal conflict which stems from recent changes in their economic life, and that these interactions further provide the opportunity for the resolution of this conflict.

Theoretical Framework

The study of interpersonal relations requires the delineation of the conceptions held by actors in a given interaction of their social position vis-à-vis others (Miller 1963). Such conceptions include a person's self-identity—his notion of his place in an interaction; his social identity—the place in the interaction he conceives others attribute to him; and his public identity—the way others actually view his social standing (Goodenough 1963; Miller 1963). This identity-interaction framework implies certain assumptions about the nature of man and the meaning of human behavior, the most basic being that a person's image of himself and of others affects his behavior and beliefs (Hallowell 1955). Second, it implies that a person's identity serves as a guide to him and others in orienting their pattern of interaction (Goffman 1956; Goodenough 1963). Further, a person's identity is formed and maintained in the course of his interaction with others (G. Mead 1934; Schwartz and

Merten 1968), and persons need to acquire information which confirms the image they entertain of themselves (Laing 1962). Finally, persons are constantly striving to bring within their orbit persons, possessions, or behaviors which confirm to them that they are indeed the persons that they believe themselves to be (Wallace 1967).

In striving to become what he believes to be a desirable person, the individual attempts to develop or acquire those attributes which serve in his society to define that identity. These attributes or features may include a certain physical appearance, the fulfillment of kinship obligations, the attainment of membership in certain groups, or the kind and quantity of personal possessions (see Wallace 1967; Miller 1963). Thus, in a given society the personal attribute of generosity may be one aspect of a favorable identity, as may the possession of such things as yams, pigs, horses, or automobiles. Given this framework the major problem posed here entails examining the social consequences of changing patterns of access to those attributes that serve to define a desirable identity, and examining the behavioral strategies adopted by persons to maintain their identities in the face of this change.

This paper will also focus on *identity-resolving forums.* Such forums are social gatherings which exhibit the following characteristics. First, they are times in the flow of community activities which are set aside for the permitting of behaviors that are otherwise disallowed (see MacAndrew and Edgerton 1969; Leach 1965). Second, they have inherent in them statements or actions which demarcate ambiguities, inconsistencies, or conflicts in interpersonal relations, in this sense resembling what Victor Turner (1957) refers to as a "social drama." Third, during such gatherings persons are permitted and encouraged to adopt poses intended to demonstrate that they do indeed possess the attributes of the identity they claim (Barth 1969). Finally, the forums serve as a time during which participants in the gathering have the opportunity to seek information to allow for the aligning of the identity they believe they possess with the identity they believe others attribute to them. In sum, such gatherings or interactions involve the enactment of behavioral strategies to permit persons to maintain, attain, or protect desired identities or social positions. Some examples of social gatherings which exhibit these characteristics are initiation ceremonies (Burton and Whiting 1965; Cohen 1964), trance ceremonies (Bourguignon 1965), ceremonial exchanges (Wallace and Fogelson 1965), and, as I propose to demonstrate, Naskapi drinking interactions.

Naskapi: Social and Economic Background

Located on the Quebec-Labrador border, the frontier mining town of Schefferville might appear at first glance to be indistinguishable from the suburbs of any large North American city. Completed in 1957, the town was built by the Iron Ore Company of Canada, supporting a Euro-Canadian population of some four thousand persons, and a native population of some seven hundred persons. The town, accessible only by rail and air, contains a department store, two supermarkets, a movie theater, two bars, three restaurants, and virtually all the other conveniences one associates with modern urban life. Located some three miles from this main residential area is what the townspeople refer to as the "Indian village," a settlement that, in fact, contains two socially distinct Indian groups: a community of some four hundred Montagnais Indians who migrated to Schefferville from the southern settlement of Sept-Iles, and some three hundred Naskapi Indians who migrated to Schefferville from the northern Ungava settlement of Fort Chimo.

The Schefferville Naskapi comprise the remnants of that group which Speck (1931) referred to as the Ungava Band, whose occupation of the area around Fort Chimo can be traced back to the mid-nineteenth century (L. Turner 1889–90). Aboriginally this group subsisted primarily on fish and caribou. Their social organization lacked any large-scale, permanent social groupings or formal political controls (Honigmann 1964*a*), with leadership and prestige being contingent upon a person's skills as orator or hunter (Leacock 1958; Rogers 1965). The only gradation in status was reflected in the number of wives a man possessed, and the number of hunting trophies he acquired, some portion of slain animals being kept and displayed (L. Turner 1889–90). In 1957 the Naskapi left a life still based on hunting, but supplemented by government relief, and migrated to Schefferville, living at present in a permanent settlement of thirty-seven government-built houses, depending for subsistence on wage labor and relief. Most importantly, wages earned at the Iron Ore Company have made available to them such Western goods as television, phonographs, refrigerators, washing machines, and electric stoves, the availability of which has had a profound effect on the character of their interpersonal relations.

Attributes utilized in a society to define a person of social worth determine not only the nature of interpersonal relations, but also the means to power, that is, the ability to influence the behavior of others, especially toward oneself. For a Naskapi to maintain or attain such power, to be, as they put it, a "good man," he must exhibit certain personal characteristics, honor his kin obligations, be a good provider for his family, and possess certain goods which are used for either display or exchange.

When asked to define the attributes of a good man a Naskapi will usually first reply that it is someone who shares what he has with others and who minds his own business. This latter attribute of reticence (see Preston 1967) makes requisite the avoiding of placing oneself or others in potentially conflict-laden situations, and avoiding the appearance of, as the Naskapi put it, placing oneself "above others." On one occasion, for example, a woman was struck on the hand with an iron pipe by a youth she was berating for his excessive drinking. The resulting injury was serious enough to require twenty stitches, but when asked for information on the matter the woman's husband merely replied, "It's none of my business." Reticence is also reflected in the evasiveness of individuals when they are asked their opinion on some matter, and in the reluctance of persons to appear in any way to be claiming that they are better than others or boasting of their exploits. In fact, the only situation in which reticence is lacking is during drinking interactions.

Generosity, the second important personal attribute of a good man, is to some extent related to the Naskapi's aboriginal subsistence pattern. Most societies in which food is scarce tend to place an emphasis on sharing because of the vicissitudes of obtaining it (see Evans-Pritchard 1940; Thomas 1959), those successful in the food quest sharing with others if only to insure a like return when they experience a food shortage. However, of more relevance in the Naskapi's present setting is the fact that sharing enables a person to obtain prestige reflected in the deference paid to the giver by the receiver of gifts. Giving or sharing is, in effect, a silent boast of success, with the acceptance of the offering affirming that success (see Ridington 1968). Not to share, on the other hand, marks an admission of failure, while the refusal of an offering indicates a negation of the giver's boast of success. Before the Naskapi moved to Schefferville, items marked for sharing or exchange were products of the hunt. However, with game now scarce and of lesser utility in the Naskapi scheme of things, items to be shared consist mostly of store-bought goods such as radios, watches, and, most importantly, alcoholic beverages.

In addition to exhibiting the requisite attributes of reticence and generosity, a Naskapi must also honor obligations defined by kinship if he is to maintain his desired identity. That all persons in the Naskapi community are kin is understood by all; however, it is also recognized that all people do not honor obligations wrought by a kin tie. Thus, the fact that a person may stand in a relationship as father to son is one thing; that he fulfills his obligations as a father is something else. Kin relationships in the Naskapi community can be divided into general types: there are those that tie together persons of equal or near equal status, or using Foster's (1967a) terms a "colleague contract"; and those in which there is some status differential between persons, or a "patron-client" relationship (Foster 1967a). Colleague contracts among the Naskapi include a man's relationship to *nistash* (older male sibling, male parallel-cousin), to *nishim* (younger sibling, younger parallel-cousin),[1] and *nistaw* (male cross-cousin or wife's brother). One illustration of this type of relationship is the tie between Joseph and Willie. They are *nistaw* to each other and both acknowledge the closeness of their tie. Their relationship is maintained by the frequent exchange of alcoholic beverages, rarely a week passing when they do not together visit one of the two local bars or exchange beer which one or the other had purchased. They frequently go hunting together, and exchange household visits virtually every day. Furthermore, they have agreed that Joseph's twelve-year-old son will marry Willie's ten-year-old daughter when both come of age. However, while the equality of their relationship is understood by both, the balance of the relationship is contingent upon the equal fortune of the two participants in the interaction, since the colleague relationship assumes that each gives to the other in like manner, kind, and quantity. In other words, if one participant in the relationship should have greater access than the other to those goods which are marked for exchange, the balance of the relationship would be disrupted and the tie between them would approach that of patron to client. There are, in fact, persons in the community who have no jobs, but who reside with *nistaw* who are employed. These relationships tend toward that of patron to client with the wage earner providing food and shelter, and the unemployed person chopping wood, carrying water, or doing other such chores. Thus, for those who are unsuccessful in wage earning it has become difficult, if not impossible, to maintain the proper balance in their colleague contracts.

There are also relationships in the Naskapi community characterized by some status difference which have been disrupted by the lack of access of persons to those attributes needed to maintain a favorable identity. Marriage, for example, generally marks the transition of a Naskapi male from boy (*nabash*) to man (*nabow*), although such a status is not recognized until the birth of the first child. At such a time a man should be able to establish a household, and assume the position of household head, one of the few roles in which a Naskapi may overtly exert authority. However, for such a status to be viewed as an attribute of a favorable identity, the husband must demonstrate that he can provide well for his family, and fulfill his marital and parental obligations. But there are some males in the community who because they do not have access to steady wages are unable to provide for their family at a level recognized by their spouse or others to be desirable. These men tend to be frequently derided by their marital partners as well as by their children. Their authority in the household is further undermined by the government practice of making relief checks out to the woman of the household, a practice initiated to prevent men from spending relief money on alcoholic beverages.

The final attribute to be treated here that is necessary for successful identity maintenance is a man's personal possessions. Thorsten Veblen in *The Theory of the Leisure Class* (1931) was one of the first social scientists to treat the importance of various forms of economic goods in the establishment and maintenance of status differences within a society, an importance that has long since been recognized by anthropologists (e.g., Mauss 1967; Sahlins 1965; Foster 1967a). A particularly lucid report on the part that economic goods play in determining social position in a hunting society is Robin Ridington's paper dealing with the Beaver Indians (1968). To the Beaver, success is measured by the amount of supernatural power (*ma yine*) a person possesses. A person's *ma yine*, however, can only be validated by his success as a hunter, for it is in the sharing of game that others convey recognition of the power of the giver, with game then serving as a trophy which confirms a person's claim to a desired identity. As was noted, hunting and the trophies it produces have ceased to be important in determining a Naskapi's social worth, since game itself is scarce, and, for the most part, they no longer accept products of the hunt as status symbols. Instead, the Naskapi now aspire to possess such items as televisions, radios, record players, and automobiles, the display of which now confirms a person's claim to a desired identity.

In sum, for a Naskapi to attain or maintain a desirable identity (i.e., "good man"), he no longer needs to demonstrate success at exploiting the physical environment. Instead, his social worth is now determined by his ability to exploit the social and economic institutions of Schefferville. His avenue to a desired identity has ceased to be through success at hunting, and now is through his success as a wage earner, since it is the goods purchased with such wages that are shared to maintain the attribute of generosity, and it is these goods that are given to kinsmen to fulfill kin obligations. Further, it is the goods purchased with these wages and the display and possession of them which mark a man as a good provider for his family.

As is the case with virtually all Schefferville residents, the Naskapi are largely dependent for wages on employment at the iron ore mines (see table 1). The Iron Ore Company began employing Naskapi workers in 1957, almost immediately after their arrival from Fort Chimo. However, as of August 1966, only eleven men were permanent employees, ten being members of the local union, a branch of the United Steel Workers of America. Two other Naskapi were at one time permanent employees, but were dismissed for job infractions. Only one Naskapi ever held a job at the company other than unskilled laborer, but his promotion lasted only one month because of his inadequate command of English. One reason for the relatively low number of permanent Naskapi employees is the hiring practice of the company prior to 1967. Company and union regulations stipulated that a person must have worked sixty-five consecutive days before he could either become a union member or gain seniority, a rule which under ordinary circumstances would have benefited the Naskapi, for, along with the Montagnais, they constitute the most permanent labor force in a community with considerable labor turnover. However, the company had a practice of employing native workers for sixty days, laying them off a few days, and then rehiring them, in this way denying their claim to seniority. Ten of the permanent employees had already accumulated the necessary time when the union was formed in 1959, so they could not be dismissed, while the remaining person gained seniority when his foreman "forgot" to report that he worked sixty-four consecutive days. In effect, these hiring rules created a situation where only a few of the adult males in the Naskapi community have access to full-time employment and the income realized from it, while the remaining Naskapi must depend on less lucrative part-time employment. While it was partly chance that ten Naskapi had worked the necessary consecutive period when the union was formed, additional factors enter into their success. They had constantly stayed on the job while others would take unannounced leaves from their jobs to go hunting or to take a vacation. They also had to limit job infractions such as appearing late to work, coming to work inebriated, or taking unexcused absences, thus quickly adapting to the norms of employment and the new temporal routine a job required.

TABLE 1. Sources of Naskapi Income for the Period January, 1965, through June, 1966

| Wage Labor | | Government Relief | | Total |
Source	Amount	Source	Amount	Income
Iron Ore Company	$115,596	Relief	$33,052	
Town	2,352	Old age insurance	7,740	
Guide	2,250	Needy mother		
Trapping		allowance	1,350	
(estimate)	1,150	Clothing		
Other	2,126	allowance	11,200	
Total	$123,473	Total	$53,342	$176,815

Part-time employment available in the mines for the rest of the Naskapi population depends upon the yearly fluctuations of labor demand, and the seasonal nature of mining operations in the North. To illustrate, table 2 indicates the number of men who worked and the number of man-hours worked by Naskapi employed on a part-time basis from 1962 to June of 1966.

TABLE 2. Days Worked and Number of Naskapi Part-Time Workers from January, 1962, through June, 1966

	1962	1963	1964	1965	1966
Number of days worked	1442	701	227	1606	377
Number of men employed part-time	20	14	6	21	12

There are few alternatives to employment at the mines (see table 1). The town occasionally employs Naskapi workers on a part-time basis, usually for snow removal, but this adds little income to the Indian community. For example, in 1964, when only six Naskapi found part-time work in the mines, twenty-two men worked for the town, but their combined income from this source was only $3200, far short of the potential income to be earned working for the company. A number of persons have been able to find jobs as guides in the hunting and fishing camps scattered in the area, but not only is this work seasonal—from June to October—it comes at a time when employment in the mines is likely to be available. The only other source of significant income is government relief. However, as noted, these payments do little toward allowing the identity maintenance of the male household heads, since relief checks are made out to the women. These payments also do little to rectify the difference in the range of household incomes (see table 3). In 1966 there were thirty-seven separate Naskapi households and while the average income over an eighteen-month period was $4774 including relief payments, the incomes ranged from a high of $10,888 to a low of $300.

TABLE 3. Range of Household Incomes from January, 1965, through June, 1966

Household Incomes	Number of Households
Over $10,000	2
$8,000 to $ 9,999	4
$6,000 to $ 7,999	8
$4,000 to $ 5,999	5
$2,000 to $ 3,999	13
Under $ 1,999	5

One key point of change affecting the Naskapi is that economic change has created greater status differences between persons than existed before the move to Schefferville: in effect, the differential between success and failure has increased. Further, there has been a scramble among persons to obtain those goods which are most relevant for identity maintenance. To demonstrate, it is only necessary to examine the way the Naskapi have allocated their income from wage labor. Money itself lacks status-conferring qualities for the Naskapi. It is not displayed, nor is it circulated outside a close circle of kin, so unless it is translated into goods which can be displayed or circulated it lacks any social value. The goods available to the Naskapi can be divided into five categories.[2] Category 1 consists of such items as food, clothing, and shelter, items which may be labeled subsistence goods. Category 2 includes such items as washing machines, freezers, refrigerators, and sewing machines, goods which have some household utility. Category 3 contains such items as guns, outboard motors, fishing equipment, and canoes, goods which, at least in the past, had considerable survival benefit. Category 4 is made up of televisions, radios, record players, and cameras, goods which are considered luxury items, while category 5 consists of such consumable luxuries as alcoholic beverages, tobacco, moviegoing, and billiards.

In terms of social meaning, none of the goods in category 1 is attended by any sort of prestige.[3] There is virtually no difference in the appearance of Naskapi homes, except, as we shall see, in the furnishings. There is little difference among individuals in dress, and little difference in types of food purchased, with slight advantage being taken of the wide variety of foodstuffs available at the two local supermarkets. Goods in category 2 would appear to function as household aids, but their utility is more potential than actual. Freezers, one of the most frequently purchased items in this category, are supposedly used to store fish and caribou, but the amount of game actually obtained and left over after sharing and consumption hardly requires a large upright freezer. Washing machines tend to be difficult to operate because the Naskapi homes lack running water. In winter, water must be carried from the adjacent lake, a trip of some twenty-five to three hundred yards (depending upon the location of the homes), and in summer must be carried from a half-mile-distant stream, the water in the lake being unfit for consumption because of a lack of sanitation facilities in the village. Furthermore, when using the washing machine, trips for water must be made twice, once for the wash cycle, and one for the rinse. While such goods are not, and cannot, be used to their full potential they may still have some utility for the women of the households, but I suspect that their prime importance lies in the status that the possession of such goods bestows upon the head of the household. Items in category 3, bush tools, were once basic items of survival, but are now recreational implements. The Naskapi still go into the bush, but rarely do such trips last more than three or four days. Goods in category 4 function primarily for display purposes, serving to demonstrate the success of the owner. Television, a popular item in this category, is purchased, although there are only fourteen hours of English-language programming each week, with few Naskapi being able to understand even them. Combination radio and phonograph consoles are purchased even though the record player portion is never used. Of the items in category 5—tobacco, billiards, moviegoing—alcoholic beverages are most important. Aside from its value as an intoxicant, alcohol serves as a source of prestige to those who purchase and distribute it.

Using the Naskapi household in which I resided as a standard of measurement, along with observation of the consumption patterns of other households, I estimate that 15 to 20 percent of Naskapi income is allocated to goods in category 1. Little is spent on housing although it is possible to invest in new homes (most being overcrowded), but such investments have not been made. The frequency of purchase of items in categories 2 through 4 is summarized in table 4. What is of particular interest is the high frequency of purchase of goods in categories 2 and 4, and the relatively low frequency of purchase of items in category 3. Cost is not a factor in this resource allocation pattern for prices of items in the different categories are comparable, a three horsepower outboard engine costing about the same as a television or freezer at the local Hudson's Bay Company store. The number of guns in the community is deceiving, since most are twenty-two caliber rifles dating back to Fort Chimo days, and few persons own higher caliber rifles useful in hunting caribou, while only two persons own shotguns for hunting duck, geese, or ptarmigan.

TABLE 4.   Allocation of Naskapi Income among Categories 2, 3, and 4

Category 2	Number of Households	Category 3	Number of Households	Category 4	Number of Households
Washing machine	24	Canoe	9	Tele- vision	19
Sewing machine	9	Outboard motor	4	Radio	18
Freezer	18	Rod		Record	
Refrigerator	1	and reel	7	player	15
Electric iron	13	Gun	34	Camera	11

The most frequently purchased item in category 5 is beer. It is difficult to gauge precisely how much is spent on such beverages since local merchants keep no records of native purchases. However, one individual stated that he spends approximately forty dollars a week on beer in addition to an unspecified amount at the local bar. This represents some 30 to 40 percent of his weekly income, and since he is not atypical in his consumption patterns one may estimate that some 25 to 50 percent of Naskapi income is allocated to alcoholic beverages.

Two things about the way Naskapi spend their money are relevant here. First, there is a marked preference for those goods which are most meaningful for distinguishing status differences within the community. Put another way, there appears to be a scramble for those goods which are most important in maintaining a person's identity or power. Second, the resource allocation pattern has effected a translation of differential income into a differential distribution of those things or behaviors needed to maintain a desired identity.

In sum, this account of Naskapi life in Schefferville reveals at least three changes in their economy which could be expected to produce changes in their patterns of interpersonal relations. First, there was a transition from a hunting economy to one based on wage labor, a shift which changed the way persons could obtain those goods needed to attain status or to maintain one's identity. All societies, of course, have some criteria for defining persons as successful or unsuccessful, whether the criteria be caribou tails or television, as well as having some way of determining who has access to these criteria. However, when there is a precipitous change in the means by which persons obtain access to status- or power-conferring goods or activities one can expect that those persons who were successful under the old system of power distribution would find their status threatened by the introduction of a new system of power distribution (see Sharp 1952). Among the Naskapi, for example, there are persons who were (and are) successful hunters, but who, for whatever reason, are not successful wage earners. These persons have seen their power and prestige decline relative to those who, while perhaps not successful hunters, are successful wage earners. Thus, in the past a leader was selected primarily for his hunting ability, but in Schefferville, all four individuals who have been elected chief since the move from Fort Chimo are persons who are permanent employees at the company, and are not particularly noted for their hunting ability.

Second, the move to Schefferville meant that status symbols were more numerous and easier to attain. The fact that such things were more numerous meant there was an influx into the Naskapi social system of what Salisbury (1962) terms "free-floating power," goods which have status-conferring qualities but which lack fixed rules of distribution. These goods, aside from being more plentiful, also are easier to obtain than hunting trophies, for whereas a hunter's access to status-conferring goods is limited by the vicissitudes of consummating a kill, a wage earner's access to such status is limited only by his ability to translate wages into goods with status-conferring qualities. One can then expect that the change in availability and quantity of status-conferring goods will result in what may simply be called a free-for-all to obtain these goods, and a scramble to obtain access to the new means by which such goods are acquired.

Third, because of the hiring practices of the Iron Ore Company after 1959 the avenues of access to power were partially closed so only some persons, those employed full-time, were able to maintain their identities at the new level required by life in Schefferville. This resulted in greater status differences between persons than one would expect to exist in a society based on a hunting economy. One may then postulate that this increased differential between success and failure would make it more difficult for some persons to fulfill obligations wrought by their ties to others.

One can deduce from the propositions enumerated earlier that any circumstance that dramatically changes persons' identities will require a reordering of interpersonal relations, and that such circumstances will promote an increase in those social interactions in which the identity claimed by a person is different from the identity attributed to him by others, relationships which Anthony Wallace (1967) terms identity struggles (see also A. Wallace and Fogelson 1965). The change in the means of access to identity-maintaining and power-conferring goods will initiate struggles between those who formerly enjoyed favored access to such goods and those whose access improved under the new system of power distribution. Further, there will develop a struggle between persons vying for the increased power injected into the community in the form of Western goods, with those who are successful in obtaining such goods asserting, in some form, what they see to be their newly acquired status. Finally, the greater status differential between persons resulting from economic change will effect struggles between persons involved in relationships in which one partner can no longer fulfill his obligations to the other.

The question that now presents itself is, if indeed one can expect the above consequences to economic change, in what form do the struggles postulated to exist present themselves?

Alcohol and the Naskapi

Social scientists have long noted a relationship between alcohol and anxiety, frustration, or failure (see Horton 1967). Graves (1967), for example, demonstrates that persons who do not have access to desired goals tend to drink more heavily than those to whom such goals are attainable. Whittaker (1963) views Sioux drinking as a reliever of tensions caused by the basic insecurities of reservation life, and Simmons (1959) sees Peruvian mestizo drinking serving as an opportunity to reduce anxiety due to a distrust and fear of others. These and other studies have tended to focus on alcohol consumption itself rather than the behavior generated by alcohol use, assuming that it is the physiological reaction alcohol is supposed to have on the person that is of prime importance. However, the utilization of this psychodynamic framework does little to explain the dynamics of Naskapi drinking, for it does not account for the fact that the Naskapi express almost unanimous satisfaction with their life in Schefferville, and does not allow understanding of the disparate forms of behavior evidenced by persons whose alcohol consumption patterns are nearly identical. Furthermore, among the Naskapi, drinking, rather than involving personal withdrawal, is preeminently a social act, guiding the person to certain types of social interaction defined by both the situation and the identity of the participants. Accordingly, the view followed here is that drinking behavior, rather than being explained by alcohol's toxic assault on the seat of moral judgment, is behavior that is culturally defined and given meaning within a given social nexus (MacAndrew and Edgerton 1969; see also Mandelbaum 1965, also in this volume). Furthermore, to understand the nature of alcohol use and drinking behavior of the Naskapi, one must focus on the social interaction accompanying the drinking act. With this in mind we will be concerned with three aspects of Naskapi alcohol usage. First, what are the different types of behavior individual Naskapi exhibit when drinking? Second, what are the social positions in a drinking interaction of the actors vis-à-vis each other, and in what way does this position determine drinking behavior? Finally, what is the nature, meaning, and significance of the social interaction that among the Naskapi accompanies the drinking act?

Patterns of Alcohol Usage

By far the most frequent beverage imbibed by the Naskapi is store-bought beer. Hard liquor can be ordered at the provincial liquor store, but the wait before such beverages are delivered—two to seven days—deters most Naskapi from utilizing that source. Hard liquor and mixed drinks are purchased at the two local bars, although the bulk of drinking activity takes place in the Indian village. Most drinking groups are small, usually from two to three persons, and on no occasion did I observe a group of more than six (see table 5). There are a number of reasons for the small size of drinking groups, not the least of which is the fact that beer is only supplied by one or, at most, two persons in such gatherings, an amount not sufficient to provide more than five or six persons. It would also be difficult, as we shall see, for the social interaction that accompanies the drinking act to be engaged in with groups of more than five or six individuals. In addition to the size composition of drinking groups, a pattern also emerges in the types of relationships between individuals drinking together. Almost half of the drinking groups I observed were composed of persons who stood as *nistaw* to each other, while 68 percent were composed of persons who stood either as *nistaw*, or as *nistash-nishim* to each other. In other words, drinking is most frequent between persons who are tied together by a colleague contract.

TABLE 5.   Size of Drinking Groups

Number in Groups[a]	Number of Times Observed
2	26
3	17
4	6
5	6
6	2
Total number of observations	57

a. The size of drinking groups did vary with time, with the above number referring to when the group was first observed.

As noted, it is difficult to determine the quantity of beer consumed by each person since local merchants keep no records of beer purchases, and even if they did one could not be certain that those who purchased it consumed it. However, except for a number of women, there are few abstainers among the Naskapi. In fact I knew of only one adult male (sixty-five years old) who claims never to drink and whose claim is substantiated by others. Furthermore, he is a virtual recluse whose most frequent interactions are with some older Montagnais who, as far as I could gather, do not drink either (see Szwed 1966). Otherwise all Naskapi males drink, and most drink heavily. But in spite of the high frequency of alcohol consumption (or perhaps because of it), virtually all Naskapi when asked their opinion will state simply that "drinking is no good." Often a person is characterized as a "good man, except when he drinks," and even persons who are frequent consumers will look askance at someone who is drinking and say, "People are no good when drinking." These negative attitudes toward alcohol consumption are reinforced from both within and without the Naskapi community. The Anglican missionary often uses church services to speak on the harmful effects of alcohol, as does the Roman Catholic missionary with his Montagnais congregation. The Iron Ore Company sends home persons who come to work inebriated, firing those for whom it becomes a repeated offense. The police reinforce these attitudes through arrests, and townspeople will usually ignore the attempt of a drinking Indian to engage in conversation. Within the community drinkers are often the subject of deprecating gossip, and it is believed by most Naskapi that drinking causes stomach trouble. Yet to focus only on these stated attitudes is misleading, for while drinking and alcoholic beverages are condemned, what is usually intended is an objection to that type of drinking that leads to socially disruptive behavior. Virtually all Euro-Canadian agencies, including the missionary and the police, express no objection to drinking in moderation, and the Naskapi themselves state that it is all right to drink to, as they put it, "get happy."

As with a number of other societies (see G. Berreman 1956; Simmons 1959; Whittaker 1963; Hamer 1965; Curley 1967), the Naskapi does not hold anyone responsible for his behavior when drinking. If a person becomes aggressive when imbibing his actions will be overtly forgotten by others the next day in the belief that he was "not himself," or was "crazy," and only when such behavior results in injuries to others will negative sanctions be applied. One person, for example, severely cut one woman with a pipe, threatened his wife with a loaded rifle, and struck another man over the head with a shovel. Only after the third incident were negative sanctions applied to him, the person's father-in-law, in whose house he was residing, asking him to leave. Nevertheless, actual injuries and the application of negative sanctions are relatively rare, surprisingly so to someone who has witnessed the frequent, apparently aggressive behavior that accompanies the consumption of alcoholic beverages.

Time and Alcohol

Any casual observer in the Naskapi community is certain to note the familiar weekend drinking spree. It is a rare Saturday night when less than fifty Naskapi adults are drinking, and rarer still when the RCMP (Royal Canadian Mounted Police) or town police do not make several trips to the village. That alcohol consumption, at least in its more socially disruptive form, is most frequent on weekends is evidenced by the fact that half of all arrests made for drinking occur on Saturday. However, there are other temporal criteria for the staging of drinking activities. At the end of the workday Naskapi mine workers will stop off at the bar for a drink or two. Paydays, and the night preceding and following a trip into the bush, signal drinking activity, as do such holidays as Christmas and New Year's. What is most apparent in this temporal distribution of alcohol consumption is that drinking is heaviest when it least disrupts the flow of everyday life.

Drinking Behavior

Naskapi males do not all react the same way to the consumption of alcoholic beverages. Nor from my observations do their reactions necessarily coincide with the amount of alcohol consumed (see G. Berreman 1956). Persons who on some occasions would show no signs of inebriation after six to ten cans of beer, would on other occasions show signs of inebriation after as little as one-half can of beer. In other instances, persons reacting aggressively to alcohol would sober up as soon as someone new entered the interaction.

The form that drinking behavior takes varies from a friendly, amicable type, to an assertive, sometimes violent type. The friendly reaction usually takes the form of the drinker loudly declaring his friendship to a drinking partner, or may take the form of a giveaway. There were frequent cases of a drinker writing checks to others for amounts ranging from five to fifty dollars, or giving away such personal valuables as radios, clocks, or wrist watches. The person exhibiting the friendly reaction will also usually insist that others share his beer with him. The assertive reaction to alcohol usually entails overt boasting by the actor. The most typical verbal statements that accompany this reaction are "me big man," or "I'm boss in my house," or simply "everybody likes me." Often such assertions will become more insistent and include the verbal downgrading of others, sometimes in their presence. On these occasions such a downgrading will lead to a like response from the accused, such interactions often culminating in physical violence.

My thesis in this article is that Naskapi drinking interactions serve as identity-resolving forums; that when drinking a person is permitted to defend an identity that has been challenged, claim an identity he believes he is entitled to, or rectify an identity that has been spoiled by failure, and that such interactions aim toward allowing the person to receive from others information which confirms the identity he is seeking. Furthermore, drinking interactions demarcate identity struggles within the Naskapi community. To give the reader the flavor of these drinking interactions I have selected four incidents involving alcohol consumption, incidents which will reveal both the regularities and variations in Naskapi drinking behavior.

Interaction 1

It was 5:30 P.M. and the bus back to the Indian village was filled with returning workers and shoppers. Bill had been drinking in town, and when he boarded the bus he shouted as he took his seat, "I been in Schefferville nine years now. Nobody push Bill around, everybody my friend." Bill is fifty years old and at one time was one of the most influential men in the Naskapi community. He was known to have been one of the best hunters in the village, but while he still spends considerable time in the bush, he realizes little income from his exploits. When he came to Schefferville from Fort Chimo he was unable to find work at the mines because a back condition prevented him from passing the company's physical examination, although he quickly informs people that he doesn't work in the mines because, as he puts it, "I'm my own boss." His major source of income is from relief, and he is reputed to be one of the heaviest drinkers in the community. Bill continued his tirade on the bus en route to the village, and soon began directing his comments to John (Bill's *nistaw*) who was returning home from work bedecked in the yellow work hat employed Naskapi wear virtually all the time. Bill shouted at him, "You no good," and continued in much the same vein all the way back to the village. John, who had stopped off briefly at the local bar, apparently tried to ignore the outburst, his only reaction being embarrassed laughter.

Interaction 2

Joseph and Tommy had just returned from town carrying with them two cases of beer which Joseph had purchased. They were joined by Moses, Thomas, and myself, and promptly opened the first case with Joseph doing the honors of distributing a can of beer to each participant. As the drinking progressed, the conviviality of the group increased. Joseph was the first to finish his can and rose and handed those present another can, although no one had yet finished their first. However, everyone readily accepted, offering their thanks to Joseph and praising his generosity. As the party continued into the fourth round of drinks, Tommy began repeating what a "good man" Joseph was, looking to the others for their nod of approval, and by the fifth round Thomas had taken out his checkbook and was writing a check for twenty-five dollars to give to Moses. By the sixth round and into the second case of beer, Thomas had given Joseph his watch and cigarette lighter.

Interaction 3

Tom had already been drinking when he came into my room and asked me to go visiting with him. He put four cans of beer into his pocket and said: "Come, we go visit George, I give him beer." George is a permanent employee at the mines, and his English surpasses any other adult Naskapi. In Fort Chimo he lived with the manager of the local Hudson's Bay Company outpost, and was once elected to the band council. However, at present, he has very little status in the community, has extremely few household possessions, and has been in frequent trouble with Euro-Canadian authorities. In Fort Chimo he threatened an RCMP officer with a loaded rifle when the officer tried to take his wife into custody to send her south for treatment of tuberculosis. When his daughter Sally was to be married, George wanted to sponsor a big feast—he approached the Roman Catholic missionary for a $1000 loan for the party—but the then Anglican missionary would not let the feast take place because Sally was pregnant. Nor would the missionary allow Sally to wear a white dress for the wedding ceremony. Whether this incident was the direct cause or not, neither George nor his wife has been to church since. In addition, the wife of the lay preacher (who is George's brother) has publicly announced that she would not allow George in church. When Tom and I arrived at George's house Tom pulled the beer out of his pocket and told me to give it to George. George accepted, told Tom to "shut up," explaining that he spoke better English than Tom. He then proceeded to tell me that he had worked at the Hudson's Bay Company store in Fort Chimo, and that he had been on the village council for two years: "We had a good chief then, better than now, but I didn't like to be councilman. The people didn't like me." Tom then interrupted: "No, George good man. Doesn't drink too much." Two days earlier Tom had told me that George drinks more than anyone else in the village.

Interaction 4

Sam and I were visiting with Willie when Sam's wife Martha came into Willie's house, grabbed Sam by the arm, and proceeded to drag him home. Sam had been drinking, and as he walked home he kept complaining that he had given Martha two checks (relief payments), one for $200 and the other for $97. "My money," he kept repeating. When they got home Martha sat Sam at the kitchen table and began making him supper. Sam said he had not eaten in two days. Martha tried to give him some water (a native cure for hangovers), but he refused saying he wanted meat. Then he began arguing with Martha, Sam repeating in English, "I'm boss in my house," and Martha repeating in Cree that Sam was crazy. Martha then cooked some Spam and gave it to him along with a cup of coffee, but Sam pushed the food aside, spilled the coffee into the plate with the meat, and proceeded to pour himself another cup. After two hours of bickering they went to sleep.

Analysis: The Drinking Interaction

In analyzing the nature of the interaction process that accompanies the consumption of alcoholic beverages it is important to note the reaction of others when a drinker adopts either a friendly, assertive, or aggressive pose. In the case of the friendly actor, the most marked response of others is one of deference. When a Naskapi offers another a drink, the recipient will usually shake his head and proclaim what a "good man" the donor is. There is also a sharp difference in the demeanor of the giver vis-à-vis the receiver. The donor tends to be more assertive in his actions, distributing beer or other goods with an obvious flourish, while the receiver tends to be more subdued and deferential. In interaction 2, for example, Joseph, who is a permanent employee at the mines, was the recipient of considerable praise for his generosity. Thomas, who works only part-time, also began to make presentations, but the check he gave to Moses was no good, and the goods he distributed to Joseph he asked for back the following day through an intermediary. One may view Thomas' presentations to Joseph (who is nistaw to Thomas) as his attempt to balance the exchange initiated by the distribution of beer. However, it is largely a fruitless effort on Thomas' part because he has got just so many watches and cigarette lighters to give away during such interactions, and he does not have a steady income with which to replenish his supply of such goods or purchase sufficient quantities of beer to present to others.

As is the case with friendly drinking behavior, the reaction of others to the assertive drinker is also marked by deference.

When a drinker begins proclaiming what a "big man" he is, or how he is "boss" in his house, others usually react with profuse agreement, nodding their heads or specifically stating that the drinker is indeed a "good man" (cf. Hamer 1969). In some cases, drinking partners will review the accomplishments of the assertive person: "He used to be councilor," or "Tom's a good mechanic." Or they may support some future ambition of the actor: "Sam is going to be the next chief." But while deference and support are characteristic of others' reaction to both friendly and assertive behavior, deference and support are, I believe, given for different reasons. In the case of the friendly drinker, the reaction of others is dictated by the real situation of the actors—the giver and receiver of gifts. In the case of the response to the assertive drinker, nothing is actually given although others react as though something had been received. Given the value that the Naskapi place on the personal attribute of reticence, the reaction of others to the assertive drinker may be viewed as their way of minimizing possible conflict, since any disagreement to the boasts of the drinker, or any appearance of remaining indifferent to them may, and often does, lead to physical violence. In interaction 3, for example, Tom reacted quickly to squash George's suggestion that people didn't like him, as well as agreeing with his boasts that he spoke good English.

When drinking behavior shifts from being assertive to being aggressive, the interaction often resembles a contest between two protagonists, each trying to convince others of their higher social standing, as I believe Bill was trying to do in his verbal attack on John in interaction 1 (see Ridington 1968). It is also significant that Bill's behavior on the bus is in marked contrast to his drinking behavior when interacting with his forty-five-year-old stepson, Pete (Bill's second wife is fifteen years older than he). Pete has rarely been employed, living on relief and income he earns collecting bottles to exchange for deposits at the local grocery stores. His wife left him ten years ago to be treated for tuberculosis, has since refused to come home to live with him, and has had two illegitimate children since she left home. When Pete does drink he often launches into a tirade against Bill, and on one occasion had to be forcibly restrained from attacking him. On this occasion Bill didn't even look at Pete, but appeared to remain completely indifferent to the attack. One can see that in this incident and in interaction 1, the person being assertive or aggressive in the interaction is someone who is less successful than the person to whom the assertions are directed, or is someone who is not able to fulfill his obligations to the other, as Sam is unable to do in regard to Martha (see interation 4).

I am proposing that in all of these interactions persons are attempting to resolve identity struggles in those interpersonal relations in which the identity claimed by the person is different from the identity attributed to him by others; that those persons who have ready access to those goods which serve to maintain a desired identity will, when drinking, attempt to elicit confirmation of their status and power through the presentation of gifts. On the other hand, those persons who do not have such access will, when drinking, attempt to defend their identity threatened by their lack of access to identity-validating goods through the use of assertive or aggressive behavior. In order to substantiate this proposition, a comparison was made of the prevalent drinking behavior of those persons with a steady income and a ready supply of identity-maintaining goods with the drinking behavior of those without a steady income, or without a substantial number of such goods. Town police and RCMP records were used for the purpose of determining the types of behavior characteristic of Naskapi male drinkers, since both law enforcement agencies do not arrest Naskapi unless their behavior becomes assertive or aggressive. Since virtually all Naskapi males drink but only those who are assertive or aggressive are likely to be arrested, we can assume that those persons with a high frequency of arrests tend to be more assertive drinkers, while those with a low frequency of arrests are likely to react to alcohol in a friendly manner. Table 6 shows the number of arrests of those persons that are employed full-time by the company and those who are, at best, part-time employees. It indicates that the average part-time employee was arrested 3 times while the average full-time employee was arrested 1.6 times. Since there are other sources of money income, a tabulation was also made of the number of arrests of persons according to gross income, but again the results are similar (table 7). Finally, since money itself does not confer a desirable identity, a comparison was made of the number of possessions owned by each household head with his number of arrests (table 8). Those persons who own eight or more such items were arrested on the average of 0.6 times per person, while those individuals with fewer than eight items showed an average of almost 4 arrests per person. In short, the above data suggests that the form drinking behavior takes for individual Naskapi is due, not to the amount of alcohol consumed, but to the social position of the actor (see Bruun 1959; Honigmann and Honigmann 1968).

TABLE 6.   Percentage of Arrests of Naskapi Able-bodied Men according to Employment Status

Number of Arrests	Part-Time Employees	Full-Time Employees
0	11%	33%
1	11%	42%
2	21%	8%
3	23%	0%
4	9%	0%
5	9%	0%
6	9%	8%
7	6%	8%
Total number	(34)	(12)
Total number of arrests	102	20
Mean	3.0	1.6

TABLE 7.   Percentage of Arrests of Naskapi Able-bodied Men according to Gross Income

| Number of Arrests | Income Category | | | |
	$0–1,999	$2,000–3,999	$4,000–5,999	Over $6,000
0	0%	0%	75%	25%
1	28%	18%	0%	42%
2	17%	9%	0%	17%
3	28%	9%	25%	0%
4	11%	28%	0%	0%
5	6%	28%	0%	0%
6	0%	9%	0%	17%
7	11%	0%	0%	0%
Total number	(18)	(11)	(4)	(12)
Total number of arrests	53	40	3	21
Mean	2.9	3.6	0.8	1.7

To summarize, I suggest that drinking interactions serve as a vehicle for the reordering of interpersonal relations unsettled by economic change; that alcohol sets the stage for persons to make status claims, claims which can only be made when drinking, since status claims in any other setting would violate the desired personal attribute of reticence. Thus, in addition to allowing persons to present claims to a desired identity (something I maintain

TABLE 8.   Percentage of Arrests of Able-bodied Household Heads according to Number of Possessions[a]

Number of Arrests	Number of Possessions		
	0–4	5–8	Over 8
0	10%	0%	44%
1	10%	12%	56%
2	10%	25%	0%
3	10%	0%	0%
4	10%	25%	0%
5	20%	12%	0%
6	20%	0%	0%
7	10%	25%	0%
Total number	(10)	(8)	(9)
Total number of arrests	39	32	5
Mean	3.9	4.0	0.6

a. Possessions used to formulate table 8 include: washing machine, clothes dryer, refrigerator, freezer, sewing machine, electric iron, electric stove, electric razor, radio, television, camera, store-purchased sofa, store-purchased armchair, and phonograph.

is inevitable given the changes in the Naskapi community), alcohol also permits the maintenance of the reticence ethic. Furthermore, status claims made while drinking demarcate identity struggles resulting from economic change with the drinking interaction providing an opportunity to resolve such struggles. Those persons whose recent success has encouraged them to view themselves as being entitled to a higher status than others recognize will claim that status while drinking by initiating presentations to others in the form of beer or other goods. Those persons who have seen their prestige decline relative to specific others, that is, who do not have ready access to identity-maintaining or identity-confirming goods, will attempt to resolve the discrepancy between their self- and public identity through the use of assertive or aggressive behavior. In this sense assertive or aggressive behavior much resembles Haitian spirit possession as analyzed by Bourguignon (1965). In Haiti, trance occurs when a person is "mounted" by a spirit or *loa* which itself is ranked in a status hierarchy. Others react to the person in trance, not according to his social standing, but according to the status of the possessing spirit. One case cited by Bourguignon is illuminating: "A.C.'s father is a mild-mannered man, generally ignored and pushed around by his kin. Yet he has one of the most powerful deities of the family, and when possessed, he is given great deference by his wife, who has left him, by his children, by his successful half brother, and by others. Significantly, his possession on ceremonial occasions appears to linger on longer than most others" (1965:53).

Economic Change and the Identity Struggle

The Naskapi usage of alcohol is not an isolated or unique adaptation to the consequences of economic change. This is not to imply that all, or even most, societies use alcohol in the way described above—although research suggests at least some do (see Hamer 1969)—but rather that in all societies in which economic change follows the lines typified by the Naskapi there will be, in some form, an increase in the frequency of identity struggles, and an increase in activities or interactions which serve in that society as identity-resolving forums. Earlier I mentioned that following the introduction of a money economy, status conflict apparently increased among the Kwakiutl, Siane, and Lugbara. I propose here to further examine these three societies to determine if economic change can account for this conflict. More specifically, I will be concerned with five questions. First, what are the major attributes by which a person's identity is defined in these societies? Second, what are the behaviors or activities in these societies by which identities are maintained? Third, what are the avenues of access to identity-maintaining goods or activities? Fourth, how has economic change affected the availability and distribution of those behaviors or things which serve to define a desired identity? And finally, has there been any change in frequency of those activities, behaviors, or interactions which serve as identity-resolving forums?

The potlatch is the prototype of that aspect of economic activities that involves the maintenance or confirmation of a social position. Codere makes this clear in her definition of the potlatch: "The Kwakiutl potlatch is the ostentatious display and dramatic distribution of property by the holders of a fixed, ranked, and named social position to other position holders. The purpose is to validate the hereditary claim to the position and to live up to it by maintaining its relative glory and rank against the rivalrous claims of others" (1950:63). In short, the potlatch is essentially competition for power, a form of activity that both manifests struggles for status and serves as an identity-resolving forum (see A. Wallace and Fogelson 1965).

According to Codere, Kwakiutl property was divided into

two categories: those things used for potlatching and "trifles" or "bad things" (1950:63–64). The former category included such items as blankets—fur and cedar before contact, Hudson's Bay Company blankets after contact—canoes, and "coppers." Trifles, on the other hand, consisted of items such as deer skins, mats, and baskets before contact, and flour, silk scarfs, and sewing machines after contact. Potlatch goods were given away or destroyed at ceremonies to demonstrate the high social position of the giver, and to humiliate a rival. One feature of these ceremonies was a hymn or chant sung by the giver relating his own self-glorification and ridiculing his opponent, statements which bring to mind the self-aggrandizing of the assertive Naskapi drinker: "I am the great chief who vanquishes. . . . I am the great chief who makes people ashamed. . . . You are my subordinates. . . . Oh, I laugh at them, I sneer at them who empty boxes (of treasure) in their houses, their potlatch houses, their inviting houses that are full only of hunger. . . . I am the only great tree, I the chief . . . " (Benedict 1959a:272).

Before contact, access to those goods which were pot-latched, and hence access to a desired identity, was determined by inherited social rank, wealthy persons apparently being heads of extended families who held custodianship over the goods of the group (Drucker 1966). However, with the introduction of a wage-money economy two changes occurred: first, goods used for pot-latching changed from locally produced items (cedar blankets, canoes) to Hudson's Bay Company products, most notably blankets. Second, the means of access to potlatch goods changed from inherited social rank to activities such as hunting, fishing, and wage labor, that is, activities through which money could be obtained (Codere 1950). With these changes persons who because of a low inherited social rank were aboriginally unable to potlatch, and hence claim a favored identity, could now improve their positions by obtaining money, purchasing blankets at the Hudson's Bay Company store, and potlatching. On the other hand, those persons who before contact had exclusive access to potlatch goods would now have their social rank threatened by those who, by the new criteria for obtaining potlatch goods, could now make status claims. The result would be an increase in identity struggles wrought by the increase in social mobility. As Codere then points out, these changes were accompanied by an increase in potlatch activity.

Among the Siane, a group of tribes in the New Guinea Highlands who until the 1930s and 1940s were virtually untouched by

Western society, the most desired identity is that of "big man." While technically anyone could attain this status—the attributes being skill in oratory, a mature age, procreation of children, and wealth—such persons are usually *yarafo*, senior members of the various generations within a lineage. The village headman, or *bosboi*, is usually a senior member of the senior generation within a lineage.

To maintain or acquire a desirable identity among the Siane, a person must have access to subsistence goods such as sweet potatoes and taros. However, for a person to rise in status and power, to become a "big man," he must have access to goods, such as pigs, which are involved in exchanges between clans on such occasions as marriage, birth, or death. When such goods are received from other clans on such occasions they are first distributed to the *bosboi* of each lineage, who then redistributes them to others, thus maintaining his high status (Salisbury 1962). Technically anyone who has a number of valuables may increase his prestige by making presentations, but the power of the "big men" is solidified by the fact that it is they who lend pigs to young men to be used as bride-price, and the debtor cannot enter into clan councils until the loan is repaid. So while a person could claim a desired identity, this identity could be confirmed only when he was free from his obligations to the "big men."

There were two stages in the change of the Siane economy. The first occurred in the form of sporadic contacts with Europeans, most often government officials, most of these contacts being made by "big men" serving as guides. For their labor these persons received goods classified by the Siane as valuables, with the result that the power of the "big men" increased further. An additional consequence of this initial contact was an inflation of bride-prices. Those groups living nearest European settlements, who hence had greatest access to European goods, would obtain these valuables and offer more in payment for women to groups living at a greater distance from the settlements. However, the outlying groups from which the women were obtained soon experienced a shortage of marriageable females, although they quickly became rich in valuables which they then used to pay greater prices for women from even more outlying settlements. As a consequence of this increase in the number of valuables (which were distributed in the same manner as before the increase), the "big man" had greater access to valuables while young men were forced to borrow even more pigs in order to pay the now inflated prices for women. In order words, the wealth and power of the "big men" grew, while the power and status of the young men remained static (Salisbury 1962).

However, this increased status differential between persons lasted only until the second stage of economic change, the introduction of indentured labor. Young men could then go to work on the coast and return with money which was classified as a valuable. This development potentially enabled the young men to free themselves more quickly from their obligations to "big men," since they could now use their wages to pay off their debts incurred in obtaining a wife. Put another way, the criteria by which a Siane could rise in status and join the clan councils changed from the production of pigs—a lengthy process—to obtaining of money through indentured labor—a far speedier process.[4] One would then expect that the young men would use their newly found riches to make status claims through ceremonial exchanges, claims which they were unable to make under the old system, and that the "big men," that is, those operating under the old power distribution system, would see their status threatened by these new developments, and, in turn, initiate ceremonial exchanges. This proposition is, I believe, substantiated by the fact that, as with the Kwakiutl, these changes in the economy effected an increase in ceremonial activities (Salisbury 1962).

The Lugbara are a Sudanic-speaking people in Uganda and what was the Belgian Congo. Their elementary social, political, and economic unit is a group consisting of a cluster of elementary or joint families, which Middleton refers to as a "family cluster" (1966:142). This unit is a patrilineage varying in composition from a dozen to as many as one hundred fifty persons. The leader, or elder, of these groups is selected for his position on the basis of his senior genealogical status in the lineage, and, ideally, has complete control over members of his family cluster (Middleton 1966). Each of these social units is further divided into status grades, a person's position in these grades being determined by his age and position of authority in the joint family. However, these status grades are extremely flexible, and there is periodic tension between persons who wish to increase their authority and prestige and those who wish to maintain their authority. These identity struggles may be resolved in one of two ways. The first involves what Middleton terms ghost invocation, and the second involves accusations of witchcraft.[5] When a Lugbara makes a status claim, and any member of the family cluster may attempt to exert authority, the claim must be legitimized by the senior members of the lineage, who, in turn, must seek statements from the dead ancestors to determine whether the person making the status claim is entitled to a higher ranking in the group. This they do by communicating with the dead through specters, omens, dreams, or, most commonly, through oracles (Middleton 1966). When someone's claim to a more desirable identity is confirmed by the dead, it follows that those of once equal status to the claimant lose prestige. Their means of rectifying this loss of status relative to the claimant is to level a witchcraft accusation against their rival, accusing him of obtaining confirmation of his new identity through witchcraft. If he is able to convince others of his charge his rival is, as Middleton puts it, "cast out from the everyday system of authority" (1966:148).

The aboriginal economy of the Lugbara was organized around the family cluster with the elder being invested with the authority to distribute the goods of the group—grain, iron objects, and livestock (Middleton 1962). The changes in this economy, as they did with the Siane, occurred in two stages. The first was marked by the Belgian practice of setting up chiefs who were paid tribute in the form of cattle and grain. These chiefs then used their earnings to acquire wives and large families, signs of high status, which increased the status differential between them and those not having the same favored access to these goods, a circumstance parallel to that existing among the Siane when "big men" acquired virtually exclusive access to European goods. The second phase of economic change occurred with the introduction of migrant labor and money. Before this change a young man could move up the status grades only by first marrying, which changed his status from "youth" to "big youth," and then by producing children, increasing his status to "man behind" (behind more senior men). This he could do only by acquiring bride wealth from his elders. But with the acquisition of money he could hasten his increase in status by using the money to buy wives or to buy beer for his seniors, becoming less dependent upon his elders in the process. In other words, as with the Kwakiutl and Siane, economic change effected a situation where the power of traditional authorities would be threatened by the newly acquired status of those having access to new status-conferring goods, as well as initiating a scramble for power among those who have access to such goods. One would then expect an increase in identity struggles, Middleton noting that accompanying these changes in the economy there was an increase in the incidence of witchcraft accusations (1960).

Summary and Conclusions

The arguments presented in this paper may be summarized as follows. First, Naskapi drinking interactions represent identity-resolving forums defining identity struggles and permitting persons to make status claims or defend an identity threatened by a lack of access to identity-maintaining goods. Second, the form drinking behavior takes among the Naskapi is determined by the identity of the participants in such interactions; those persons experiencing success at wage earning attempt to gain confirmation of what they see to be their increased status through the use of the friendly reaction to alcohol, while those who have been less successful manifest assertive or aggressive behavior when drinking to defend an identity threatened by their lack of access to identity-maintaining goods. Finally, Naskapi drinking interactions represent but one form of a class of phenomena that accompany economic change: Given a situation where economic change results in an increase of free-floating power, and a change in the means of access to things, persons, or behaviors which serve to maintain a desired identity, there will be an increase in identity struggles. These struggles will stem from either a threat to the power of established authority, contention for power among those for whom the status system has opened up, or from the uneven distribution of goods among those of once equal status. Further, the increase in identity struggles will produce an increase in the frequency of those activities or behaviors which serve in a given society as identity-resolving forums.

The extent that such forums permanently resolve identity struggles, however, is another matter. A person may give a potlatch, make a witchcraft accusation, or become assertive when drinking, attempting to resolve a contradiction between his view of himself and the way others view him, but may in the process threaten others who, in turn, may feel it necessary to give a potlatch, or make a witchcraft accusation. So while a person may resolve, at least temporarily, discrepancies in some of his social relationships, the whole process may lead to a steady spiral of identity struggles for the community at large, and hence lead to a steady increase in the frequency of those activities that serve as identity-resolving forums.

I began by drawing a parallel between those conditions that promote millenarian movements and those that promote increases in identity-resolving forums. It appears, however, that there are at least two differences in the antecedents of the two types of phenomena. First, in millenarian activities all participants are denied access to identity-confirming information (cf. A. Wallace 1970*b*), whereas when there is an increase in the frequency of identity-resolving forums only some members of the group are denied such access. Second, in millenarian activities the reference point from which participants measure their identity tends to be external to the group partaking of such activities. Put another way, the reference point tends to be the dominant group (see Burridge 1969). On the other hand, when one finds an increase in the frequency of occurrence of identity-resolving forums, one finds that the reference point for measuring identities lies within the group. If a New Guinea native includes within his field of competition the whites he has recently come into contact with, then his perceived failure at such competition will likely lead him to millenarian activities and beliefs. If, on the other hand, his field of competition includes only those of his own society or group then he will likely take recourse in competition manifested in those activities that serve in his society as identity-resolving forums. The Naskapi, for example, appear to be competing only with other Naskapi, and not, as yet, with Euro-Canadians or, for that matter, the more acculturated Montagnais, a proposition that is substantiated by the fact that only rarely do they engage in assertive or aggressive behavior with nonmembers of their community.

Finally, the hypothesis presented in this paper suggests we further examine economic aid programs, for, rather than introducing economic or social stability, they may, in fact, promote social instability and conflict by the mass introduction of new goods and resources, or by changing the means of access of persons to goods and activities vital in identity maintenance. If this is indeed the case we need to be able to determine the form this interpersonal conflict will take, and what cultural mechanisms will be used to resolve it.

Notes

1. The term *nishim* denotes both male and female younger siblings, and male and female younger parallel-cousins, although colleague contracts refer only to male relationships.

2. I was unable to obtain a native classification of goods available in Schefferville (if one, indeed, exists), so the scheme used here is based primarily on my observations of how goods were used.

3. This may be changing. The Naskapi now appear to be taking an interest in purchasing mail order clothing such as suits with the explicit aim of "dressing up."

4. My analysis of the effects of economic change differs somewhat at this point from Salisbury's (1962) analysis, for he states that indentured labor did not reduce the status differential between "big men" and others. I am assuming that since young men could free themselves from their obligations *sooner*, that the status differential was, in effect, reduced.

5. Actually, the two methods, distinguished by Middleton, appear to be complementary aspects of the same phenomenon with the same native term, *ole rozu*, applying to both.

IV. Alcohol Use in the Pacific Islands

Forms and Pathology of Drinking in Three Polynesian Societies

Edwin M. Lemert

Introduction

Studies of drinking by primitive peoples have ranged from descriptive treatment in single societies to large-scale uses of statistical data exemplified in the cross-cultural method employed by Horton (1943), and more recently by Field (1962). For those who prefer to move beyond a descriptive emphasis yet seek to keep generalizations about drinking within a societal context, the modern comparative method offers a possible alternative meeting ground. In any event it seems well adapted to inquiries as to how or to what degree drinking practices get integrated into whole cultures.

Bunzel (1940) initiated anthropological interest in the problem with her detailed comparison of "alcoholism" in two Central American cultures, concluding that drinking was a pivotal mechanism of social integration for one, the Chamula (Mexico), but for the other, the Chichicastenango (Guatemala), largely a symptomatic response to conflict-producing situations of extraneous origins. A number of single-culture studies, including those of Honigmann and Honigmann (1945), Mangin (1957), Lemert (1958), Heath (1958), Sangree (1962), and Field (1962), have stressed the integrative function of drinking in primitive societies along with considerable recognition of its importance in primary group formation and continuity. On the other hand, Gerald Berreman (1956), from his observations of drinking among Aleuts concluded that drinking can be integrative or disintegrative, tending to be a byproduct or symptomatic of the same factors which make for social disorganization.

Ullman (1958) proposed that rates of alcoholism, in the sense of addictive drinking, will vary indirectly with the degree to which drinking customs are well established and consistent with the rest of culture. The reciprocal of dissensus on drinking customs and values among different segments of society is ambivalence on the part of the individual towards his own drinking, which becomes the immediate causative agent in alcoholism. Simmons (1960), from his investigation of drinking among Peruvian villagers, found support for the first part of this hypothesis but not for the second. In other words, there may be a high degree of integration of drinking in a culture, a low rate of alcoholism, yet substantial ambivalence of attitudes towards the use of alcohol.

One of the difficulties complicating the study of integration of drinking practices in culture is the lack of an explicit meaning for the term *integration*. Thus Bunzel (1940) stated that the Chamula did not regard their drunkenness as a problem, but she herself did so regard it. Apparently she was impressed by the costs of their drunkenness in a different way than were the Indian drinkers, for she notes that they recognized and to some extent deplored the costs of their indulgence. This, together with the fact that ambivalence may coexist with culturally integrated drunkenness, suggests two significant perspectives from which drinking can be described: (1) the form and behavioral consequences of drinking as seen by the detached observer; (2) the situational valuations placed upon these by drinking participants and by those affected in the society, resulting in a kind of cost assessment.

Lemert (1962) argues that all that we know about alcohol use indicates that while it is socially integrative in the sense of bringing people together in ritual and convivial groups and useful to individuals for anaesthetizing psychic ills, nevertheless, certain costs are created thereby not only in economic terms but also in terms of threatening or destruction of societal and individual values. These costs, theoretically estimable in time, energy, and psychic stress, can serve as a measure to which drinking is culturally integrated or, conversely, nonintegrated or pathological.

It is a reasonable assumption that human beings at whatever cultural level become aware of costs of satisfying their values but that the action they take to minimize such costs is variable. Thus social control, not only to lessen insobriety, as Horton (1943) saw it, but to change the form of drinking or drunkenness, must be reckoned with as a factor in accounting for the integration or nonintegration of drinking in culture. The conditions under which social control of alcohol use emerges, the availability of means of control to those whose values are threatened, and the motivations and ability of individuals to utilize controls, are all important aspects of the complete analysis of cultural integration and drinking.

In this paper I will present some descriptive and interpretive materials on forms and pathology of drinking in three Polynesian societies which represent a historical continuum of contact and experience with alcohol and which, in my estimation, approximate a "series" in regard to its cultural integration. These are Tahiti and Bora Bora in the Society Islands; Aitutaki, Rarotonga, and Atiu in the Cook Islands; and Upolu and Savaii in Western

Samoa. With these data I hope to illuminate some of the possible relationships between forms of drinking, cultural values, costs, and social control, together with certain tentative conclusions in regard to addictive drinking.

The Historical Setting

Historical sources are unequivocal that Polynesians, like most of the Indians of America north of Mexico, were without alcoholic beverages in their pristine state. Liquor was first brought to Polynesians by European voyagers in the middle and late eighteenth century. While the original reaction to liquor was one of distaste, this soon changed to avid liking, and a lively trade grew up in many areas. Around 1800, escaped convicts from Botany Bay in Australia taught Hawaiians how to distill a highly potable liquor, *okole hao*, from the fructose sugars of the *ti* root. Hawaiians in turn carried their skills to the Society Islands, where the consumption of locally distilled liquor from *ti* root and breadfruit underwent a period of efflorescence and then decline. It was replaced by *ava anani*, a crude wine made from the juice of oranges, perfected by enological experiments conducted with a kind of early technical assistance program of whaling crews. In 1848 traveling Tahitians carried the techniques of brewing and drinking "orange beer," as it came to be called, to the Cook Islands, where much to the discomfiture of the missionaries, it quickly became established in a distinctive pattern of drinking known since 1910 as "bush beer schools."

While alcohol consumption quite early spread throughout most of Polynesia, Samoa in western Polynesia remained as a kind of brooding citadel of sobriety until quite recent times. Samoa, even more than the Pueblo Indians of our Southwest, stands as a classic case of cultural conservatism in relation to the readily diffusable and utilizable cultural item of alcohol.

Prototype Drinking

The prototype for patterns of alcohol consumption in all areas of Polynesia except New Zealand is found in the kava circle. Kava, an astringent infusion made from the root of the plant *Piper methysticum*, was everywhere drunk in sacred, ceremonial, and secular contexts. Drinkers customarily sat cross-legged in a circle and were served in a common cup from a fixed point by one or two persons charged with responsibility for its preparation. Drinking was pretty well confined to men, and it tended to be monopolized by chiefs and priests. In western Polynesia, especially Samoa and Tonga, kava drinking became a sacred ceremonial distinguishing titled from untitled persons and symbolically validating status differences between chiefs.

The linguistic continuity between Polynesian kava terms and those used for alcoholic drinks is unmistakable. At the same time, a common overlay of European influence is apparent from the use of such terms as *tuati* and *barmit* to designate the man given control over the drinking group, these being Polynesian conversions of steward and barmaid. In part, the older tendency to reserve distilled liquor for use by the ruling class has been perpetuated by "permit" systems which were set up by colonial administrators to control the distribution of imported liquors, to which chiefs and high ranking natives as well as white persons are allowed access.

Forms of Drinking—Festive

For purposes of description I have used a threefold classification to differentiate drinking in the three areas under consideration: festive, ritual-disciplined, and secular. These do not exhaust all of the forms of drinking in the areas but rather call attention to what I regard as the dominant patterns.

The earliest drinking in Tahiti and Bora Bora, on which there are data, was essentially festive in form. Fermented orange juice was added to food as an item around which feasts were organized, or by itself became the basis for festive indulgence. Festive drinking in Tahiti and Bora Bora took place during the orange harvest season, spring and early summer. While brew was made and drunk by families, the more spectacular fetes were collective enterprises of the village under the direction of one of several brewmasters called *aito* ("champions"). The work was done by ten to twenty-five helpers called *rima tauturu* ("hand helpers") who peeled and cut the oranges with a split bamboo knife and squeezed them through a cloth into a large barrel, which was then covered with a spray of leaves and buried for three to five days, depending upon the presence or absence of active dregs from previous brewings. When the brewmasters found by testing that two glasses produced intoxication, they pronounced it ready. The barrel was then hoisted by a sling and brought to the village for drinking.

Drinking was on a come-one-come-all basis but confined to married adults. Youths under twenty years were roughly driven away from the area and single women discouraged from attending. Drinkers sat in a circle around the barrel, with women in the front rows, to "show respect," and were served or helped themselves with a common coconut cup. Choral singing and dancing to the accompaniment of nose flutes and drums took place either in the vicinity of the barrel or in nearby houses. Festivities continued as long as *ava anani* remained in supply, which could mean several days. There was also an effort to program the brewing so that drinkers could move from one village to another on a rotation basis, and prolong the fete into one or several weeks.

On certain occasions, twice during the orange season according to one informant, drinkers from one or several villages retreated to an upland grove for nightlong drinking and dancing. At a critical point, drinkers were served small amounts of *namu*, distilled coconut toddy made for the occasion (possibly learned from Marquesans), which became a signal for the beginning of nude dancing and promiscuous sexual pairings. Such fetes were ended by passing out, exhaustion, or both. In some cases they were ended by the appearance of *mutois*, village police, for increasingly towards the end of the nineteenth century the French authorities actively sought to repress these drinking rites.

Although beverages, time, and place of drinking have changed, Tahitian drinking remains essentially festive in form. A blight on the orange groves and the dying off of foremost native brewmasters in the influenza epidemics of 1918 pretty well put an end to orange-brew making. In 1920, wine and beer were made available to Polynesians who were French citizens, and penalties against brewing were severely applied. Along with this, native drinking was structured by administrative manipulation of dispensing outlets and encouraging festive celebrations during July and at Christmastime.

The work week and increasing dependence on a money economy have further shaped drinking in the Society Islands, weekend drinking becoming commonplace, together with periodic small-scale recurrences of village type festive drinking when money becomes available to families from vanilla and copra crops. Society Islanders have a decided preference for beverages of low alcoholic content, especially beer at the present time, which undoubtedly is meaningful in terms of achieving desired physical and psychic states associated with their singing and dancing. Plateau drinking, or the "long slow drunk," in my opinion, aptly describes the ideal pattern of alcohol consumption for these people. Many Tahitians have indicated their dislike for strong liquor on grounds that it makes them *"très fatigués,"* or makes them go to sleep. As one cogently put it, "Two drinks of whiskey and you are no good."

Ritual-Disciplined Drinking

While festive drinking similar to that in Tahiti and Bora Bora appeared in the Cook Islands, the latter are noted for the growth of highly ritualized drinking. Indeed, the most distinctive patterns of drinking in all Polynesia are found in the so-called bush beer schools on the island of Atiu and, to a lesser extent, on Rarotonga and Aitutaki.

On Atiu, during the orange season, drinking was a daily occurrence and brewing a highly organized activity, tokened by the sound of the conch shell summoning the drinkers. One steward, a cook, and three helpers are delegated on a rotation basis to prepare and squeeze oranges while the rest of the group carries on its libations. Drinkers are ranged around the beer barrel, which until recent times was a hollowed-out base of a coconut tree called a *tumunui*. The drinkers numbered from six to twenty men, although jumbo groups of forty or sixty are not unknown on Sundays. The rule against female participation varies but it is very strict on Atiu, on the grounds that a drunken female is a highly disruptive and unesthetic element. Single men above twenty years are the core of the group, with older men and married men being the marginal participants. Drinking groups tend to get organized along kinship lines.

A drinking session on Atiu ordinarily begins with a single round of drinks, which is followed by a prayer and a church hymn. Then the *tuati* delivers a speech urging those present not to fight and to be careful on going home not to cause trouble. He then announces that the time has come for a good time and starts the coconut cup on its periodic rounds. There is considerable pressure on the individual to drink, although he may pass up a round. He may not, however, sip the drink, and if he tarries too long, the steward makes a quick stamping movement which scatters sand over the reluctant drinker.

Informal conversation covering sex, politics, fishing, and crops accompanies the drinking. Genealogies may be recited, and, even more distinctive, choral singing and the chanting of *utes* takes place. These utes deal with historic events, often those of drinking itself. If the beer barrel is a new one, it is dedicated by a specially composed ute, which heralds its great size or importance, in some cases by comparing it to cargo boats which have visited the islands.

Drinking is disciplined in a very real sense, for the *tuati,* who remains sober, has complete control over the session and may determine when a person has had too much to drink. When thirsty strays or roamers from other groups approach, he alone determines if they may join the drinkers. Troublemakers are evicted from the group and by common understanding are blacklisted by other groups. They remain on probation for a month or year, after which they are eligible for readmission to a school. The system works well enough, particularly on Atiu and the outer islands.

The Secular Drinking of Samoa

For purposes of describing and discussing drinking in Samoa I have employed the term *secular.* This classification is residual because Samoan drinking lacks all but the basic elements of patterning, is without ritual, and seldom if ever has it been the basis of village- or district-wide festive behavior. While it indirectly expresses some of the values of Samoan culture, it is much more conspicuously a mechanism or device through which individuals in group settings find release for a variety of unintegrated feelings and impulses. It has evolved under conditions of continuous prohibition.

Some surreptitious drinking was indulged in by Western Samoans under German rule, but the great mass of Samoans learned their brewing and drinking from New Zealand troops and government workers who took control of the island after 1914. American soldiers stationed on the islands during the last war also gave a big impetus to brewing through their willingness to pay extremely high prices for almost any kind of alcoholic drink. There has been very little use of native sugar-bearing fruits or plants for brewing. Imported ingredients, malt, hops, sugar, and yeast have been relied upon almost from the first to concoct brew. This, known in Samoan as *fa'amafu,* has a quite high alcoholic content, ranging from 12 to 18 or even 20 percent, suggesting its frequent fortification by the addition of spirits. Besides fa'amafu, Samoans consume considerable amounts of methylated spirits, which are "purified" by boiling in various ways.

Fa'amafu is manufactured in Samoan houses, *fales,* or in the bush, depending on the current degree of risk. It is made by women as well as men and there is an extensive illegal trade at a going price of two shillings per bottle. Some notion of the scale of brewing is gained from the situation in a village near Salailua, on Savaii, where there are at least twenty brewmakers for an adult male population of two hundred fifty. At least one of these brewers averages an output of two hundred twenty-six-ounce bottles per week. The brewer usually sells his surplus to finance his own drinking; women brewers supply their drinking spouses and sell the rest to meet family expenses.

Drinking takes place either in the bush or in unused fales in the back part of the villages. Drinkers sit in a circle, and the host who has made or bought the beer serves, sometimes using one glass, sometimes several. While some etiquette is observed, it is quite generalized. Guitar playing and singing occur but drinking interaction more commonly is in the form of discussion and gossip. Large groups, such as are sometimes found in the Cook Islands, are absent because of the risk of arrest. Participants generally are young, untitled, single men, and one of the impressive facts about Samoan drinkers is the extremely young age at which they have begun. In one village on Savaii, a sample poll showed that 66 percent of the *taulelea* had begun to drink before the age of fifteen. Beyond a few exceptions in the Apia area, Samoan women do not drink—not because of any rule to the effect, but because they find liquor distasteful or unappealing.

In both the Cook Islands and Samoa, liquor is an indispensable means of recruiting labor for certain kinds of work. In Samoa it has been found that money will not induce workers to carry out tasks of clearing and planting on small plantations. Workers for this are usually rounded up by a foreman with the promise of *mea miti*, "something to sip." This takes the form of several bottles of brew for a four o'clock drinking session after the day's work has been done.

Drinking Pathology

In keeping with my introductory statements, drinking pathology here refers to drinking which is costly to society and costly to the individual, costs taken to be the extent to which other values are sacrificed in order to satisfy those associated with drinking. In this broad sense drinking pathology does exist in Polynesia, although care must be taken to specify whose value hierarchies are being invoked when the costs of drinking are assessed.

French authorities in Papeete are convinced that drinking is a very serious problem among their Polynesian peoples, primarily because they see earnings of the native population going for heavy weekend drinking and periodic, fete-type indulgence instead of into housing and other forms of material self-improvment. They are also distressed by the growing number of traffic accidents and injuries in the Papeete area which are traceable to intoxication. Yet it is doubtful that Tahitians see their expenditures for liquor as sacrifices in the same sense as do the French, largely because as yet their commitment to material values is still quite tenuous. In fact, it can be argued that many Tahitians work or grow crops to obtain money for the indulgent pleasures it makes possible. Thus when one informant was asked why his fellows use their money for liquor instead of better housing and furniture, he laughed and said the Tahitian is likely to say: "If I spend money for those things I won't have any for beer and wine." Even when Tahitians are motivated to spend money for material improvement, they are compelled to put first the hospitality claims which relatives and others have on the products of their land or earnings, which often means that it goes for a communal drinkfest.

Intoxication does lead to quarreling and fighting among Tahitians, which run contrary to their values, but the overt aggression involved is mild, being mostly verbal, or random pushing and slapping. Stones or weapons are never used. Fights between drunken Tahitian women are far more spectator-inspiring than those between men, and women are not reluctant to tackle a male they find offensive. This reveals some of the essential personality characteristics of males who, when sober, are quiet, shy, and almost timid. It also suggests one of the main motivations for male drinking—to overcome shyness sufficiently to make sexual approaches to their women. This, in turn, is probably related to residual sacred values which sexual communion has for Society Islanders under certain circumstances.

As in other societies, drunken quarrels between spouses are common, but the wife can usually give a good account of herself in these. Both the husbands and the wives are apt to vent their hostilities towards one another by seeking out another sexual partner rather than through physical combat. This is capriciously interactional, but eventually the two are reunited, usually through the offices of a pastor. In the background of this are older cultural values disapproving of sexual jealousy.

Intoxication or its effects does run directly contrary to health values and to important native values of excelling in sports and physical prowess, and this may be one of the more important psychic stresses created by drinking. It is significant that fairly successful organized programs of sports have been instrumental in decreasing drinking in certain areas, particularly where there is a strong authority figure, such as a church pastor. This usually operates through an older movement of nineteenth-century European origins, the Blue Cross, which prescribes a self-imposed taboo on drinking for given periods of time. The agreement is ordinarily written out on a piece of paper in the presence of a priest, pastor, judge, or a doctor. This strongly resembles an individual variant of the old technique by which chiefs tabooed scarce food items to allow for a period of retrenchment.

I conclude that drinking and intoxication have been and still are reasonably well integrated with the basic values of Society Island peoples. Liquor undoubtedly is instrumental in the periodic satisfaction of esoteric values which natives can only vaguely phrase as *la vie tahitienne*. Central to these is the value of psychic rapport overtly symbolized by collective eating, singing, dancing, and sexual communion. The preference of Tahitians for low or moderate alcohol beverages and slow drinking suggests an adaptation of the pattern of drinking to achieve or preserve physiological states compatible with these values. While the results of intoxication contravene certain of their values, these people seem to have a technique for bringing them under control which, at least in certain contexts, appears to be effective. Their drinking, of course, is contrary to the demands of a wage-work economy, and, as they are more drawn into such an economy, the form of their drinking can be expected to change, presumably in a more secular direction.

Drinking Pathology in the Cook Islands

Drinking by natives of the Cook Islands is now and has been illegal for many decades. Quite early it was condemned by the dominant Protestant mission or church of the islands. In earlier years drinking and drunkenness were the main expression of anticlericalism and cultural reaction, clearly indicated by missionary references to their native opposition as the "drunken party" in their writings. At one time youthful bush drinkers, influenced by Tahitian migrants, conducted military drill, which hinted at more than symbolic resistance to the new religion. This led to a historic compromise between the recalcitrant drinkers and a perceptive missionary, James Chalmers, 1903, who was an early advocate of cooptative philosophy not unlike the American idea: "If you can't lick 'em, join 'em." In effect, an organizational syncretism grew up in which, according to a Rarotongan proverb, "The church was taken as a lap child on one knee." The missionary church was transformed into a native institution, and, while formally repudiating the use of liquor, at the same time allowed for the evolution of a patterned evasion of Christian temperance ideology (Lovett 1903).

Cook Islands society, in my estimation, represents an equilibrium or a contrapuntal balance between Christian, Western values and many of the older values and organization of native society. Patterned evasion of the law has been facilitated by a continuity of experience in the life history of the male adult, which permits a conventionalized inconsistency between creed and action. Thus, many church members—even deacons and occasionally pastors—have youthful histories of participation in beer schools. Today it is not unusual for a married man to attend church on Sunday morning, then change his clothes and join a beer school for the rest of the day. Respected church members are known to cooperate in supplying *kava ainga*, beer for work gangs on their plantations.

Most of the police in Rarotonga and elsewhere in the islands are church deacons and they have an espionage system which keeps them well apprised of brewing and drinking activities. Until 1950 fines for brewing were divided three ways: one part for the government, one for the church, and one for the arresting officer, who sometimes split this with informants. This suggests that law enforcement in relation to liquor offenses was in reality a taxation system, in which the church had a stake. It is also known that brewing and drinking by persons with high status seldom has resulted in arrest or fines. This is consistent with older feudalistic exploitive patterns and notions of monopoly of liquor for chiefs. Status is protected in other ways; thus the wife or relative of a man caught brewing often pleads guilty in his place. Arguments in court usually concern who is guilty rather than whether the illegal act occurred.

A somewhat idyllic illustration of the spirit of compromise between drinkers and law agents occurred in Atiu during the orange season about ten years ago. Getting sufficient oranges to fill the cargo vessel was imperative if it was to be induced to call again. Yet orange beer drinkers threatened to consume the oranges as fast as they ripened. Consequently the resident commissioner asked all the beer school stewards to bring their tumunui to police headquarters, with the promise that they would be returned after the cargo was made. The arrangement was dutifully observed on both sides and drinking resumed after the ship had sailed.

Unquestionably, Cook Island drinkers are much more aggressive than those in the Society Islands. Disputes often arise in drinking sessions over women, land, and genealogies, and they not infrequently end in fights with fists or with sticks. Men become hungry when they drink and mistreat their wives when they wander home late and food is not immediately made available to them. Sometimes wives retaliate by informing on their husbands, which aggravates the quarrels.

The men of Atiu are even more hostile and aggressive when intoxicated than are those from the other islands, reflecting something of the history of their reputation as invincible and ruthless warriors. A fair number of brutal assaults and murders have followed drinking sessions on their island. At the same time, it is to be noted that their drinking discipline is stronger and their rule against female drinking stricter than elsewhere. One gets the impression that male Atiuans enjoy their warlike image from the past and may see the assaults and murders as its contemporary validation.

Drinking Pathology in Samoa

Western Samoa most clearly exemplifies a Polynesian society in which the consequences of intoxication directly threaten or destroy cherished values which are central to the *fa'a Samoa*, the "Samoan way." This was frequently captioned in statements made by paramount chiefs and the minister of police during my last visit, who stated in several ways and on different occasions that "drinking is the most serious problem we have."

Samoan society differs from that of the Society and Cook islands in that it successfully absorbed Christianity, resisted foreign domination, and maintained its village-based social organization relatively intact. Its conservative emphasis is revealed by the values placed on conformity, acceptance of group decisions, ceremonial compliance, and politeness in interpersonal interaction. The dominance of these values is guaranteed by a prompt and rough system of social control, administered by the *matai* ("chiefs"). Respect for the matai who make and carry out decisions is crucial to its continued functioning.

It can be expected that this kind of system, particularly inasmuch as it makes no place for direct contradiction and openly symbolized hostility, will develop a deep substratum of aggression in its members which readily comes to the surface with intoxication. The focus of drunkenness and aggression appears among the *taulelea,* the young, untitled men, upon whom fall the greatest demands for silent conformity and respect. It is also true that their aggressiveness is in part culturally inculcated, that it is encouraged in certain kinds of structured situations.

A fairly common occurrence is for a drunken taulelea to stand at one end of a village and shout drunken defiance and challenge to any and all who wish to test him in combat. This, even when not motivated by hostility towards the matai, is nevertheless a desecration of Samoan custom, an insult to the whole village and particularly to the *matai.* In other instances drunken young men parade in front of the chief's house, which is sacred ground, shouting insults and threats. In some cases *matai* have been attacked physically.

Samoan aggression differs from that met with in Tahitians and Cook Islanders in being cumulative, slow burning, and explosive. In some forms it comes very close to the psychiatric concept of "free-floating" aggression, subject to hair-trigger release. A Samoan may brood for weeks over what he regards as an injustice and then with an apparently trivial provocation burst into a murderous rage. Moreover Samoans often fight with rocks in their hands or with bush knives, which cause serious injuries and deaths. Such offenses cannot be handled easily through village justice; they bring the offenders to the attention of central authorities, thus adding a further dimension of stress to the system. The problem has been sufficiently distinctive that a local jurist has proposed legal recognition of criteria of provocation differing from those applicable to Anglo-Saxon societies (Marsack 1959).

Rapes, in which drunken Samoans beat up a man and take away his girl, are not uncommon. Rough beatings of wives by drunken husbands also occur, and children may be harmed. A frequent form of drunken aggression against wives is the destruction of all the furniture in the fale, and I encountered cases in which a man's drunken rage had led him to burn down the fale. Wives are far from acquiescent in the face of such treatment and the economic deprivation drinking causes. A substantial number have left their heavily drinking spouses and sought divorces.

While there are Samoan villages in which brewing and drunkenness are effectively controlled, there still are periodic outbreaks of disorder. This usually happens when a split or a cleavage appears among members of the village council. Most villages have their "drinking matai," who sit solemnly in council, pass rules against drinking, and fine liquor offenders. These same matai at times may be found drinking with taulelea or be driven to buy brew from them. This gives a further impetus to the slow erosion of their authority already at work from other intrusive forces.

Conclusion

It seems clear that cultural conservatism has importantly shaped the forms of drinking in the three Polynesian societies under consideration, although it has asserted itself in quite variable ways. Undoubtedly the perspectives and decisions of administrators from the wine-drinking culture of France have helped give form to drinking in the Society Islands, especially in the light of their willingness or conscious efforts to preserve native cultural practices through organized fetes. The replacement of Protestant Anglo-Saxon missionaries by Catholics beginning in 1840 likewise tempered the climate of drinking. Beyond these factors, a variety of others, ecological, those of physical isolation, and perhaps sex ratio of the population, have had a bearing on the permutations of drinking in these islands. While the persistence of Tahitian values requires a more complete explanation, there is little question that intoxication has had a significant function in their recurrent expression and validation.

The drinking group in the Cook Islands, originally a collective reaction to institutional stresses, evolved into a form which also serves to maintain continuity with older cultural values and to preserve certain types of organization. Some of my data suggest that kinship patterns are articulated and probably strengthened through drinking experiences. Despite extensive study by legislative committees in recent years, no significant changes have been made in the church-government system of control of drinking in these islands.

In both the Society Islands and in the Cook Islands, the more intimate drinking situations serve to promote in-group solidarity by releasing symbolic aggression against governing elites, although in true Polynesian tradition it is linguistically subtle and well concealed. I do not regard it as a central element in the drinking in either area.

In Western Samoa the determination by traditional native elites to maintain the old way of life in the face of increasing contact and interaction with the outside world had made it difficult for the government to entertain alternatives to the makeshift permit system of liquor distribution which denies it to all save a few native Samoans. The situation has been complicated by hostility towards Europeans and the half-caste population who have strongly advocated liberalizing the law. When pushed too hard on the issue, Samoan leaders have spoken ominously of prohibition for all, a threat which today has pretty well silenced the voices of thirsty Europeans in Apia.

Everywhere the form of drinking shows evidence of the close association which exists between drinking and cycles of work and play in Polynesian society. The heaviest burden of work rests upon young, unmarried males, and even from aboriginal times it may have had qualities of exploitation and anomie. Entrance into the money economy and wage work have imposed daily and weekly routines and goals which are alien and tension-creating for Polynesians. As this increases, heavy weekend drinking and periodic indulgence, coupled with absenteeism, can be expected to figure large in the labor problems of these people.

Numerous data reveal that control of drinking can be and has been successfully organized in the three societies under consideration. However, status rivalry, which is endemic in Polynesia, complicates control by producing cleavages in authority. This does much to explain the so-called outbreaks of drunkenness commented on in historical accounts of these societies and currently observable in Samoa.

Alcoholism in the sense of addictive drinking, with complex personality changes and serious organic pathology, such as cirrhosis of the liver, is nowhere found among full-blooded Polynesians. The only such case I was able to locate, despite persistent and careful inquiries, was that of a noble in Tonga, and his was clearly that of a deviant. At the same time cases do occur in all areas, but especially in Samoa, of persons who have drunk very heavily—to the detriment of their family life—and have beginning physical complications such as gastritis. In addition, I met a few on Savaii who told me they got sick if they didn't drink, by which they meant that their hands would shake. Yet equally impressive is the large number of heavy drinkers who have successfully stopped their drinking.

One fact which may be important to note in understanding the absence of organic pathology among heavy drinkers in Polynesia is that, in contradiction to patterns of drinking found in our urban society, indulgence stimulates appetite. It is not unusual for a late-carousing Samoan to disturb the whole household rummaging around for food before he goes to sleep. Food and the well-rounded belly stand high in the order of Polynesian values, with at least as much anxiety surrounding eating as drinking. This may help explain why the development of gastritis and interference with food assimilation by drinking become a motive for giving up liquor in some cases.

Another relevant paramount value for Polynesians is that of psychic rapport with one's fellows. Destructive drinking ultimately thwarts the desire for this state by isolating the drinker from relatives and friends; it may cause him to lose his wife, and above all, his children, through divorce. Yet Polynesian ideology and institutions provide no support for "living alone and liking it." The pleasures of solitary drinking, which is almost a contradiction in Polynesia, are poor recompense for the isolated drinker's losses.

A final consideration is that guilt over drinking or drunkenness does not seem to develop in Polynesian society. A person is in no way disadvantaged by a history of drunkenness, particularly after renouncing drinking. Samoans, when they think on the problem, objectify liquor; typically they ask the question as to whether "this liquor is good for *me*?" or "for Samoans?" They seldom think in terms of whether it is morally right or wrong to drink or get drunk. Such attitudes, I believe, leave Polynesians relatively free to utilize what we would regard as naive methods to stop drinking. They are, however, consistent with the system of overt avoidances and compliances which seem to be characteristic of Polynesian education methods and social control.

The Samoan case clearly is a negative one insofar as Ullman's hypothesis is concerned, for here is a society in which drinking practices are unintegrated culturally and disruptive in extreme, yet addictive drinking has not developed. At most it can be said that individual Samoans develop relatively serious drinking problems; however, they do not eventuate in organic pathology and psychic deterioration of the sort characterizing much alcoholism in Western societies. I am inclined to explain this on the basis of the kinds of values contravened by intoxication, the possible physiological effects of values on the form of drinking (eating), and the ways in which a particular kind of social organization confronts the individual with the costs of his intoxicated behavior.

In general, my survey indicates that values are a crucial factor in understanding the forms, cultural integration, and pathology of drinking. It also argues that the study of values must be supplemented by study of social organization and social control in order to determine which values and costs become dominant in a society or are brought to bear in drinking situations. In societies in which moralistic concepts of drinking and stigma-management problems of drinkers are absent, a value-cost model may explain the absence of addictive drinking in individuals as well as be useful to account for the collective forms of drinking. Possibly it may have uses in understanding how drinking histories are interrupted or truncated short of addiction in our own society.

Holy and Unholy Spirits:
The Effects of Missionization on
Alcohol Use in Eastern Micronesia

Mac Marshall and Leslie B. Marshall

A frequent theme in Pacific history is the well-known antipathy that existed for much of the nineteenth century between missionaries and other foreigners residing in the islands. Although this antipathy was especially pronounced between missionaries and beachcombers, it also existed between missionaries and a variety of other expatriates—for example, blackbirders, traders, and whalers.[1] The antagonism between missionaries and the beach communities has been variously attributed to the missionaries' Puritanism; to the hypocritical and narrow-minded morals of the missionaries; to the lawlessness, degeneracy, and debauchery of the beach communities; and to economic conflicts of interest between the two groups. While all of these matters undoubtedly contributed to the mutual animosity that existed, they do not offer—singly or collectively—a satisfactory explanation of the rancor so frequently expressed on both sides.

Focusing on the Congregationalist missionaries of the American Board of Commissioners for Foreign Missions (ABCFM) who went to Micronesia, and on the beach communities that existed in the eastern Caroline, Gilbert, and Marshall islands in the nineteenth century, the antipathy between these two groups is here explained as a fundamental clash in life-style and values that reflected a similar clash occurring at home in the United States. Each group viewed the other as a threat to its prestige, power, and position, and the issue was thus joined as a political struggle for control over the future of the island communities. As in most political contests, symbols became critically important for distinguishing one side from the other. In the case at hand it is argued that alcoholic beverages became the primary symbol which the Protestant missionaries used not only in their struggle with the beach communities, but also in their struggles with local political elites and foreign colonial governments: one either supported the missionary cause (the cause of the Holy Spirit) and abjured alcoholic beverages or one supported the cause of 'evil' and embraced unholy spirituous liquors. One was either a good Christian or one was not, and one's faith was measured by one's abstinence from alcohol.

Sustained foreign contact with the islands of eastern Micronesia began in the 1820s, accompanying the expansion of the whaling industry in the "on-the-line" and "off-Japan" whaling grounds. Sporadically at first, whalers began to call at some of the islands for provisions, and the number of such visits grew rapidly in the 1830s. During the 1830s and 1840s the continued growth of the whaling industry in the western Pacific led to increased contacts between whalers and Micronesians. By 1844 the American whaling fleet alone consisted of 675 vessels, crewed by sixteen thousand men, most of whom were in the Pacific Ocean. This fleet grew to over 700 ships by 1846, and "the eight years between 1846 and 1854 transcended all others in Pacific Sperm whaling" (Dakin 1934:65, 107). Whaleships were so numerous in Micronesian waters during this period that they "spoke" to each other almost daily, and several ships would put into a single island at once for supplies and "recreation." When this occurred, a hundred or more men would be loosed on the local populace and the resulting carouse often wrought havoc in the local community. In addition to simultaneous visits by several vessels, some of the whaling bases would be "blessed" with extended stays by a single ship of up to four months (Jones 1861; Borden 1961).

The brunt of this onslaught in Micronesia was borne by the high islands of Guam, Kusaie, and Ponape because they offered more to the whalers than the atolls in terms of food, wood, water, and room to roam. All three of these islands also possess excellent deep-water, sheltered harbors in which the ships could safely anchor. Truk, on the other hand, acquired an early reputation for ferocity that caused whalers to shun it, and which delayed missionization and the establishment of resident traders until the 1880s (Hezel 1973). It has been estimated that an average of thirty whalers a year called at Guam from the 1820s to the 1850s (Doty 1972). The report of the missionary "voyage of exploration" to Micronesia in 1852 states that at that time Kusaie received an average of twelve ships a year; from 1852 to 1856 seventy-five ships visited Kusaie, and "at the beginning of October [1856], twenty ships were anchored at Lele" (*Missionary Herald* 1853; Lewis 1967:31). Ponape hosted even greater numbers of whalers during the 1840s and 1850s. So heavy was the traffic—especially visits by American whalers from New England—that Kiti in Ponape and Port Lele in Kusaie became known to whalers as "the little Bangor and New Bedford of the South Seas" (Borden 1961:42).

Concurrent with the whalers, beachcombers began to move into the islands of eastern Micronesia in the late 1820s. By 1830 a few such men had established themselves on Ponape and Nauru, and the first known beachcombers in the Gilberts, Robert Grey and John Kirby, landed respectively on Makin in 1834 and on Kuria in 1838 from English whalers (Maude 1968*a*; Wilkes 1845). By the late 1830s the beachcomber colony on Ponape had swelled in numbers to between twenty-five and thirty, and there were thirteen Europeans living on Nauru (Maude 1968*a*). When Wilkes picked up Kirby and Grey in 1841 Kirby stated that there were six other Europeans living in the Gilberts: "An Englishman and an American reside on Nukunau. . . . The other four are on Peru Island" (Wilkes 1845:106–7). In the same year, "upwards of sixty" beachcombers were said to be living on Ponape, and this number seems to have remained relatively stable until 1846 (Simpson 1844:103; Cheyne 1852). The small atoll of Ngatik, south of Ponape, had "four Englishmen and about twenty Bornabi [Ponape] natives, male and female, residing there [in 1846]. They rear pigs, which they sell to the whale ships" (Cheyne 1852:123). According to published accounts in *The Friend*, Captain Calott of the *Hobeoricock* found four foreigners on Kusaie, and Captain Hull of the *Romulus* estimated that "about 150 foreigners" were resident on Ponape in about 1850 (*Friend* 1850:68). At approximately the same time "an estimated sixty" beachcombers were scattered throughout the Gilberts (Maude and Doran 1966:275).

From tabulations of the number of beachcombers reported for Ponape in different years supplied by Maude (1968*a*), Riesenberg (1968*a*), and Shineberg (1971), and from scattered data for other islands, it is clear that Ponape was indisputably the beachcomber "capital" of eastern Micronesia in the first half of the nineteenth century. From 1840 to the mid-1850s, Ponape supported at least four times as many foreign residents as any other island in the vicinity excluding Guam.[2] The number of beachcombers on Ponape seems to have peaked around 1850. By 1855 they had dwindled to twenty-five, although in 1877 there were fifty whites on the island including missionaries (O'Brien 1971; Westwood 1905).

Just as the beachcombers overlapped with the whalers, so the traders overlapped with both groups. As noted above in reference to Ngatik, many beachcombers engaged in barter trade with the whaleships—particularly on Ponape, Kusaie, and in the Gilberts. Nevertheless by the 1840s full-time traders began to come on the scene and trading companies began to make their presence felt (Maude 1968*b*; Shineberg 1971). The first resident traders in the Gilberts, Richard Randell and George Durant, set up shop on Butaritari in 1846, and soon thereafter "the firm of Smith, Randell and Fairclough was formed and a regular shipping line established between Sydney and Butaritari" (Maude and Doran 1966:276). While Andrew Cheyne failed to implement his grand scheme for organizing the trade on Ponape in 1843, his influence in the area was maintained as he continued to trade extensively in Micronesia for the next twenty years (Shineberg 1971).

Most trade in eastern Micronesia north of the Gilberts remained in the hands of beachcombers until the 1860s. Trading vessels plied Micronesian waters, to be sure, but resident traders were not yet established in the islands. Persons who are often referred to as 'traders' in the literature (e.g., Kirkland on Kusaie in 1852), actually were nothing more than settled beachcombers and were not in the employ of any of the companies that eventually came to dominate Micronesian trade.

No later than 1864 resident traders began to move into the Marshalls and eastern Carolines. The German firm of Stapenhorst and Hoffschläger in Honolulu placed Adolf Capelle on Ebon to purchase coconut oil in 1864 (Finsch 1893), and Capelle later founded his own firm on Jaluit. By the 1870s resident traders were widespread over the eastern Micronesia region. Most of these men were in the employ of five major trading firms: the German enterprises, Hernsheim and Company and Godeffroy and Son; the American businesses, Crawford and Company and Wightman Brothers; and the British firm of Henderson and MacFarlane.

Trading companies in the Gilberts centered on Butaritari. Morrell reports that Godeffroy failed there in the 1870s, "and in 1883–4 the Sydney firm of Ong Chong and Company held first and Hernsheims second place" (1960:272). Morrell also notes that Henderson and MacFarlane was present in 1883 and that by at least 1886 Wightman Brothers also was represented. Interestingly, both MacCallum and Stevenson, who were on Butaritari in 1889, mention only the presence of Crawford and Company and Wightman Brothers, although MacCallum (1934) informs us that there were white traders on all islands in the Gilberts except Abemama (and, presumably, its satellites Kuria and Aranuka) in that year. Whatever the case, at the time the British established a protectorate over the Gilberts in 1893 Crawford and Company had gone bankrupt and ceased trading, and Wightman Brothers and the Jaluit Gesellschaft (formerly Hernsheim and Company) had abandoned the Gilberts trade, with the result that the field was left solely to Ong Chong and Company until after World War I when the Japanese Nanyo Boeki Kaisha began trading on Butaritari and Makin (Maude and Doran 1966).

In the Marshall Islands a major entrepôt was built on Jaluit Atoll, beginning in the mid-1870s. Hernsheims and Capelle and Company were represented by 1877, and Crawford and Company had a store there by at latest 1884 (Bridge 1886; Finsch 1893; Humphrey 1887). In the mid-1880s, it was said of Jaluit that "one may buy almost any object of the civilized world . . . from sail needles to sewing machines, from ship's bread [biscuit] to Strasbourg goose liver patties" (Finsch 1886:2–3). Henderson and MacFarlane had their major station on Majuro at this time, and other traders were known to be on Arno, Likiep, and Namorik atolls (Bridge 1886; Dana 1935; Moss 1889; Dewar 1892; Westwood 1905).

George Westbrook represented Henderson and MacFarlane on Pingelap for more than a year in 1878–79, and on Mokil for several months in 1879–80. He also mentions a trader, James Currie, resident on Nukuoro in 1880, and traders named Jack Reece and George Barrows are reported for Kapingamarangi in the late 1870s and early 1880s (Dana 1935; Westwood 1905). There was already a trader living on Lukunor Atoll when the first missionaries went there from Ponape late in 1873, and soon thereafter John Westwood began a six-year sojourn (1877–83) on Lukunor trading for Henderson and MacFarlane (Doane 1874; Westwood 1905). In the valuable account of his adventures, Westwood (1905) mentions traders on Satawan in 1878, on Namoluk, Puluwat, and Ulul in 1881, and another trader in competition with him on Lukunor (representing a German firm) in 1882. Narruhn, Nedelec, and Hartmann, the first traders to enter the long-dreaded islands of Truk Lagoon, did so in the 1880s, and in 1887 Japanese firms activated trade in the eastern Carolines. By 1891 Japanese traders were settled ashore on Truk and Ponape (Purcell 1971). Thus while traders began to replace beachcombers in the late 1840s, the process required twenty to thirty years before it was completed.

It is important to have this perspective on the commercial and contact history of the area in order to understand the situation encountered by the first missionaries who moved into eastern Micronesia in 1852. Micronesians, by that time, had had thirty years of ever-accelerating contact with Europeans, from whom they had learned many things, suffered many things, and about whom they had formed decided opinions. Standard patterns of inter-ethnic relations had evolved, and crucial to these were the major trade items of the day: tobacco, firearms, and alcoholic beverages. The beach community life-style and the modus operandi that they had developed for interacting with the islanders were anathema to the missionaries.

By almost any measure the beach communities of the Pacific in the nineteenth century were composed of a tough, brawling lot. The islands represented a frontier situation,

> . . . perhaps the ultimate frontier where the European cultural streams moving west via America met those moving east via Australia—and the beachcombers were the spearhead, the first pioneers, of these streams; the counterpart of Turner's Indianized hunters, trappers and squawmen living beyond the pale of western civilization. [Maude 1968a:161]

Although whalers and traders did not live "beyond the pale of western civilization" in the same way as the beachcombers, they too were frontiersmen in the Pacific in a very real sense: they explored and mapped much of the frontier and they were the major source of outside contact for many Pacific Islanders during the nineteenth century. Unlike beachcombers, however, most traders and whalers were not absorbed into island societies, and they continued to rely on the outside world for physical and psychological support. Missionaries and government officials, representing "civilization," generally came to the islands later than members of the beach communities, and they usually came from a very different stratum of society. The difference in class backgrounds of these two groups at home (principally in the United States and in the British empire) was a major reason for their clash on the Pacific frontier, just as their attitudes and values came into conflict in the American West.

While voices occasionally were raised in defense of the beach community, most observers were repulsed by its excesses. This is so even if we discount the writings of the missionaries (see Bridge 1886; Moss 1889). Several themes run repeatedly through this commentary: the beach communities were characterized by frequent fighting (and occasional homicide), sexual indulgence with island women, rough language, and above all hard drinking.

The importance of alcoholic beverages in the beach communities is emphasized over and over again from the earliest descriptions through to more recent accounts. Discussing his observations at Nauru in 1843, Captain Simpson of the *Giraffe* provides the following sketch of life ashore:

> This island, and many others in the Pacific, are infested by Europeans, who are either runaway convicts, expirees or deserters from whalers. . . . They live in a manner easily to be imagined from men of this class, without either law, religion, or education, to control them, with an unlimited quantity of ardent spirits which they obtain from distilling the toddy that exudes from the cocoa-nut tree. This spirit is not very palatable, but it serves, to use their own expression, to tickle the brain; when under the influence of intoxication the most atrocious crimes are committed by these miscreants. [1844:101]

Alcohol was an integral part of nearly every social occasion in the beach community. Jones mentions a visit in 1852 to Butaritari aboard the *Emily Morgan* in which they discovered the crew of the bark *S.* of New Bedford already ashore: "The crew of this vessel, including the captain and officers, with ten or twelve beachcombers, were engaged in making coconut rum, and all hands, natives included, were as drunk as rum could make them" (1861:249). MacCallum describes the meeting of the *Emma Crawford* and the *Equator* at sea in the vicinity of the Gilberts: in response to a request to carry a letter to San Francisco, "the captain's answer was, Sure, if you have anything to drink aboard, I haven't tasted a drop of liquor for two weeks. We lowered a boat, and the old man went aboard the bark, with a case of square face gin, which was joyfully received by the crew of the Crawford" (1934:302). Even when wrecked on an island far from home, the crew of a ship lost in the Marshall Islands wasted little time in salvaging a case of gin and becoming roaring drunk (Mahlmann 1918). Accounts also exist in the literature of men in the beach communities suffering from delirium tremens, and of men occasionally drinking themselves to death (Dana 1935; Mahlmann 1918). Whether the port was Lahaina, Apia, Papeete, or Ponape, sailors who had been cooped up at sea for weeks or months on end looked upon shore leave as a time of total release. At such times seamen often "ran riot in drink and debauchery" (Wood 1875:51).

Alcohol played a leading role in blackbirding, or the "labor trade" as it is more politely known. Scarr maintains that "few abstemious masters sailed in the labour trade" and he recounts several examples of blackbirders unable to manage their ships properly when under the influence of alcohol (1970:234). Worse yet, Wawn (1973) reports a labor recruiter committing suicide from the effects of drink, and Bromage (1892) and Speiser (1913) specifically mention alcoholic beverages used to entice islanders aboard to be kidnapped or as payment for recruits. That black-birders were active in the Gilberts until the 1890s is widely known, but they also carried out their depredations elsewhere in eastern Micronesia, for example, the Mortlocks, Pingelap, Nuku-oro, and the Marshalls (Doane 1874; Dana 1935; J. Alexander 1895; Wood 1875).

The evidence is overwhelming that Micronesians lacked alcoholic beverages at European contact. While the islanders might obtain an occasional bottle of gin or rum from a passing ship, they did not learn to manufacture their own strong drink until foreigners settled among them. Beachcombers lost no time in teaching the islanders that fermented coconut toddy made an alcoholic beverage that could be increased in potency through distillation, and the techniques of manufacture were well known all over the Gilberts and on Ponape and Kusaie by the 1850s. Marshallese apparently did not learn the process until the 1860s and 1870s, and Trukese had no locally produced alcoholic beverages until at least the late 1880s and possibly the 1890s (Marshall and Marshall 1975). Teaching the islanders to manufacture alcohol from coconut toddy was widely assailed as the worst legacy of the beach community in Micronesia (e.g., J. Alexander 1895; Cheyne 1852; Crawford and Crawford 1967; Simpson 1844).

Alcoholic beverages remained very important in the beach community long after traders replaced beachcombers as the major influence in the islands. As trading centers became established on such islands as Jaluit, Ponape, and Butaritari, bars or "grog shops" sprang up to cater for the men of commerce, and, of course, for those islanders who had the money to frequent the saloons (Humphrey 1887). An infamous American black, known as "Black Tom" Tilden, ran a saloon on Jaluit (after he was forced to give up trading on Arno by the local populace) from the late 1870s until well into the 1880s (Dana 1935; Humphrey 1887; Kurze 1887). A second grop shop, run by a man named Sanders, also existed on Jaluit in 1884, and one of the two saloons had a billiards table (Humphrey 1887). Butaritari boasted two saloons when Robert Louis Stevenson visited the atoll in 1889, each operated under the aegis of one of the two trading companies then present on the island. These two taverns were frequented by a very different clientele: The Land We Live In, a Crawford and Company enterprise, was tended by an American black named Williams and catered for ships' crews; the Sans Souci, operated for Wightman Brothers by "Norwegian Tom," served ships' captains, officers, and other "aristocrats" (MacCallum 1934; Stevenson 1971). Such a division of accommodation was not peculiar to Butaritari. Ralston, for example, writes that in Honolulu in 1824, "there were numerous shanty grog shops kept by runaway sailors but there were others 'fitted up in a superior style, for the exclusive accommodation of Yeris [chiefs] and ships' officers, admission being refused to Kanackas and sailors' " (1970:91). Even in what was by then the missionary stronghold on Ponape Captain Narruhn ran a saloon in 1898 (*Missionary Herald* 1898). While some of the drinking in these bars was probably restrained, much of it was very rowdy. Jaluit was described in the 1880s as "the place where they say that they always know when Sunday comes round, from the people being worse drunk than in the rest of the week, and I think it is true: but I never saw them sober any day" (Churchward 1888: 102–3).

The traders did not restrict their drinking to their periodic visits to the commercial centers such as Jaluit, however. Trading vessels that called from island to island always carried a large stock of liquor to treat the traders on the outer islands, and, one presumes, to increase their profits at the traders' expense by getting them drunk (MacCallum 1934). In outfitting his ship for such a journey from Jaluit, John Cameron, trading for Crawford and Company, stocked one case each of Scotch, bourbon, and brandy, two of gin and beer, a basket of champagne, and few bottles of bitters. This was necessary because the traders "would refuse to deal with vessels that brought no liquor; invariably the first order was for gin or whisky" (Farrell 1928:334). Cameron also tells us of men replaced in their jobs because they drank too much.

Not only did traders indulge themselves in alcohol, often to excess, but they also supplied it to the islanders in exchange for copra and other island products (Farrell 1928:333–34). Cheap gin was the standard trade item, and "by the end of the 1870s the Marshallese, Gilbertese, and Caroline Islanders had become accustomed to ship's biscuit, beer and Schnaps, as well as the usual cotton and iron goods" (Firth 1973:13). But if fault is to be found for supplying alcohol to the islanders, blame cannot be laid solely on the traders.

As a voluminous literature suggests, alcohol long had served as a mainstay in the trader's bag of goods among Indians on the American frontier. Similarly, almost from the beginning of a

British settlement at Port Jackson in Australia in 1788, Yankee traders found a ready market for rum-running (*Australia* 1964; Strauss 1963). Thus as the frontier was pushed into the islands of Oceania from America and Australia in the late eighteenth and nineteenth centuries, alcohol went right along. Writing of Tahiti in the 1820s, Morrell notes that "American whalers had no scruple in peddling rum for island produce" (1960:58), and Strauss (1963) mentions that pearl divers in the Tuamotus often were paid in whiskey or rum. There is even mention of land, the Pacific Islander's most prized possession, being "sold" for a "case of gin and a musket" (St. Johnston 1922:85). Clearly, then, traders who swapped liquor for copra in Micronesia in the last third of the nineteenth century were simply following a long commercial tradition in the islands. In fact, in many cases island chiefs upstaged local traders and reserved the sale of liquor to their subjects as their own prerogative (Wright and Fry 1936).

Whatever the history of alcohol and trade in Micronesia, there is little question that the islanders actively sought liquor. Koskinen's general statement about Pacific Islanders applies equally well to the specific case of the islanders of eastern Micronesia: "As a result of their craving for drink the natives were prepared to give up almost everything to obtain alcohol. Irresponsible traders exploited this desire with a complete lack of scruples" (Koskinen 1953). Just as along the Northwest Coast, the dispensing of liquor quickly became an essential concomitant of trade and a means of ingratiating traders with the island populations (cf. Lemert 1954). So much was this the expectation that when the *Morning Star* called at Ngatik in 1889 the people asked the missionaries for gin and tobacco (*Missionary Herald* 1889b).

Thus alcohol was not the only new drug that the islanders rapidly came to demand. At least as important in trade was tobacco, usually the variety called "Niggerhead." The people of eastern Micronesia seem to have become inordinately fond of it almost from their first acquaintance with it. Stopping briefly at Nauru in 1843, Simpson observed that "they were exceedingly anxious to barter for trinkets, beads, pipes, and tobacco; the latter were most in demand" (1844:100). In the Gilberts at about the same time Wilkes repeatedly mentions the extreme fondness of the Gilbertese for tobacco: "Their chief desire was to obtain tobacco . . . it was their constant request, and whilst in their canoes alongside, or on deck, the cry was constantly 'tebake' " (1845:49). Later Wilkes expresses revulsion at the Gilbertese craving: "In the use of tobacco, they are truly disgusting, for they eat it and swallow it, with a zest and pleasure indescribable. Their whole mind seems bent upon obtaining this luxury, and consequently it will command their most valuable articles" (1845:62). So much did the Gilbertese desire tobacco that they would follow a ship for miles in their canoes, often out of sight of land (Gulick 1932; Jones 1861).

Not to be outdone by the Gilbertese, the Marshallese also were strongly attached to tobacco (Finsch 1893; Humphrey 1887). Smoking was firmly established on Ponape and Kusaie when the missionaries arrived in 1852. Loomis (1970) has written that the Ponapeans would do anything, no matter how laborious or degrading, for a "plug" of tobacco, and she notes that despite their opposition to smoking the missionaries were forced to use tobacco in paying native builders in order to have houses of their own erected when they first arrived. The Trukese and Mortlockese were similarly habituated by at latest the 1870s. Echoing a familiar refrain, Bollig (1927) describes the Trukese as holding smoking dearer than food and drink. Thus, while the beach communities played the major role in spreading alcoholic beverages and tobacco throughout eastern Micronesia, and while most members of the beach communities partook themselves of these substances, they hardly had to force them on unwilling islanders.

The role persons in the beach communities played as dispensers and consumers of liquor and tobacco, as slavers and fighters, and as "ravagers" of native women earned these communities an unsavory reputation in the Western world. They have been described as "scoundrels who disgrace humanity" (Sterndale 1874:24), as men who taught "only the power and unscrupulousness of the white man" (Blakeslee 1921:174), as "men of the very worse description" (Simpson 1844:101), as men who "left behind them a train of sin and debauchery and unchekt crime" (Crosby 1899:13), and as men whose "intellect is of a low order" and whose morals are "very lax" (H. Cooper 1880:99). Although there may be some truth in these characterizations, it is important to remember that the men who made up the beach communities of the Pacific were no better and no worse than many of their contemporaries at home. While some of the early beachcombers were indeed escaped convicts from New South Wales, the majority of men in the beach communities had not been criminals. Moved by adventure, avarice, lassitude, or simply circumstances, they took up their lives in the islands and lived them with gusto. They taught many things to the islanders—both good and bad—and, as Maude has noted, while they were often "drunken, profligate and quarrelsome," they were "still essentially human and tolerant" (1968a:169). The ABCFM missionaries who followed them often lacked this tolerance for the island way of life.

Following the successful evangelization of Hawaii beginning in 1820, the ABCFM missionaries, along with native Hawaiian teachers sponsored by the Hawaiian Missionary Society, expanded their activities into the islands of eastern Micronesia commencing in 1852. That year saw the beginning of mission stations on Ponape and Kusaie, the former under the Reverends Albert Sturges and Luther Halsey Gulick and their wives, and the latter under the Reverend and Mrs. Benjamin Snow. On their arrival at Ponape and Kusaie, following a brief stopover at Butaritari, the missionaries discovered members of the beach community already firmly entrenched; and from the very first moment the *Caroline* touched at these two islands, the missionaries began to have dealings with them. On Kusaie they were met and piloted to a safe anchorage by an American, Mr. Kirkland, who was one of three foreigners then living on the island. At Ponape a Portuguese named George May, who claimed to have lived there for seventeen years, met the ship, accompanied by another foreigner, and steered them into the harbor at Madolenihmw. Already at this first encounter the missionaries were sizing up and making judgments about members of the beach community. John Gulick (Luther's brother), who accompanied the voyage in order to report to the Hawaiian mission, says of the foreigners who had boarded them at Ponape, "They seem to be rather a hard set, though two or three are, I think, of rather a better stamp" (1932:81). Given the backgrounds of the missionaries themselves, and the history of missionary-beach community relations in Hawaii and elsewhere in the Pacific at that time, such judgments seemed inevitable.

Gulick, Sturges, and Snow were all college-educated men from middle-class or upper-middle-class backgrounds in the United States, and Gulick was a medical doctor as well. Their wives were of similar genteel upbringing, though they did not match their husbands' educational accomplishments. Fired by the evangelical spirit of the times, these couples had responded to a call from the American Board for volunteers to carry the gospel to Micronesia. They shared a strong belief in God and an equally strong belief in matters of right and wrong. The success of the ABCFM in Hawaii was their model for Micronesia, and the rightness of their calling and of their opinions on matters of morality were, to them, beyond question.

Both Protestant and Catholic missionaries had been at work in Polynesia for half a century or more at the time the ABCFM moved into Micronesia. During this period Protestant missionaries in particular had taken strong stands against the use of alcohol and tobacco by islanders and by members of the beach community. Although initially the Wesleyan and London Missionary Society (LMS) clergy had no objection to the moderate use of alcohol and tobacco, the growth of the temperance movement in the United States and Great Britain in the 1820s and 1830s was reflected in a striking change in attitude toward alcohol by missionaries in the Pacific. Where once many missionaries imbibed, it soon became essential that aspirants to missionary posts be teetotalers; where once missionaries sometimes drank so much that they became alcoholics, it soon became a major sin even to taste "ardent spirits" (Gunson 1966).

It is of significance in understanding the attitude of the ABCFM missionaries toward alcoholic beverages to know that the Calvinist ministry of New England was at the forefront of efforts to reform American drinking habits in the early nineteenth century. "The first national Temperance association, the American Temperance Society (founded in 1826), was led by Congregationalist and nonevangelical Presbyterian ministers of Federalist commitment" (Gusfield 1963:41). This movement had had strong repercussions among the ABCFM missionaries in Hawaii during the 1830s and 1840s. As the missionaries in Hawaii gained a stronger foothold, they began to speak out ever more boldly against the traffic in intoxicating drinks. In January 1843 the mission began publishing a newspaper entitled *Temperance Advocate* in Honolulu, under the editorship of the Reverend Samuel C. Damon. Eventually this newspaper took the masthead *The Friend, A Journal devoted to Temperance, Seamen, Marine and General Intelligence,* and it became an influential voice in Hawaiian politics for many years. Indeed *The Friend* was instrumental in gaining the tariffs on alcoholic beverages imported into Hawaii that led to military intervention by France in 1849 in what Murphy (1973) has called "the great brandy caper."

By 1852 the ABCFM gave no quarter in its struggle with spirituous liquors and tobacco. Both were sinful, but the greater of these was alcohol. It is hardly surprising, then, that the missionaries to Micronesia spoke so approvingly of "King George" of Kusaie's effort to impose prohibition on his island (Crawford and Crawford 1967; Gulick 1932; Loomis 1970; *Missionary Herald* 1853). Nor is it any more surprising that on their second day at

Ponape, returning from Kiti to Madolenihmw aboard the *Caroline*, the following incident should occur: "George May who went with them got a bottle of liquor while at the other harbor [Kiti], and was drinking on his way back till Mr. Sturges got his bottle and kept it" (Gulick 1932:87). Already the stand against alcohol was taking shape and the potential clash with the beach community over this issue was becoming apparent.

The vastly different views of the missionaries and the beach communities in the Pacific regarding alcoholic beverages were already well known to both parties. LMS missionaries had established a temperance society in Tahiti in 1833, followed by a prohibition law in 1834 (Morrell 1960). Soon thereafter, such organizations and laws against alcohol spread throughout the missionized portions of Polynesia. That many of these laws were ineffective is beside the point. The important issue is the firm stance of the church against liquor in the islands, and the continuing efforts by the missionaries to prohibit its use. Not unrelated to this issue in Polynesia was the undertaking of the LMS missionaries "to bring native customs into line with the prejudices and social behavior then characteristic of English Protestantism. . . . Monogamous marriages were insisted upon and the use of tobacco and alcoholic beverages forbidden" (V. Thompson and Adloff 1971:184). The same effort to impose a style of life and a system of morality on the islanders and on members of the beach community also characterized the ABCFM mission in Micronesia.

As might be suspected, initially neither the islanders nor the beach community took kindly to these missionary efforts. Details are given later of the consequences of these clashes for all parties involved. But it is of immediate interest to see how missionary efforts to impose their own morality were viewed by others.

While praising the Reverend Robert Logan (the first ABCFM missionary to Truk), Moss has harsh words for the native Christian teachers and for many missionaries who ignored the white settlers on the islands and "appear to regard themselves as sent exclusively to preach to the heathen" (1889:70–71). Moss also laments the rigidity of the missions and the "want of healthy mental recreation" for the islanders (1889:186). Some foreigners viewed the missionaries as too sanctimonious on the alcohol/tobacco issue. For example, concerning a visit to Kusaie, Dewar writes in exasperation:

> The native missionary tried to sell me some sweet potatoes. I had
> previously learned from the trader that the proper price was three
> cents a pound; but this self-righteous individual, who would have

been scandalized at any of his converts drinking a glass of beer or smoking a pipe, was not above trying to cheat me egregiously, for he asked $3 for a barrel which could not have held more than 50 lb., and when I asked to have them weighed he pompously declined to agree to this. [1892:420]

Bridge grants that the success of the missions has been very great, "but great as it is, I think its magnitude has been exaggerated" (1886:564). Apropos of this point, Bridge and Finsch speak of missionary efforts in the Marshalls by the 1880s and 1890s as "not very significant" (Bridge 1886:555–56) and of Christianity as having "scarcely taken root" (Finsch 1893:13). Despite this negativism, some, like Fletcher, laud the "simple earnest men following a definite line of duty as missionaries in various islands" (1970:128).

Five years after the ABCFM established itself on Ponape and Kusaie, mission stations were set up on Ebon in the Marshalls and on Abaiang in the Gilberts. In 1858 the mission gained a foothold on Tarawa, and in 1864 on Butaritari. Not until 1873 were Ponapean Christian teachers sent to the Mortlocks, and it took another seven years to make the move to Truk. Thus it took nearly thirty years for the mission to spread throughout the eastern Micronesia region, and in those thirty years numerous conflicts occurred with the beach community and with local political elites over the issue of prohibition.

From their first day ashore on Ponape the missionaries made it clear that their attitudes toward alcohol and tobacco were the opposite of those held by members of the beach community. In a visit to the Nahnken of Kiti, in which the missionaries sought permission to establish a station in his dominion, the Reverend E. W. Clark (using George May as an interpreter) "gave an account of the results of the Sandwich Islands mission, showing our position in regards to matters of government, and the sale of tobacco and stimulants" (*Missionary Herald* 1853:88). Mention was made of the church's stand regarding alcohol and tobacco by way of explaining to the Nahnken their refusal of his friendly offer of fermented coconut toddy to refresh themselves. Right from the beginning, then, the missionaries began to use the symbols of alcohol and tobacco to set themselves apart from other foreigners in the islanders' eyes. The message was simple and clear: we are different people with a different purpose.

While the missionaries opposed alcohol and tobacco on several grounds, their major objection to the former was the association they saw between alcohol and "wickedness": crime, physical violence, and indiscriminate sex. It was particularly the association they saw between liquor and lasciviousness that led them to preach against strong drink. But the missionaries were also astute enough to have realized that in the islanders' eyes all Westerners were pretty much alike. The missionaries must have sensed that to obtain a hearing for their teachings they would have to violate many of the established patterns of interaction between outsiders and islanders that had developed over the years. Fortunately for the missionaries, this was not hard to do since they viewed nearly all of these patterns as sinful.

For the missionaries of the ABCFM who went to Micronesia, matters of morality were stark black and white; there could be no compromise with evil. Christian men and women sought to be good and do good in the world, but more than this they also endeavored to save others from their own wickedness. This evangelical zeal was carried not only to the heathern islanders, but to the "fallen" men in the beach communities as well. In the missionary view, such men had educated the islanders in vice: they had taught Micronesians to make and to drink alcoholic beverages, and, while under the influence of these spirits, to behave in all sorts of unchristian ways. The missionaries held the beach community responsible for the islanders' drunkenness, lax sexual morals, and petty thievery. The solution was obvious to the missionaries: they must supersede the beach community in influence with the islanders and teach them a better, Christian way of life.

When they first arrived in Micronesia the missionaries had to rely on members of the beach community for all sorts of assistance, from piloting their ship to anchor to translating their wishes to the islanders. Many in the beach community responded to the missionaries' needs with warm hospitality. On both Kusaie and Ponape members of the beach community opened their homes to the missionaries until the latter could arrange to have their own dwellings built. The Snows lived for a month with Kirkland on Kusaie at his invitation, and he continued to assist them in numerous ways. Another foreigner, resident in Kiti, Ponape, by the name of James Cook, "was not going to need his home for awhile and offered to let the missionaries use it temporarily," and the Gulicks remained in his house almost seven months. Despite initial suspicions that he "might be difficult for them" another member of the beach community on Ponape, Louis Corgat, who "had a reputation for his vicious habits," became "almost indispensable to the missionaries," and they were greatly saddened by his death in 1853 (Crawford and Crawford 1967:46, 61–62). Thus even though they opposed many aspects of the beach community's way of life, the missionaries were served well early on by many of its members.

But a reconciliation between the two groups was not to be. In spite of their indebtedness to some in the beach community, as their local contacts with the islanders increased and as they began to learn the language and hold study classes the missionaries began to rely on other foreigners less and less. Furthermore, they were sensitive to "malicious attempts by foreigners and native priests" to slander them, and they were upset by the continuation of intercourse in sex and ardent spirits between the beach community and the islanders. The more they felt their own motives and morals called into question, the more they withdrew from friendly interaction with other foreigners.

Even before the missionaries had arrived on Kusaie, foreigners had told the king and chiefs "that missionaries would interfere in governmental matters, and that he would lose his authority over the people," and the missionaries found it "very remarkable, that all the endeavors of unprincipled seamen to prejudice the King against missionaries have had so little effect" (*Missionary Herald* 1853:86). Such was not the case on Abemama in 1868, when Tem Baiteke refused to allow the missionaries ashore. Trading captains had warned him that "if you let those missionaries come on shore upon your islands, in less than a year you will not be master over your own people" (Moss 1889:103–5; cf. Maude 1970). From incidents such as these the missionaries came to view members of the beach communities as antagonists rather than allies, and there was little trust given on either side.

Although the missionaries spoke out forcefully against alcohol, the business of distilling rum on Ponape was carried on pretty extensively at times, and was mostly in the hands of foreigners (*Missionary Herald* 1857a); and foreign vessels calling at the islands continued to provide the islanders with liquor (Crawford and Crawford 1967; Dana 1935; *Missionary Herald* 1854, 1860a, 1868, 1886a). Though faced with such opposition from other foreigners, the missionaries resolutely sought to draw the islanders away from alcohol. Again and again they mention their successes and failures in inducing islanders to give up liquor consumption and persuading chiefs to declare prohibition (*Missionary Herald* 1856, 1869b, 1876, 1882; Wetmore 1886). The friction between the beach community and the missionaries over the issue of temperance was succinctly put by the Reverend E. T. Doane writing from Ponape in 1870: "This is what most of the whaling vessels do, visiting Ponape. They deal out death and desolation, or that which causes it, and then, when the missionary tries to teach the natives how wrong the use of such drink is, they *curse* us" (*Missionary Herald* 1870*b*). The missionaries were not sorry at the deaths of foreigners who opposed them. Commenting on the recent demise of three such men on Ponape, Sturges said, "We cannot help feeling that our teachings will now have clearer way, since positive opposition has pretty much ceased" (*Missionary Herald* 1860*b*). Unfortunately for the mission, this prediction proved premature.

The special conflict between the beach community and the mission over alcohol was not restricted to Micronesia. In his review of missionary work all over Oceania, Koskinen observed that "the beachcombers naturally realized that the advance of missionary work could only mean the end of their influence and therefore they generally tried to prevent missionary influence from establishing itself and spreading" (1953:40). Koskinen goes on to note that most white men in the islands were "scarcely Sunday School types," and that even those favorably disposed to the mission were put off by the "narrow-minded morals" and "uncompromising attitude" of the missionaries; "even the more respectable white residents were accustomed to consume strong liquors" (1953:128). Added to this were a number of factors that strained relations between the missionaries and the traders. Koskinen maintains that the traders felt the missionaries obstructed their work (and vice versa), and "there was no lack of traders who considered conversion and education as harmful, since they prevented the making of big profits. A common symptom, apparent before long, was that missionaries and traders were mutually antagonistic" (1953:134). Such antagonism resulted in definite campaigns by some large trading firms in the Pacific against mission work. Fletcher contends that the house of Godeffroy, for example, instructed its traders "to oppose and obstruct missionaries at all points" (1970:128).

Profits from trade may have been the underlying reason for the antagonism between the missions and the beach communities; but alcohol and tobacco became its symbols. Thus Yanaihara writes: "The traders and whalers were antagonistic to the missionaries partly because the missionaries from Boston preached against the use of intoxicants . . . [and] forbade smoking" (1940:15). When the missionaries in Micronesia wrote home about the misdeeds of foreigners, they were sure to mention alcohol, if not tobacco, as the cause. The widespread animosities between these two groups seem to have come to a head on Ponape. Visiting that island in the late 1880s Moss exclaimed, "In no place does the unfortunate antagonism between missionary and trader seem stronger than at Ponape. In no place could their cooperation be more beneficial to the natives" (1889:189).

Whatever their opposition to the mission may have been, members of the beach community unwittingly performed it an important service; as Maude puts it: "By their contempt for the local gods and apparent inmunity from the consequences, they created a general spirit of scepticism—a readiness for change" that paved the way for the missionary. This service, revealed by historical hindsight, was not apparent to the missionaries at the time, and they found it expedient to use the beach community as a scapegoat in their reports home. A stereotype of the beachcomber as a "renegade from civilization" served to galvanize public support for the mission's work in the home countries, and the missionaries' "published views had a major effect in forming public opinion in England and America" (1968a:163, 164).

The struggle between the beach community and the mission was essentially over by the mid-1880s. Though occasional skirmishes continued to flare up for the next quarter of a century, "by the middle '80s, the American missionaries had come to be the strongest influence in the Eastern Carolines, the Marshalls, and probably in the neighbouring Gilberts as well" (Blakeslee 1921:175). Even though they gave up their stations to the Liebenzell Mission in 1907, Bascom could write nearly fifty years later that individual Protestant missionaries were fondly remembered by name on Ponape, and that "there is no question of their good intentions even among Catholics and those who have not given up smoking or drinking kava and alcohol, which were condemned along with many other practices" (1950:142).

Concurrent with their efforts to wrest influence with the islanders from the beach communities in Micronesia, the missionaries also embarked on a struggle to convert island political elites to their point of view. This struggle was waged vigorously for half a century or more, and, again, a few basic symbols became critically important for delineating one side from the other—namely alcohol, tobacco, and, on Ponape and Kusaie, the indigenous beverage kava, made from the roots of *Piper methysticum*.

The political power of traditional elites in eastern Micronesia varied widely. In general terms, leaders on Ponape and Kusaie had the greatest power over their subjects in this region, although they were followed closely by Marshallese chiefs. All of the Gilberts at contact, and the islands in what is now Truk District, were marked by a fundamental egalitarianism in which chiefs had little actual power to force their wishes on their followers.

Many traditional elites derived special benefits from having one or more members of the beach community under their jurisdiction. The latter served the chiefs as traders and translators in exchange for safety and often considerable status in the island community. Thus beachcombers and traditional elites were often in a symbiotic relationship which the missionaries worked to upset. In the latter half of the nineteenth century, however, many island chiefs took the bull by the horns and actively sought to compete with outsiders in trade. "Many islanders were concerned in the supply trade, including local alcohol, but their participation was often curtailed by jealous chiefs anxious to monopolise the trade" (Ralston 1970). A few of these chiefs purchased their own ships for such competition. Most famous, perhaps, were those owned by the "Kingdom of Abemama": Tem Baiteke had a four-gun, sixty-ton schooner in 1871, and his successor, Tem Binoka, owned both the ninety-five-ton brigantine *Coronet,* which was wrecked in 1882, and a smaller schooner, the *Sunbeam* (Ralston 1970; Dana 1935; Farrell 1928; MacCallum 1934). A number of Marshallese chiefs also acquired vessels in the 1880s and 1890s; "King John" of Ailinglapalap maintained the twelve-ton schooner *Lotus* in 1884, and in 1895 "chief Kabua" and "chief Loiala" acquired the *Jaluit* (twenty tons) and the *Laurak* (twenty tons) respectively, both of which were built at Likiep (Humphrey 1887).

That the chiefs on many Micronesian islands took such an active role in trade in the nineteenth century helps explain some of the animosity they felt toward the missionaries. On some of the islands, for example Abemama, trade in liquor and tobacco was strictly controlled by the chief (Stevenson 1971). Tem Binoka would periodically lift the prohibition against drinking and permit his subjects a spree, but normally they were forbidden to possess liquor or to manufacture fermented toddy, and they were only allowed to receive tobacco "from the royal hand." Since alcohol and tobacco were in great demand by the islanders such a trade monopoly gave the chiefs considerable leverage over their followers, and missionary efforts to eliminate the use of these substances were seen by the chiefs as a direct threat to their power.

Other factors enter into this matter as well, however. Drunkenness frequently led to violence and unsettled conditions in the islands of Micronesia, and chiefs sometimes tried to control such behavior when they believed it presented a threat to their

positions. The most striking instance of this was Baiteke of Abemama's prohibition law:

> The drinking of sour toddy was regarded as a threat to the political
> structure on the same footing as sedition, and the same punish-
> ment was provided for both: staking the offender spreadeagled on
> the lagoon beach for a maximum of forty-eight hours, scorched by
> the equatorial sun during the day and eaten alive by mosquitos at
> night. It was said that few survived the sentence and that those
> who did invariably went mad. [Maude 1970:211]

A final related matter is that the chiefs were often the only islanders who had the means to purchase alcohol. Finsch says
drunkenness was not widespread in the Marshalls because only
the chiefs could afford this vice "which the Mission was not able
to eradicate, and for which they displayed a great fondness"
(1893:18). Apparently island political elites recognized quite early
in the contact period that alcohol and tobacco were important substances (symbolically, if not physiologically) over which they must
assert their authority.

That many Micronesian political elites viewed alcohol as an
important symbol of their station in life is revealed clearly in the
literature. Tem Binoka demanded to be served Hennessy's brandy
or champagne by those foreigners who wished to do business with
him (Dana 1935; MacCallum 1934). The Nahnmwarki of Madolenihmw had come to expect gifts of rum from visiting ships' captains as early as 1833, and the Nahnken of Kiti required "a tribute
of schnapps" in consideration of his rank from "all the foreign
captains who come into the harbor" (Riesenberg 1968b:8; Spoehr
1963:91; cf. Wood 1875). Many local leaders stockpiled alcohol
and tobacco as a sign of their wealth; this practice also permitted
them to dole these substances out to their followers as the occasion demanded. Tem Binoka of Abemama kept an amazing cache
of wine, liquor, brandies, etc. (Moss 1889), and Wood recounts
that the chiefs on Ponape "are very fond of buying small boxes of
American tobacco. . . . These they never open, but store in their
houses, and, in fact, look on them much as we should on old and
valuable china" (1875:147–48). It seems likely that such stockpiles
of alcohol and tobacco were built up by local elites to be consumed in competitive feasts such as happened among the Indians
of the Northwest Coast (Lemert 1954). While we have found no
specific mention of this in Ponape, where competitive feasting
was a fundamental aspect of local status rivalry and political mobility, Bollig (1927) mentions the use of beer and liquor in competitive feasts on Truk during early Japanese times.

With very few exceptions (e.g., Baiteke of Abemama), traditional political elites, like members of the beach communities, initially welcomed the missionaries. Local leaders were anxious to have missionaries reside with them, presumably in the hope that they might control and exploit them as they had other foreigners who had lived among them. Jones writes that "King George" of Kusaie "appeared to have taken quite an interest in the missionary" in 1852, noting that the king had given the missionary "a large piece of good land, built him a nice substantial house, and assisted him in all his power" (1861:252). But it did not take long for many chiefs to realize that the missionaries did not recognize their authority over them. O'Brien has argued that "the first efforts of the missionaries were directed towards remaining independent and apart from the island society's [Ponape's] well-defined system of authority and tribute" and that "Sturges and Gulick were determined as far as possible to set themselves apart from and above chiefly authority" (1971:54). As soon as the chiefs understood what the missionaries were about they usually withdrew their assistance and, in some cases, began to actively oppose mission efforts. The primary symbol of this opposition to missionary presumption of authority was alcohol: drunkenness communicated clearly to the missionaries that the chiefs rejected missionary claims of authority over them.

Examples of Micronesian leaders expressing opposition to the missionaries by flaunting the symbol of alcohol are legion. The Nahnmwarki of Sokehs was a continual thorn in the side of the mission. He attempted to force those of his subjects who professed Christianity to drink rum as a symbol of their continued subordination to him, and when drunk he "kidnapped" a young girl who had joined the church to add to his "already large harem" (*Missionary Herald* 1870a). When Doane sought to reason with him over this latter event, "the king told us plainly why he acted as he did. It was because I would not let him pray and talk in our meetings, but passed by *him* and asked common natives. Was he not the king? he would not allow the common people to be raised above him" (Coale 1951; *Missionary Herald* 1869a, 1870a). A few years earlier, the friction between the Nahnken of Kiti and the missionaries had led the Nahnken to set fire to the church in his district while, of course, drunk (*Missionary Herald* 1865). Although the king of Butaritari was for a time friendly to the mission, by 1867 he had stopped attending meetings and visiting the missionaries and "had become very dissipated, drinking heavily" (*Missionary Herald* 1854, 1867). Even "good King George" of Ku-

saie, whose famed prohibition law had so impressed the missionaries at first, was not above imbibing alcoholic beverages when he
could, although he seemed sufficiently cowed by the missionaries
to do so largely in secret (Hammet 1854).

While alcohol became the primary symbol of the missionary-
traditional elite struggle for power in eastern Micronesia generally,
kava became an equally important one on the islands of Ponape
and, to a lesser extent, Kusaie. Widespread in Polynesia, kava was
used only on Kusaie and Ponape in Micronesia, where it was an
important symbol of chiefly authority and the major means of communication with island deities. For these reasons the missionaries
fought passionately to eradicate its use (Coale 1951; O'Brien 1971).
Gulick and Sturges were particularly alert to the importance of kava
in Ponapean religion, and they saw that to supplant "pagan worship" with Christianity they would have to oppose kava drinking
(*Missionary Herald* 1855). Beyond this, though, the missionaries
equated kava with alcohol as an unholy spirit that deprived men of
their reason:

> Religious components of the culture were assiduously hunted
> down and combated. *Kava* drinking bore the brunt of this attack.
> Being a slightly narcotic beverage, its evil effects on the body
> were equated to those of alcohol by the strongly prohibitionist
> missionaries. [Coale 1951:51]

Although kava drinking seems to have been widespread on
Kusaie up until the coming of the missionaries (Jones 1861), its
open consumption appears to have ceased almost coincident with
their arrival, and the kava ceremony has not survived on that island. Ponapeans, however, were much more deeply attached to
their "national beverage," and in spite of more than a century of
Protestant missionary opposition to its use they have clung tena-
ciously to their kava customs (Glassman 1950; McGrath 1973;
Ward 1974). Today kava consumption is so popular on Ponape that
a number of "*sakau* [kava] bars" have opened in the center of
Kolonia (Demory 1974).

O'Brien has argued that the missionaries on Ponape made
membership in the Christian camp a direct challenge to the authority of the chiefs by forbidding tribute to them through feasting
and kava. She goes on to assert that "the attack on kava was much
more than the general missionary dislike of alcohol. The missionaries were far less concerned with prohibiting coconut toddy or
rum. Kava was singled out for special attention because of the
important position it held in native society" (1971:55). If we restrict our attention only to the struggle for power between the

missionaries and local political elites on Ponape, what O'Brien says is essentially correct, although she perhaps underestimates the importance of the simultaneous missionary attack on alcoholic beverages. But if we take the larger view of missionary struggles with traditional leaders all over eastern Micronesia, then it is clear that alcohol was the primary symbol employed to separate Christians from heathen. In the Micronesian mission generally, the primary symbol of allegiance to the church was to forsake alcoholic beverages and tobacco; and kava was simply added to this list on Ponape. As Coale has correctly observed, "The reports in the *Missionary Herald* [for Ponape] decrying the use of alcohol were several times as frequent as those noting the use of kava" (1951:68).

So much did the missionaries inveigh against kava on Ponape that Moss has recorded a scene worthy of the temperance movement in America.

> At Kite the heathen natives were in great tribulation. Their Christian brethren, impelled by a burning zeal in the cause of temperance, had just come in force and rooted up all their plantations of the 'Piper Methisticum', from which . . . kava . . . is made. . . . Had the heathens been strong enough, they would certainly have resisted . . . but their Christian fellow-countrymen were the stronger and did what they thought the work of the Lord in their own way. [1889:206]

Such incidents make it evident that by the 1880s the struggle was largely over and the Christian converts and missionaries were becoming the major political power on Ponape. By 1873 Wood (1875) noted that the Christians had physically separated themselves from the heathen at Kiti by dwelling apart, and by 1876 the missionaries had succeeded in getting the Christian chiefs to appoint policemen to enforce their wishes. Significantly, the first business of this police force was a crusade against liquor (*Missionary Herald* 1876).

That the mark of Christianity in eastern Micronesia was abstinence from alcoholic beverages is well demonstrated in a story concerning islanders adrift at sea. A British trading ship picked up a Gilbertese canoe with five survivors aboard (out of an original twelve) six hundred miles from the Gilberts from which they had drifted over a month before. When the nearly unconscious islanders were rescued, "the crew of the rescue ship, *Northern Light*, with Captain Slocum, tried to revive the helpless natives by offering them some brandy, but they refused it saying that they were Christians and could not drink" (Crawford and Crawford 1967).

The islands of what is now Truk District presented the missionaries with a different challenge. When they arrived in the Mortlocks in 1873, and again when they carried their work to Truk Lagoon in 1880, they found no alcoholic beverages present. Doane wrote of the Trukese eye as "round, black and lustrous, not dimmed by the use of ava or toddy from the cocoa-nut blossom" (*Missionary Herald* 1881:209), and this observation was later confirmed by Logan who noted that the Trukese "make no use whatever of anything intoxicating" (*Missionary Herald* 1886b). This lack of alcohol and kava presented the missionaries at Truk and the Mortlocks with a dilemma: what symbol could they employ to differentiate Christians from non-Christians? The answer was not long in coming. Avoidance of tobacco, which had been opposed with much less vehemence than alcohol and kava in the other islands of eastern Micronesia, here became the major symbol for demonstrating obedience to God. So much was this the case that when Logan opened a school at Anapauo in 1885 some of his young scholars "clung to tobacco and had to be dismissed" (*Missionary Herald* 1886b).

The importance of having a ready symbol for distinguishing Christians from heathen was not perceived by Moss, who observed that the prohibition against tobacco in Truk and the Mortlocks "tends to make Christianity burdensome to a people to whom smoking is the chief luxury" (1889:165). Moss wondered why the mission did not instead oppose "the dirty habit of smearing their bodies with tumeric and oil, or of twisting their hair into unseemly chignons on the top of the head" (1889:166). In fact the mission also made concerted efforts to lead Trukese converts away from these practices, and thus tumeric, long hair, and dancing (all of which were caught up with indigenous religious worship) also came to symbolize pagan status.

In the late 1880s Spain and Germany began to actively assert their claims to hegemony in the islands of eastern Micronesia, following the papal arbitration of 1885 that awarded the Marshall Islands to Germany and the Carolines to Spain. As these countries sent contingents of soldiers and colonial officers into eastern Micronesia to enforce their claims, they inevitably came into conflict with the American missionaries. In the case of Germany in the Marshalls, the mission had already been engaged in a running battle for several years with German trading firms over the issue of trade in liquor and tobacco. Once again, as in the mission's struggles with the beach communities and with local political elites, the symbol of alcoholic drink was employed in their quarrels with the Spanish and German colonial regimes.

The strategy in this case was to brand Spain and Germany as "soft on alcohol" in the hope of drumming up support in the United States for diplomatic reprimands to these two countries and in the fainter hope of convincing the United States to move forcefully to claim territory in eastern Micronesia (see Blakeslee 1921). The ABCFM missionaries also feared that the Spaniards would force them out of the Carolines in favor of the hated Catholics.

The Spaniards concentrated their colonial efforts on Ponape in eastern Micronesia, and they did not seriously interfere with the mission's work elsewhere in the Carolines. On Ponape, however, the missionaries and the Spaniards were continually at odds. In broadcasting this clash to the faithful in the United States, the missionaries repeatedly accused the Spaniards of undoing their good work by encouraging prostitution, the manufacture of alcoholic beverages, and a return to the kava ceremony. Doane spoke of the Spanish governor's headquarters as "the centre of liquor influences, houses of ill-fame, and other evils" (*Missionary Herald* 1889a: 545), and Crosby quotes another missionary of the period visiting on Ponape (Price) in the following way: "The people have all the weaknesses of the other islanders, with the added vice of intemperance. The latter is most destructive, and the center of the devastating work is the Spanish colony" (Crosby 1899:17). In like manner, it was claimed that the Spaniards encouraged the Ponapeans "to return to the cultivation and use of the kava plant, from which in the days of heathenism they had made one of their intoxicating drinks, a practice which . . . had under the missionaries become well-nigh obsolete" (Laurie n.d.). Moreover, as if kava were not bad enough, the islanders were encouraged to manufacture intoxicating drinks, since any hindrance to the making and selling of such beverages was ostensibly viewed by the Spaniards as a serious interference with trade. Such evil influences by the Spaniards even caused one chief who was a deacon in the church to return to his cups. More threatening to the mission's work than this, however, was the fact that the Spanish party that arrived in Ponape in March 1887 included six Capuchin priests (Laurie n.d.; Crosby 1899). The Protestant missionaries smugly rejoiced that "none or next to none of the natives go near them; none have gone to their faith; liquor was freely given, tobacco freely passed out, but all ends in a perfect failure" (*Missionary Herald* 1888). Significantly the Spanish Catholics chose to do battle for men's souls with the American Protestants by flaunting the very symbols of conversion to New England Protestantism.

Even after the Spaniards left Ponape following the Spanish-American War, the Ponapean Protestant leader, Henry Nanpei, wrote that "they left the island as they came, viz. in a drunken, brawling, disorderly manner," and he averred that the Spaniards "have succeeded in making many good young Christian men and women drunkards and common harlots" (*Missionary Herald* 1900). Although he had earlier accused the Germans of being largely responsible for the liquor traffic on Ponape, Nanpei ex-ulted following the German takeover from the Spaniards on Po-nape that the German governor's "first order was to prohibit the use and sale of all intoxicating liquor to the natives. . . . This cursed liquor nuisance is what we have been trying for years and years to put down" (*Missionary Herald* 1900).

While Nanpei might rejoice at the German prohibition law on Ponape, however, matters were not so smooth in the Marshalls. As in the conflict between the mission and the beach communi-ties, once again the crux of the problem was trade. The German colonial government in the Marshalls, which was for all practical purposes the Jaluit Gesellschaft, would brook no interference with trade. This included traffic in liquor and tobacco. Moreover, the Jaluit Gesellschaft was heir to many of the same unfavorable atti-tudes toward the missionaries that had been widely trumpeted by Godeffroy and Son (cf. Fletcher 1970). The upshot of this was repeated clashes between ABCFM missionaries and Germans in the Marshalls.

As with the accusations made against the Spaniards on Po-nape, the medium of protest was the German position regarding liquor and tobacco:

> Our missionaries and the Christian natives themselves have . . .
> taken a firm stand against the use of beer and strong drink and of
> tobacco. But the German commissioner denounces such rigidity.
> Restrictions upon trade he will not allow, and he demands permis-
> sion from all to drink beer and buy tobacco. [*Missionary Herald*
> 1893*b*]

Although the mission was initially cheered by the efforts of Mar-shallese chiefs to maintain prohibition on their islands, it soon became apparent that the Germans would only honor such laws in the breach. This realization led to renewed efforts by the mission-aries to have their wishes met. They were appalled that the Ger-man commissioner "had even been on a tour through the [Mar-shall] islands teaching the natives that it was right and proper for them to drink beer, use tobacco, and labor on the Sabbath," and such episodes led to repeated visits to the commissioner's office on Jaluit by the missionaries to plead their case (*Missionary Herald* 1893a:234; 1891).

German commercial and military might proved stronger than the mission's position in the islands, at least in the short run, and the immediate consequence of this struggle for power was that the ABCFM handed the Micronesian field over to the German Liebenzell mission in 1907. At least one German viewed this apparent triumph with satisfaction, although he acknowledged that "the influence of the Boston Mission . . . was great and will not disappear quickly" (Deekin 1912). The truth of this prophecy—particularly regarding the belief that good Christians do not use alcohol or tobacco—may be seen today throughout the islands of eastern Micronesia where the ABCFM held sway.

In his incisive analysis of the American temperance movement, Gusfield has argued that drinking and abstinence became important symbols of social status in the United States during the first half of the nineteenth century. The rural, native American Protestant in particular supported temperance ideals: self-control, hard work, and impulse renunciation were in high repute, and sobriety was considered virtuous. As the temperance movement increased in size and influence during the 1830s and 1840s, "abstinence was becoming a symbol of middle-class membership and a necessity for ambitious and aspiring young men. It was one of the ways society could distinguish the industrious from the ne'er-do-well; the steady worker from the unreliable drifter" (Gusfield 1963:5–6).

It was precisely at the time that temperance ideals were ascendant in the United States and Great Britain that sustained contact with the islands of eastern Micronesia began. But the Westerners who moved into the islands were anything but temperate! Indeed, they stood for the opposite of all that was held dear by the ever more powerful middle class in their home countries. They exhibited little self-control, avoided hard work if they could, and gave free rein to their impulses to drink and fornicate. These members of the beach communities provided Micronesians with their first opportunity to observe Westerners at close hand for a sustained period of time. Their behavior when drunk on the alcoholic beverages that they taught the islanders to make provided Micronesians with a model of drunken comportment that was largely unrestrained, and in good measure this reflected their working class origins in the United States and Great Britain (cf.

MacAndrew and Edgerton 1969; Maude 1968*a*). Standard patterns of interaction evolved in which island systems of values, religion, and morality remained largely intact, and in which trade in alcoholic beverages, tobacco, and firearms played a significant part. Then, in 1852, the missionaries came.

Subscribing to the temperance ideals of the times, the deeply religious missionaries, from middle-class rather than working-class backgrounds, were appalled at the behavior of the "ne'er-do-wells" and "unreliable drifters" that they found in the islands, and they set themselves unmistakably apart from such people. Alcohol became the primary symbol that separated the forces for good from the forces for evil and very quickly the islanders learned that Christians abjured its consumption. In eastern Micronesia, as in the United States, the temperance ideals of the middle class fervently supported by the Protestant churches in time became the dominant values of the groups in power.

In pressing their crusade the missionaries were concerned not only with teaching a new religious doctrine to the islanders, but also with altering the very fabric of their society to bring it into accord with the values of middle-class American nineteenth-century Protestantism. To bring about such a fundamental change, the missionaries found themselves in competition with local political elites for the allegiance of the common people. Once again the missionaries employed the powerful symbol of abstinence to press their cause. Christians were prohibited from drinking liquor, smoking, or chewing tobacco, or, on Ponape and Kusaie, pounding kava. Chiefs encouraged their supporters to do all these things in defiance of missionary claims to authority. Those who relapsed into drinking or smoking were systematically dropped from church membership. The missionaries slowly eroded the power base of traditional political leaders as more and more converts were won. They opposed dancing, nakedness, polygamy, long hair, and tumeric—anything that offended their own brand of morality. But while they preached against all of these evils, they reserved their strongest sermons for demon rum.

The ABCFM missionaries to Micronesia firmly believed that drink was sinful and its appearance a sign of defective character. Their ascetic ideals left no room for behavior that failed to improve and perfect man's ability to improve and perfect himself (Gusfield 1963). By attacking alcohol and tobacco, however, they did not simply strike at the beach community life-style. These substances occupied such an important place in trade, both for members of the beach communities and for island political leaders, that by advocating their elimination the missionaries threatened an important mode of livelihood as well.

From their arrival in the islands of eastern Micronesia, then, the ABCFM missionaries engaged in a series of struggles for political power, first with the beach communities and island leaders, and later with foreign colonial governments that moved into the area. While they were victorious against the beach community and traditional elites, they eventually were forced out of the Micronesian field by German colonial efforts. Nevertheless the values they sought to implant, especially regarding alcohol, tobacco, and kava, have survived to the present day on islands where missionary influence was strongest (see Bascom 1950; Riesenberg 1968a; Schaefer 1975; Severance 1974).

Members of the beach community taught Micronesians that alcohol had commercial value and that its effects were to be sought to increase "bravery" and decrease inhibitions. Members of the church taught that alcohol was sinful, and drunkards denied a place in heaven. Attitudes learned from both of these groups may still be found in eastern Micronesia in a marked ambivalence toward spirituous liquors, and while the Protestant churches working in the islands at present continue to preach against the use of alcoholic beverages, the battle engaged over one hundred twenty years ago by the men of the ABCFM has yet to be completely won.

Notes

1. For the sake of convenience all nonmissionary foreigners will be referred to collectively in this paper as members of "the beach community" (cf. Ralston 1970).

2. Because Guam was under firm Spanish colonial control during this period it was not a haven for beachcombers.

Sardines and Other Fried Fish: The Consumption of Alcoholic Beverages on a Micronesian Island

James D. Nason

Even the most remote islands in Micronesia have now undergone social and cultural changes as a result of foreign contacts. In some instances these changes are of a relatively minor order, e.g., the introduction of foreign tools or materials, whereas in other instances foreign contact has led to significant alterations in many sectors of traditional native life. Some theorists of social change have suggested that one consequence of extensive sociocultural change is a period of societal disruption. Such disruption comes about as a result of significant alterations in traditional attitudes, values, and normative behaviors, particularly those associated with social organization and social structure (Smelser 1963). One facet of this period of heightened social stress is the emergence of dissociable behavior in interpersonal relationships. This behavior may occur in the form of sharp generational breaks between parents and their children or as disputes between elder and junior members of the community (e.g., Marshall 1975). Indicative of such behavior would be transgression of traditional proprieties, defiance of established contemporary laws and customs, and the like.

A specific indication of social instability is the misuse of alcoholic beverages, particularly drunkenness and associated behavior that are negatively viewed by the community at large or, alternatively, by the senior segment of the community.

This study will examine the use of alcoholic beverages in a Micronesian community that has undergone rather extensive sociocultural changes during the past hundred years. I will attempt to show that while the consumption of alcoholic beverages is viewed as dysfunctional and negative behavior by some elements of the community, the perception of the community as a whole is that drinking serves to maintain and even reinforce traditional community values and attitudes that are positively regarded.

The History of Drinking on Etal Island

Etal Island is a small, remote coral atoll located in the southern portion of Truk District, United States Trust Territory of the Pacific Islands. The Etal people, known as traditionally good navigators with trading experience in both Truk and Ponape districts, were almost certainly acquainted with Ponapean kava, *sakau* (general term for alcoholic beverages), and with fermented coconut toddy, *achi*, prior to Western contact. The word *sakau* is also used to refer to the state of drunkenness, originally that produced by the drinking of fermented coconut toddy. It seems likely that the English loan words for whiskey and wine, *wiski* and *uain*, were introduced into the Mortlock Islands via Ponape, where American and British trading and whaling ships began to visit in increasing numbers after 1831 (Riesenberg 1968*a*). By the mid-1850s, Ponape was a center of foreign activity in Micronesia. The Reverend Sturges, for example, reported in 1856 that there were three brothels on Ponape and that the natives were producing a distilled coconut beverage under the direction of foreigners (*Missionary Herald* 1857:4). By that time at least some foreign vessels had called at the Mortlock Islands. In 1828, for instance, the Russian explorer Lutke treated the chief of Lukunor Island, Selen, to strawberry jam, English biscuits, and madeira, "which the savage liked very much" (Nozikov 1946:136). The only other alcoholic beverages to enter the local scene were beer, *pio,* and a fermented yeast drink, *yiis.*

Both yeast and beer, according to island informants, were known during the period of Japanese administration (1914 to 1945) but neither was drunk because of fears that the Japanese would whip or otherwise punish those found drinking or drunk. This prohibition was also clearly in accord with the teachings of American and, later, German Protestant missionaries active in the area. Protestant missionary activities began on Etal Island in 1872 and have stressed the importance of not using either alcoholic beverages or tobacco. Catholic missionary endeavors, which began on the island in 1911, have never prohibited either indulgence. Of the present-day population, approximately 86 percent are Catholic and 14 percent Protestant, with some Protestants becoming "Catholic" for a day or two to indulge in drinking parties (just as some Catholics temporarily become "Protestant" in order to obtain a divorce).

As an autonomous island municipality in Truk District, Etal Island has a law in effect that prohibits the sale or consumption of any alcoholic beverage on the island, including *achi,* palm toddy. Because of this law, traders who come to the island on the periodic interisland trading vessel are unable to sell any such beverages. What is available within the community, then, is either palm toddy or yeast. Palm toddy was made on the island by young men who tapped old trees for the necessary sap until the fall of 1968. The production of toddy stopped in 1968 apparently because some young men were using trees which did not belong to them. The result was the imposition of public fines (i.e., work details) on two young offenders and the cessation of toddy production.[1] At the same time most of the men decided that it was better to have bearing coconut trees in order to make copra (dried coconut meat used for its oil) to sell in exchange for yeast and other goods than it was to use the trees to make toddy. (The tapping procedure usually killed the coconut trees.) Yeast, then, became the sole alcoholic beverage drunk on the island.

The drinking of yeast first began after the arrival of American military personnel at the end of World War II. On Etal Island, yeast is made by combining a large metal tin of dry active yeast powder with a five-pound bag of sugar and water. A normal batch of some two to five gallons is either drunk as is or flavored with uncooked ground coffee, coconut water, or occasionally some canned fruit juice. Three types of yeast are known and used: (1) a four-hour yeast, not usually drunk on Etal because of dangers to health; (2) a twelve-hour yeast, ordinarily for "spur-of-the-moment" occasions and not highly regarded; and (3) a twenty-four-hour yeast, the type most commonly prepared and imbibed. The only difference between these types is the varying degrees of time allotted for the yeast to "work."

Patterns of Yeast Drinking, 1968–69

A total of twenty-five yeast drinking parties was recorded during a five-month period from October 1968 to January 1969 and from April 1969 to June 1969 (table 1). These probably represent anywhere from 50 to 75 percent of the parties that actually occurred during the same five-month period. Thus the number of parties that might take place during a year would be approximately fifty, based on the rate of known occurrences, and about seventy to one hundred based on the estimated occurrences. These estimates are founded on unverified rumors about parties that had taken place the day before and take into account the fact that some parties are continued by latecomers as separate events in secluded bush locations after the initial party has broken up. Most of the parties known to have occurred took place on a weekend. Of the twenty-five known parties, ten were on a Saturday, nine on a Sunday, three on a Wednesday, and two on a Thursday.

Only men participated in these yeast parties. On only two occasions did a man leave a party to take his wife a cup of yeast, and both of these were instances in which the woman was playing bingo close to the location of the party. The exclusion of women from drinking (and for the most part smoking as well) appears to be a long-established pattern. No early historical accounts mention women drinking except in foreign ports, and no explanation was ever given except that drinking was for men and not women.

All yeast parties involved primarily younger men, i.e., men in their twenties and thirties. Most also included at least some

TABLE 1.   Occurrence and Participation in Yeast Drinking Parties, Etal
Island, October, 1968, to June, 1969[a]

Date of Party		Number of Participants	Average Age	Occasion[b]
27 October	1968	9	38	F
2 November		5	27	F, V
3 November		10	35	F
9 November		7	32	P
17 November		13	41	V
20 November		15	35	F
15 December		16	36	F
18 December		10	39	F
21 December		18	37	F
22 December		8	34	F
29 December		7	32	V, P
1 January	1969	26+	37	P
2 January		10	32	P
25 January		9	38	V
26 April		8	38	F
3 May		10	35	P
4 May		7	32	P
10 May		12	39	P
17 May		15	34	F
18 May		10	39	F
24 May		6	33	F
25 May		27+	37	F
29 May		15	37	V
7 June		18	34	V
7 June		18	34	V
Total, 25		309+	35	

a. Field research was suspended from mid-February to mid-April 1969.
b. F = visit of a field-trip ship; V = arrival of visitors from neighboring islands;
    P = a public event (including a funeral, feasts to celebrate the dedication of a
    public building, New Year's and Christmas, and Law Day).

men in their forties or early fifties (table 1). In general, however,
most older men rarely frequented such parties and some never did
so since to do so would jeopardize their positions in the community as religious, social, or political leaders. It was considered
foolish for an older man to engage in drinking unless his indulgence was moderate, infrequent, and associated with some special
occasion where his social presence was de rigueur. Conversely, it
was not at all foolish for young men to drink with some regularity

since to do so was public affirmation of their masculinity, particularly masculinity as demonstrated by acts of derring-do. Men
under the age of thirty-five or forty were not considered to be
"settled" and fully responsible adult men. Instead, they were perceived to be somewhat irresponsible and carefree, in accordance
with the traditional attitudes about young men. Thus while older
men sometimes initiated a party or supplied the necessary ingredients, it was usually the younger men who acted as the sponsors
or who actually prepared the drink. This is illustrated by the data
in table 1, which show an average age of thirty-five years for all
participants in known yeast parties (range, twenty to sixty).

The size and duration of yeast parties varied considerably.
The twenty-five known parties had a total of 309 participants, or
an average of 13 men at each party. A small party, one that would
be considered to be rather secretive, might have only 5 to 7
drinkers, while a large party might have 25 or more men at any
one time. Interestingly, there is a correlation between size of
party, day of occurrence, and nature of occasion for the party. Of
the sixteen parties with 10 or more participants, twelve occurred
on a Saturday or Sunday. Of the nine parties with fewer than 10
participants, all occurred on a Saturday or Sunday. Nine of the
large and four of the small parties coincided with the visit of a
field-trip ship, four and two with the arrival of visitors from
neighboring islands, and four and two with public events of island interest.

There was much less variation in the duration of parties.
Most lasted only three to five hours regardless of the occasion.
However, very large parties with twenty or more men could continue at several locations in sequence for as long as thirty hours.
(Two known parties lasted this long.) The estimated rate of consumption at most parties was about one gallon of yeast per hour by
a group of six to eight men, although it varied tremendously depending on who actually was present and what drinking style was
used. If a man was just passing by a party and had not been
originally asked to join, he would ordinarily be entreated to take
part. However, the obligation of the drinkers to share with such a
passerby was met after a cup or two, and the casual visitor might
not be offered any more or might be otherwise made to feel less
than fully welcome, particularly if he had no close friends or kinsmen among the drinkers. This behavior toward uninvited participants was indicative of the contemporary stresses in interpersonal
relationships within the community, particularly in relation to tra-

ditional attitudes toward the sharing of goods. In the past, there had been a pattern of generalized sharing on request of both goods and services among community members. While this was most pronounced among members of the same or allied clans, it also encompassed patterned sharing between nonkinsmen on a reciprocal basis. The entry of the community into the market economic system and its use of liquid currency had altered this by placing a superordinate value on many goods and services, especially imported goods. Preeminent among imports were cigarettes, and the supply obtained through the sale of individually produced copra never lasted out the interim between ship visits. Cigarettes were an important feature of drinking parties, and participants were expected to bring and share whatever cigarettes they had. The actual extent of such sharing depended on the supply and the closeness of the interpersonal (usually kin) relations of the participants. Since the core group of any drinking party usually comprised close friends and kinsmen, the sharing of individually obtained and owned goods of value presented no difficulty. But many of the casual visitors to parties were neither close friends nor kinsmen and they were not usually encouraged to stay beyond a short period of polite participation since otherwise those present would be obligated to include them in the pattern of sharing a scarce valued commodity.

The locations of drinking parties were also related to traditional island social ideology. Of the twenty-five parties, fifteen occurred in a *fal* (a men's or canoe house), eight in village houses in the absence of women, and two in the bush outside the village area. The location of most drinking parties in a canoe house further emphasized their masculine orientation, since such structures were traditionally off limits to women and essentially remain so today. Only five large, old-style canoe houses have survived on the island, although in the past each clan owned at least one such structure devoted entirely to the activities of men. Canoe houses were the most significant public structures of the village. That a majority of parties took place in these open-sided structures indicated that, in spite of the prohibition law, very little effort was made to conceal a drinking party. Indeed, the boisterous behavior at such parties would have made them difficult to conceal, even if the participants, particularly the younger men, had not publicly demonstrated their drunkenness. This public drunken comportment, and the general noisiness of such parties, made their concealment in dwelling houses also difficult.

The timing and sponsorship of yeast drinking parties was directly related to the economic affairs of the island community. Most parties occurred during or shortly after the arrival of a field-trip ship, which offered the only significant transport link with Truk, the district center, and provided the islanders the opportunity to sell their copra and purchase goods, including yeast. It also brought the paychecks for islanders who were employed by the district or local island governments; most parties were sponsored by these men.

The arrival of the ship is a time of general relaxation and fun. The ship comes to Etal about every three or four months. Its arrival is probably the most significant event to interrupt the otherwise calm and somewhat monotonous daily round of activities. The island may be notified only a few days or weeks in advance of the ship's intended arrival. Until it is announced men do not begin to produce any copra, since the island lacks proper storage facilities for processed copra. Men work long, hard hours just immediately before the ship's arrival. After the transfer of copra has been accomplished, there is always a general letdown that includes one or more yeast parties. Eleven of the twenty-five known parties, for example, were held within the first three days after the arrival of the ship. Other occasions that warranted a yeast party included a variety of public celebrations or events and the arrival of visitors from nearby islands. In some instances the rationale for holding a party was multipurpose. One party, for example, marked the first birthday of a sponsor's first child as well as the visit of island neighbors, while another occurred during the winter holidays in honor of visitors to the island. In some cases the rationale changed at the last moment. A planned party that had been intended for men who had worked on the newest island building became instead a spur-of-the-moment drinking session to relieve the depression following a funeral. Ordinarily, however, drinking parties denote a festive occasion. In line with the general feeling of festivity that accompanies these parties is the occurrence of gambling, usually bingo or blackjack. Of the two forms of gambling, blackjack is considered the more appropriate. First, women do not play blackjack but do play bingo; i.e., blackjack is a male activity like drinking. Second, as a form of gambling blackjack is considerably more daring than is bingo because of the local modifications of the rules of the game, which are oriented toward increasing the odds against winning. This aspect of risk taking is also indicative of the general style of any yeast party and, in general, of drinking itself.

Social Attitudes toward Drinking

The foregoing data have brought out several general points about drinking behavior on Etal. First, drinking was a strictly male activity always carried out by a group. There are no data (even rumors) to suggest that individuals sought to drink alone. Second, drinking was a public phenomenon even though a law prohibited drinking on the island. Third, drinking parties were always primarily associated with events of a public nature—e.g., the arrival of the field-trip ship or of visitors from neighboring islands, and the celebration of public occasions. Parties were only rarely associated with personal events, and then only as a secondary factor. And, fourth, drinking was primarily a young man's endeavor rather than a pattern of behavior consistently or regularly associated with older men, particularly after the age of forty-five or fifty. These data do not, however, inform us as to the specific reasons that lay behind drinking nor about the style of drinking and associated behavior.

The matter of style is one that is very apparent in drinking parties. Every party began as a festive occasion of good times and good will. In addition, there was always a presumed element of daring. Everyone was aware that they were breaking the law—either the island law that prohibits drinking or, for some, the Protestant "law." This sense of daring was reinforced by the occurrence of several other activities also associated with yeast parties. Blackjack was one form of risk taking. It was not uncommon, for example, to see a man lose all of his recently purchased cigarettes, losing because of the exorbitant risks taken during play. The rules of the game did not make it necessary to take unusual risks, but they permitted variations where the odds against winning were very high. Most men took such risks—particularly the younger men. Moreover, there appeared to be as much satisfaction for the player and his comrades in taking high risks and losing as in taking them and winning. It was assumed, of course, that a young man who did lose would do so with good grace and would not lose heavily or frequently. In other words, his status as a virile and reckless young man was not enhanced by consistently taking foolhardy risks, but was affirmed by his demonstration of willingness to risk all that he had occasionally. Such risk taking also showed a man's economic worth since only young men who earned wages or owned copra-producing land had the means to take risks. In this sense, then, taking risks at blackjack was an indicator of the "up-and-coming" status of younger men.[2]

In a quite different way there were other risks associated

with drinking. First, each party began with someone, not always the sponsor, specifying what kind of drinking would be done, either "American cup" or "Indian cup." Evidently, sometime shortly after the end of the Second World War an American Western film was shown on the island, in which both American Indians and cowboys were shown drinking. The cowboys, or "Americans," sipped their liquor slowly, while the Indians gulped or "chugged" their liquor. Thus, an especially daring yeast party was one where Indian cup had been established at the outset as the kind of drinking that everyone would do. It was daring because after gulping down eight to fifteen cups (holding from eight to ten ounces) in a half hour or so a man was in danger of disgracing himself by vomiting, passing out, or performing some other unusual act that warranted the hilarious jibing of the assembled company. Most parties at least started out as Indian cup parties, but usually did not continue as such beyond the first hour or so.

Regardless of the kind of drinking that ensued, yeast parties included other risk taking, i.e., behavior that would not be tolerated in any nondrinking circumstance. The singing of songs was one example. A variety of songs was loudly shouted out or sung at a yeast party. The songs were usually of two types: World War II Japanese songs and Trukese love songs. The singing of World War II Japanese songs was made to seem rather risky for the singers because of my presence. They assumed that an American would not approve of the islanders' remembering the Japanese times so well as to be able to sing songs that were then current. A great many Etal men believed that Americans do not like the Japanese and that any reference to the Japanese period in Micronesia would be offensive to an American, who might retaliate by spreading bad stories about the singer. The singing of Trukese love songs was quite another matter. As Fischer and Swartz (1960) have pointed out, love songs in Truk are usually sung in very soft tones because singing loudly for an audience or displaying heterosexual affection in any form in public would be embarrassing to the singer. Moreover, such songs are inherently risky since they can be construed to have been composed for adulterous liaisons. In local customary law, to be caught at or suspected of adultery could result in heavy losses of land and other goods, not to mention status as a clever and accomplished man. During a drinking party, then, love songs were sung with abandon and with no thought of the consequences.[3]

There is another sense in which drinking was a form of risk taking. The predominant pattern of party behavior was jocular and festive in an atmosphere of happy camaraderie. Everyone knew, however, that any party might have one or more exceptions to this usual pattern. Persons who became argumentative, abusive, and either verbally or physically aggressive were known as "sardines." This was a serious matter since the island community was noted for its rather striking ethic against any form of verbal or physical aggression (Nason 1970). A sardine was someone who had lost his head (just as the canned sardines imported to the island have no heads) and who was therefore temporarily beyond the pale of normal behavior. A sardine would wrestle with his companions, lose his temper and attempt to fight others, pound on houses, throw rocks or sticks aimlessly or at others or at houses, and cry or shout until he was subdued or stopped of his own accord. Normally, a sardine would not be stopped unless the ruckus created became great enough to draw neighbors or kinsmen to the scene or unless there was an imminent threat of physical or personal damage to others or to himself. Thus, sardine behavior was not only a striking departure from normal drinking behavior, but also a significant transgression of the community's attitudes toward aggression or disruption.

The Etiology of Drinking and Drinking Behavior

Drinking is continued and even generally countenanced on the island, in spite of the law, because it is ordinarily associated with relaxation and pleasantry and because yeast itself is a pleasing change from the normally available beverages such as coconut water or, occasionally, sugared coffee. Moreover, even though drinking and getting drunk had associated risks, the act of drinking had positive merits that warranted its continuation. To explain this I shall briefly review some of the social changes that have altered life in the community.

Before 1935, Etal citizens were members of one or another of the eleven matrilineal clans. These were named, exogamous, and corporate units that served to define clearly and unambiguously an individual's social position in the community—at least for marital and social-exchange purposes. Clans also provided the framework for the accomplishment of a variety of group tasks, e.g., house building, fishing, gardening, and buying large canoes. As one of my informants put it, the most important thing about clans was that their members were a cooperative body, mutually supportive of all members. This support manifested itself in many ways, including economic activities, child rearing, litigation, warfare, and even in marital difficulties. This notion of clans as social units altered as a result of changes in island life brought about by missionary activities, the inception of German and then Japanese political changes, and the introduction of a market economy based on liquid currency with wage labor and export trade. In a meeting held in the mid-1930s, community leaders decided to do away with the corporate ownership of property by clans. Up to this time, most of the land on the island was owned by clans which gave individuals usufruct tenure to clan lands. This decision led to further changes in the system of interpersonal relationships, changes particularly related to Christian and market-economy notions of individual labor and individual responsibility. By 1968 the result of these social and economic changes in the traditional pattern of island life was a community in which clans acted only as markers for incest and marriage regulations, but had no other significant social role. As one informant put it, "Cooperation is obeying what the clan chief says to people and working together on things. No one does this anymore. I do not see any cooperation anymore in clans so everyone should just think about their own family" (Nason 1970:298). By 1968 there were no longer any tasks being performed by groups of individuals united by kinship in clans or by other traditional patterns of reciprocally defined and systematic rights and obligations. Instead, individuals worked for wages for one another or for the government, or solely on the basis of very close kinship ties (e.g., within an extended family or on the basis of sibling ties, real or fictive). This was a social situation that was frequently and readily bemoaned as entirely wrong. All island leaders, including the now virtually powerless and roleless clan chiefs, would entreat the community at island meetings and feasts to cooperate with one another, not to engage in gossip or other bad actions against each other. The practical effects of such entreaties were not clearly observable in the day-to-day events in the community.

In this context, then, drinking can be seen as a process whereby men actually did join together for a common purpose in good fellowship. It was always a group phenomenon, most frequently occurring in the remaining structural vestiges of clans, the canoe houses. Drinking parties, aside from being the only recurrent occasions on which groups of men assembled, also emphasized and promoted the continuation of traditionally valued behaviors such as sharing between kinsmen and acts which reaffirmed and reinforced ideals of masculinity.

The changes in island social organization also introduced a new set of interpersonal stresses, which were most readily observable in the increasingly bitter and frequent conflicts over land rights between sibling co-owners, each of whom was competing with the other in the economic sphere, and in the relationships between young men with wage-paying jobs and their in-laws. In the first instance there was a considerable strain because of the maintenance of customary laws about how siblings should make land-rights decisions, e.g., whether or not to sell a given piece of land or how to pass land rights in inheritance to their children. In the event of a dispute, the traditional attitude was that the matter should be amicably settled by discussion of the problem as a private family matter. The concept of discussion as the proper means to settle disputes held and still holds true as a general pattern for most island litigation. If for some reason the dispute did become public knowledge, i.e., was brought into the public arena via a shouting match outside a village house, it would almost certainly be settled by court action in the island or district court system. In the instance of interpersonal conflicts over the sharing of wages or other income with in-laws (or, for that matter, parents and other kinsmen), or in any inter-kin dispute, customary law specified that a private settlement through discussion should prevail—unless, of course, the matter was somehow brought into the public domain. All disputes of any sort were known to virtually all members of the community. The village was highly nucleated and its members operated on the basis of almost total and up-to-date biographical and genealogical knowledge about each other. Disputes might be known but not publicly discussed or recognized until and unless one of the disputants chose to make it a matter of public record by some very public act. While private discussions about a dispute could continue for some time, even generations, the transformation of a dispute into a matter of public concern forced the disputants to settle.

The existence of these new interpersonal problems and their escalation due to new social conditions provide one possible way to interpret sardine behavior. The men who became sardines at a yeast drinking party were invariably known to be in the midst of some wrenching interpersonal dispute with another islander, usually a kinsman. For instance, a carpenter angry over the non-payment of services in building a house attempted to attack the debtor at a party; a young man angry with his father-in-law because of the latter's demand for a major portion of the former's wages threw stones at the father-in-law's house while crying and shouting out his anger and its cause; or, a young man angered by his parents' refusal to turn land over to him beat his mother's house with a stick, crying and shouting, and ran through the house upsetting its contents. In other words, a sardine could express his anger and frustration publicly (and in the process force or attempt to force the issue to some resolution) and do so in a context of rather sympathetic public regard. He was excused on the basis that he was drunk and therefore temporarily "out of his mind," and thus he did not realize the seriousness of this breach of common proper behavior. A sardine could not be fully blamed for bringing a dispute into the public domain, even though he had to apologize to the injured party for his breach of good behavior. If nothing else was accomplished, there was always the fact that the sardine had released a good deal of negatively regarded aggression in a manner that did not redound to his immediate and thorough discredit in the eyes of the community.[4]

The enactment of other kinds of risk-taking behavior at drinking parties represents something quite different from that of the sardines. Murdock (1965) has commented on the possibility that baseball, as played on Truk proper, is a substitute for warfare. By the same token, I suggest that yeast parties, with their gambling, singing, and other forms of risk-associated behavior, provide men—particularly young men—with a substitute for a host of dangerous and risky endeavors which used to define the proper male role, especially that appropriate to younger men, such as warfare; being a navigator, captain, or crewman on a long-distance voyage in outrigger canoes; and becoming an *itang*, a specialist in magic and military matters. Even though these tasks were no longer performed, the associated role concept that young men are carefree, irresponsible, devil-may-care types has not completely disappeared and may be validated by risk taking at yeast drinking parties.

Summary

Drinking on Etal was a male-dominated group phenomenon associated primarily with concepts of risk taking. Insofar as it was group behavior, it was not considered, even though illegal, a particularly bad or improper enterprise. The use of alcohol fulfilled the requirement for a reasonable adaptive substitute for traditional male roles that were no longer possible. Drinking parties also provided the community, especially younger men, who are caught in the bind between traditionally defined social responsibilities and contemporary notions of individualism and economic reality, with an interim means of handling anger and frustration. Drinking parties were, in this sense, an inefficient bridging mechanism between outmoded customary law and proprieties and contemporary problems. It is irrelevant to ask whether the men who became sardines were conscious of their actions, although one could argue either way from the available data.

Drinking did, then, serve useful ends in contemporary Etal society. At the 1968–69 levels of consumption, it did not represent a significant economic drain on community resources, nor did the rate and nature of the alcohol consumed present any real likelihood that men would become "alcoholics." A final question is why the prohibition law was maintained in the face of such flagrant and regular violations by a majority of adult men. It is clear, I believe, that to remove the law would be to remove one small component of the risk-taking aspect of drinking, whereas to maintain it, even though nonsensical legally, is to enhance those attributes of drinking that make drinking a matter of positive merit within the community.

Notes

1. This action was in keeping with the traditional pattern of avoiding potential conflicts by the removal of the source. At one time, for example, the island grew its own tobacco. Thefts of leaves, however, led to the tearing up of all tobacco plants.

2. A more cynical view would be that the younger men would lose all of their cigarettes or money in any event to older male kinsmen who could legitimately borrow all or most of either in the possession of a young man.

3. No penalties were levied against a man for having committed adultery during the research period, although such cases had taken place in the years just prior to the research. No man would, in the usual case, accuse another man solely on the basis of songs, although the songs could be one point of evidence.

4. There is, obviously, a corollary danger that real violence or irreparable damage could occur. This possibility is well known, and thus every attempt was made to restrain and calm any one who had become a sardine, even if this meant taking a few blows in the process. If restraint were not successful and some real damage was done, then the guilty party would be shamed and find himself in a poor social position.

Drinking and Inebriate Behavior in the Admiralty Islands, Melanesia

Theodore Schwartz and Lola Romanucci-Ross

In the course of a study of culture change in the Admiralty Islands (Manus) of northwestern Melanesia, we had the opportunity of observing the initial public use of alcohol among natives. We noted behavior associated with the "drunken" state. Integration of alcohol use into the "contact culture" involved behavioral patterns based on colonial circumstances of the contact situation and on traditional native concepts and institutions. At the "first drinking party" it was possible to observe the development, the communication, and "crystallization" of behavioral cues for the drunk and the sober, the performer and the audience. Most striking was the accommodation of the consumption of alcohol to the prestige system, and to the uses of altered states of consciousness along with folk explanations of such altered states. Interpretations are suggested that fit behavior fragments, such as "drunken comportment," into the behavioral repertoire of the cultural-historical moment. Our observations and descriptions of initial alcohol use were informed by long-term anthropological investigation of the total cultural context.

Background

In November of 1962, a prohibition on the legal sale of alcoholic beverages to natives was replaced by antidiscrimination laws that guaranteed their right to purchase and consume such beverages in hotels and other licensed premises, or to buy beer for consumption off premises. A year later, this law was modified to permit the purchase of any alcoholic beverage for off-premise use. Although we made many observations between 1963 and 1966 in towns, in hotels, and in bars, this analysis is directed in particular to patterns of public drinking in two native villages, Mokareng and Peri.

The Admiralty Islands lie about one hundred fifty miles north of New Guinea. They constitute a small archipelago at 2° south latitude and 147° east longitude. The population in 1963 consisted of about twenty thousand natives from approximately twenty linguistic groups as recognized by natives. A few hundred "Europeans," mainly Australian, and some Chinese of Australian citizenship, lived in the administrative town of Lorengau on the main island of Manus, or at the nearby naval base, Lombrum.

Mokareng village is a few miles from the naval base and the airfield. Peri village is on the south coast of the main island, a day's trip by sailing canoe from Lorengau or the naval base.

Natives of the Admiralties classify themselves into three groups. The Manus formerly lived by fishing and trade, and they formerly inhabited pile-house villages over the shallow lagoons between fringing reefs and the shore. (Since 1948 they have rebuilt their villages on the beaches.) The Matankor are people of various linguistic groups who lived on the small islands around the Great Admiralty Island and combine fishing with the cultivation of tree crops and/or gardening. The Usiai formerly were exclusively gardening people from the interior of the Great Admiralty Island.

Admiralty Islanders have had sporadic contacts with ships since the sixteenth century, but there were no established bases until the nineteenth century. German administration begun in 1884 was replaced by Australian administration in 1914. We are not aware of German policy on native use of alcoholic beverages, but with the Australian administration, laws prohibiting its consumption and sale to natives were in effect.

From the 1880s to the present, Admiralty Island natives have served in European employ, working on ships, in towns, and on plantations. Though contact with Christian missions came during German times, permanent missions were established under Australian administration. Peri village became Catholic in the early 1930s; Mokareng had been converted to Catholicism earlier.

In 1942 Australian rule was interrupted by the Japanese invasion. Two years later the American invasion restored Australian rule and led to a massive occupation by American forces. An air strip several miles long was cut through land belonging to the people of Mokareng. The people of Peri had not been as close to the bases but, as in Mokareng, most of the men had worked for each of the successive occupying forces.

In 1946, certain religious and political events occurred which evoked highly contrastive responses in the two villages. Mokareng joined an attempt with the North Coast people to petition the Americans to take over administration of the Admiralties from Australia. On the South Coast, Peri was the site for an abortive local movement (one of a series in other South Coast villages) to discard tradition, particularly economic and ceremonial exchange systems. These local movements proved unsuccessful but their leaders gained a following mainly among young men. A movement with broader goals was begun toward the end of 1946 by Paliau, of Baluan, who was attracting young men to his meetings from all over the South Coast and beyond. In the excitement of this rapidly growing movement, and in the impatience with its secular program (which involved such features as starting native plantations), the coming of the *cargo* was proclaimed. This cargo was to appear within a week brought by ships filled with European goods.

Mokareng, by contrast, was one of many North Coast villages that did not join the Paliau movement. Rather, one large village faction became part of a militant opposition to the cult and the movement. The people of Mokareng retained a hostility to the Australian administration, which they had wished to see replaced by the Americans; but they remained loyal to the Roman Catholic mission and thereby somewhat secondarily supported the administration. Thus, for almost fifteen years, Mokareng and other North Coast villages refused to join the native local government council. Whereas both Peri and Mokareng contained internal village factions, factionalism was particularly characteristic of Mokareng where there was a deep cleavage, going back many generations, over the legitimacy of a series of oblique successions to land and chieftainship (Romanucci-Ross 1966). Indeed, the village headman, who represented this line of succession, and his faction had long been sympathetic to the Paliau movement and the council, but he could not swing the village as a whole to the movement.

The setting for deprohibition was not exclusively influenced by the cultures and social situation of Admiralty Island villages. After World War II, New Guinea became a trust territory under the United Nations. As decolonization swept through the world, pressure increased for Australia to prepare New Guinea for self-government. During the 1950s, Australia began an intensive educational effort and took steps toward the development of local government through councils, as well as through the formation of a representative body for the whole territory. The older lines of racial discrimination became increasingly embarrassing as more and more natives came to occupy jobs at status levels equivalent or superior to those of many Australian personnel. By the time of deprohibition there were native doctors, higher clerks, elected politicians on district and national levels, and school superintendents, some of whom supervised European teachers. Such people, although formally integrated with whites of their status, were not able to drink with them. Some Australians drank heavily but, more important, they made extensive use of alcohol in the symbolism and ceremony of sociability and acceptance. Like many of the enlightened policies of the postwar administration, discrimination in all forms that could be legally influenced was ended.

The deprohibition act of 1962 was greeted with the utmost skepticism by the majority of the white population, including local administrative officers and journalists who predicted the dire consequences of permitting natives to drink. In the first years of legalized native drinking, journalists reported frequently on native drinking behavior in hotels and bars in the towns. An increase in violent acts was alleged by some. Others complained about bad behavior. Broken bottles and glasses were said to lead to gashed feet and with the frequent requirement that footwear be worn in bars, native entrepreneurs reportedly went into the business of renting shoes for such use. There were "reports" that natives behaved badly in bars, sometimes urinating in public, drinking to the point of vomiting or unconsciousness, fighting, or angling for drinks and not taking their "shout" (buying their own round of drinks). Still others told of the great increase in business at bars and hotels as natives in towns flocked to enjoy their new privileges in these highly prestigious places, where they previously had entered only as servants.

There was much concern with the economic effects of urban drinking on the native domestic economy. Beer, rum, gin, and whiskey were expensive in the territory, even for Europeans. Many an Australian civil servant spent a large portion of his salary on "grog." There seems little doubt from what we observed in various towns, that on payday many natives used much of their weekly wage to buy alcoholic beverages. For the unskilled urban worker not in the civil service, a day's wage bought less than three bottles of beer. There were protests from some women that they were getting too little money from their husbands to feed their families.

It is probable that one effect of this heavy investment in alcohol was to exacerbate the sense of disparity in wealth between natives and Europeans. Journalists pointed out that giving natives the right to drink in hotels and bars did not eliminate segregation in drinking. In the hotels there tended to be informal zonal separation into different drinking areas. Often, as natives moved into the hotel bars, some whites abandoned them in favor of still-segregated private clubs. What was overlooked in the negative accounts of the results of eliminating segregation and legal discrimination, however, was the many private and administrative functions at which mixed groups of natives and Europeans were now able to drink together.

From the outset, missionaries and the many mission sects opposed permitting natives the use of alcohol. Many missions lobbied against deprohibition, preached against it to their congregations, and prohibited use of alcohol by their members. Various Protestant groups began a pledge campaign for voluntary abstention. The Catholic mission, which seemed the most tolerant toward the idea of native drinking, preached moderation. The Seventh-Day Adventists marked off their religious communities by strict taboo on three of the things for which natives had a particular liking or addiction: tobacco, betel nut, and pork, and long before deprohibition they had preached against the evils of alcohol. They drank grape juice as "unfermented wine," claiming that this was the wine spoken of in the Bible and drunk by Jesus. Paliau set himself in strong opposition to native use of alcohol, much as he had long unsuccessfully opposed gambling as a waste of the money and energy needed for native development. His opposition was entirely on these grounds, not on religious grounds expressed through his native separatist church. Campaigns by the Australian administration also were conducted, almost from the start of deprohibition, by such means as posters showing a drunken and disheveled native, bottle in hand, with ragged and starved wife and children in the background accompanied by the warning that "this could be you."

It is important, then, that the legal public use of alcohol came in accompanied by many preconceptions, including the notion that this was the European's vice, an expensive, addictive activity for males, with certain highly expected behavioral effects, possibly sinful, and in any case wasteful and perhaps socially destructive. But it also could be prestigious and gratifying in the "identification" that it permitted (Ogan 1966) though many Europeans were known to be either nondrinkers or temperate. It was gratifying and prestigious in other ways related to traditional culture, as well as the contact culture. With the introduction of drinking, a compensatory position of self-righteousness was prepared for the nondrinker as well.

Prior to the presence of Europeans, natives of the Admiralties, as elsewhere in Melanesia and New Guinea, had no knowledge of fermented, alcoholic drinks. Betel nut (in combination with powdered lime and pepper leaf) was chewed in much of Melanesia and lowland New Guinea as a stimulant that could seemingly be habit-forming. It is said to promote wakefulness and the ability to sustain work effort. Natives had reported dizziness and light-headedness from excessive use. We have heard it referred to, by natives, as "the native's whiskey." In the Admiralties, betel nut had many herbalistic, ceremonial, and symbolic uses. The large clusters of nuts from the betel palm could be divided, used for counting contributions to a feast and for making token distributions. Betel nut was divided and sent by important men as a message to members of their dispersed networks in their own as well as other villages, to announce and elicit, in its acceptance, a commitment in entrepreneurial feasts, ceremonial exchange, or warfare. Use of betel nut in magic, sorcery, and curing is connected to the notion of its "strength," its "bite," and burning sensation as it is chewed, and the bloodred color of the expectorate.

Kava, a nonfermented infusion prepared from the roots of *Piper methysticum*, was used only on the islands of Baluan, Lou, and Rambucho. Drunk in all feasts as part of ceremonial exchange, or in a mourning feast for an important person, the infusion was prepared by straining water through a mass of kava roots that had been pounded in stone mortars. The soil in which it grew was not to be washed from the roots, so that one drank large bowls of muddy kava through cane straws. Garden workers often chewed the root for refreshment. It is reported to be mildly intoxicating, inducing a drowsy state of well-being. (We noticed no effect from several cupfuls but felt the mouth to be anesthetized by chewing the root itself.) Use of kava did not diffuse beyond this group to the other linguistic groups of the Admiralties with whom the kava users were in intensive interaction. Before deprohibition, tea, coffee, and soft drinks had begun to replace kava at Baluan feasts. There was no equivalent to kava in the feasts and exchanges of the other peoples who comprised the majority of the Admiralty Islanders.

Native experience with alcohol may have begun with visiting ships or with traders during German times, but there is no memory of this. During the German administration, natives began to work for Europeans and began to observe European drinking as "houseboys" serving the drinks or caring for drunken masters. During the German period and particularly around Rabaul, New Britain, where so many Admiralty Islanders have worked throughout this century, Chinese merchants have sold bootleg liquor to natives. But most natives came to try alcoholic drinks as domestic servants, or from contact with the Japanese or American armies during World War II. Others took part in the fairly widespread experimentation with the drinking of methylated spirit, particularly after the war when spirit (ethyl and methyl alcohol) was the most generally available form of alcohol. The "spirit," as it is known to natives in Pidgin English, was used throughout the territory to preheat kerosene-burning pressure lamps and stoves. For many years natives were constantly warned against its poisonous effects, but its illegal use continued. It remained the cheapest available means to intoxication. There was no prestige attached to its use since it was known that Europeans did not use it. When other more expensive and prestigious forms of drink were used, however, the "spirit" was kept in reserve or used as an additive to assure that the desired effect could be reached. Natives had come to expect that as one drinks, one becomes loud, abusive, and feisty, and that sometimes one vomits, walks unsteadily, sings loudly, or passes out and needs assistance. It was also known that the most common outcome of drinking is simply that of somewhat freer sociability than is considered normal or proper. Terms that can be glossed as "crazy," "dizzy," "confused," and "sick" were used to describe the inebriate state.

Drinking Parties

The first public drinking party held in Mokareng after deprohibition in 1964 was a "finish-time" party, given for a man who returns home after having been away a long time at work or in jail. On this particular occasion Popolu, a young man whose marriage had recently been celebrated with a major ceremonial exchange in surprisingly traditional form, had just been released after a month in jail. Popolu, attempting to board a freighter to make a purchase at the canteen, had been stopped by a native policeman whom he punched after alleged rough treatment. Others joined him in fist fights with police.

This "finish-time" party followed the Admiralty-wide pattern for all rites of passage, which serve as markers for a series of stages, such as naming and (the now-discontinued) ceremonial occasions such as ear or nose piercing. Such ceremonial in the Admiralty Island cultures, from birth through the events mentioned, betrothal, marriage in various phases, the birth of children, mourning, and finally commemoration much later, are all part of the long event cycle of affinal exchange. The essence of this exchange pattern is the giving of valuables by the groom's side, once dogs' teeth and shell beads (now mainly cash), and a return by the bride's kin in consumables, foodstuffs (now prestigiously including imported food) (M. Mead 1934; Schwartz 1963). Mead saw one function of such exchanges as a stimulant to the production of usable consumables in quantities above those required for immediate subsistence. Coconut oil, sago, and other consumables could be used gradually over months or shunted, as was often the case, into other exchanges. Generally only a small part of what was given was to be consumed at the feast itself. Most was given uncooked to be brought home by the recipients. Thus, consumables were also converted into stored obligations. Alcohol now occupies a favored position among the consumables. The context in which alcohol is used conditions drinking behavior and its effects.

On this first occasion, Lokowa, as Popolu's mother's brother, and Pokumbut, his mother's mother's brother, gave the feast in honor of his return from jail. Traditionally, this feast was seen in terms of affinal exchange. This was a continuing exchange in the marriage of Popolu's deceased parents, and Lokowa, as the principal to the mother's side, was the giver of consumables, aided by Pokumbut, his own mother's brother. At the same time, Lokowa was engaged in exchanges with the relatives of Popolu's bride from whom he had just received a large consignment of consumables. Popolu's bride's party helped Lokowa in this new exchange. The recipients in the "finish-time" feast were relatives of Popolu's father. The principal on the father's side was Potihin, the aged but vigorous headman under the precouncil system to which Mokareng still adhered. Mokareng was a village deeply riven by factional conflict between the groups represented by Pokumbut, head of the clan descended from the original Matankor people of Mokareng, and by Potihin, who represented the immigrant group of Usiai that was dominant in the precolonial period. This particular feast, then, marked another in a long series of exchanges in competitive validation of the statuses of these "big men." But this feast, for the first time with Pokumbut and Lokowa giving a large and expensive quantity of alcohol, not only provided an obligation to be discharged at the later date, but the alcohol had to be consumed at the feast itself, almost immediately, as it was phrased, to be "pissed away," leaving nothing but the debt and the momentary perturbation of the self. For this reason, we suggest, alcohol is the ultimate consumable. It cannot serve as it did in the past, as a gradually consumed or retransmitted commodity compensating the groom's side for their amassed money and valuables.

Lokowa provided ten bottles of gin and rum and nine dozen bottles of beer. In addition, in the previous "modern tradition" he gave eighteen small drums of rice and six dozen carbonated drinks. A very large feast of cooked food was provided, served formally at tables in the village clearing, along with the drinks. Lokowa proudly said that there was plenty of whiskey and so there would be no drinking of methylated spirit, but at least one of the guests on the receiving side had brought a bottle of "spirit."

Following the customary long speeches by the host and recipients, Pokumbut spoke of the marriage of Popolu, "a good Catholic marriage," Potihin dissented sotto voce, countering that the mission had spoiled many good marriage customs such as polygamy and divorce, making it difficult for a man to dispose of a lazy or barren wife. Pokumbut then directed school children to sing several hymns in English. He went on to mention the fight that led to Popolu's arrest. He deplored the violence that jeopardized their carving industry, but then expressed sentiments that more truly reflected group feelings. He thanked those who had been bloodied, who had fought the police, who had had to pay fines. Other speakers repeated these points while food was served in European style. Food at feasts was traditionally distributed for home consumption with bowls marked for return. Betel nut used to be distributed to "clear the record" as to what and how much was given. Now a written record was also made by both sides, of every item, including the amounts of all beer, whiskey, and food. This record would be used to distribute the later cash payment by the present recipients of consumables. Pokumbut, Lokowa, and Popolu, the main members of the donor group, abstained from drinking, explaining that it would not be right for them to consume the gift. All of the recipient party drank except Potihin, since abstinence was one of the various taboos he imposed on himself. His strength "required" the constant use of tobacco and betel nut, but he would not take alcohol because of the effects he had seen it produce in others, European and native. He was, by his own admission, afraid to experience this disturbance of the self. At none of four parties in Peri and Mokareng did we see any attempts by people who were drinking to induce others to drink, or to drink more.

After the meal, strong tea with large amounts of sugar was served to all who were seated. Women were not served alcoholic drinks. Some of the principals (Lokowa and Popolu) said they could not be seated with some of the donors because of avoidance rules applicable to some affinal kin. One woman substituted for the bride who could not eat among tabooed affinal relatives.

Three violations of avoidance by inebriates were noticed during the evening, two considered humorous and one shocking by the onlookers. The last occurred between brother and sister. The son of Kapur, a New Guinean who had settled in Mokareng, wanted to fight, and was shouting and challenging everyone. As his sister tried to restrain him he tore her dress. Since normal behavior between brother and sister is one of reserve, almost avoidance, this caused much comment.

In this "finish-time" party there seemed to be two phases of intoxication. The first phase was two or three hours after the party had begun, the other was toward morning, just as the party was breaking up and as the audience was renewed by the awakening village. During the early part of the evening the party seemed gay, the audience large, the drinking open and conspicuous. Until after midnight there were about eighty people taking part at any one time, most of whom, if they were not directly involved in the core groups of the exchange, did not drink. Most of these persons went to sleep and returned in the morning. The host and his wife made several remarks that made their aims explicit. Lokowa referred to the bottles as "bombs." For the first drinking exchange he wanted to see if he could "lay waste" the guests, demonstrate how great a quantity of liquid wealth was being consumed, and have a small amount left over after having reduced everyone to intoxication or unconsciousness so that it could be said that all that he had provided had not been consumed.

By morning Lokowa's "bomb" had taken effect. One powerfully built young man from another village was still dancing to ukulele accompaniment as the village children rejoined the party on their way to school. As the sun rose this young man removed his shirt and began dancing with an adolescent boy. Eight men "passed out" and were now sleeping. Kapur's son, bellowing in agony, shouted obscenities, as he ran and walked about in a pattern of inebriate behavior known as "big mouth" (not previously encountered, but to be heard again in Peri and from inebriates coming home on the road from drinking in Lorengau). He had been restrained by the sober, a useful function quickly taken up by abstainers. Now he was being watched at a distance by villagers with fearful seriousness and expectancy. Several young men, still awake, were sitting in a stupor. Others, despite the heat, were still wandering about in their dance finery, the best of whatever European clothing they had, including heavy Navy sweaters. One of the speechmakers of the night before who kept the written record for the recipients, assured us that he was "all right" because he had not drunk spirit. He passed out shortly afterwards. We saw no sign of further drinking once the sun had risen. A schoolteacher had been sitting dazed. He jumped up with a loud yell, ran to the road, vomited violently, and collapsed there. Another, Potihin's son, spoke heavily and deliberately indicating that the trouble with the rest of them is that they have not learned the taboos that go with drinking, such as not mixing drinks. He had learned around Europeans, he said, that one must stick to the same drink all night; he had had only gin and whiskey. A visitor from a nearby island in the Admiralties was lying on his back on the ground surrounded by a group of onlookers. He was speaking unintelligibly to all. Everyone was listening to his utterances. It seemed incoherent speech in his own language, admixed with meaningless words. He was "speaking in tongues," a behavior that occurs in Admiralty Islands religious cults in which Mokareng and this man's village had not participated. The rapt interest of the onlookers, as if each word might be oracular, was strongly reminiscent of what had been observed among cultists. Toward morning, a number of inebriates had begun saying things in English, watching in particular the reactions of their guest (L.R.). The use of English (by unschooled adults) is taken as very funny, and is sometimes heard on other occasions, unassociated with drinking. Men shout mock orders to each other, in English in a European manner, often with obscenities that are also incorporated in Pidgin English.

The party was considered to be a great success, and Mokareng was to become known for its weekend drinking parties (mainly of the second type described below). Lokowa's pride and satisfaction over the imbalance of the prestige were evident.

The second party in Mokareng, also in 1964, was given by a group of about fifteen young men, six of whom worked in Lorengau. The composition of such informal recreational gatherings usually included young married men as well as bachelors, men working out of the village, work buddies from other villages or ethnic groups, and invited guests. Eight bottles of rum and gin with some methylated spirit as "backup" impressed villagers with the high bottle-to-man ratio. The party began late in the evening and, in native tradition, it had to continue until after sunrise. The windows of the scrap iron house were filled with a constantly changing group of assorted onlookers. Women, including those belonging to the household, did not enter the party room itself, nor did they drink. We heard some expressions of resentment about the exclusiveness of this party, but some village men simply entered and were offered drinks. Mwaka, and Kapur, the New Guinean in his late fifties who had married into the village thirty years earlier, drunkenly provided excitement by dancing all night and at intervals the latter challenged his two sons in a European pugilistic stance. Some drank and danced to ukulele and guitar music until morning, while others drank, joked, chewed betel, smoked cigarettes, both ready-made and those made from strong trade tobacco and newspaper. Some slept from time to time. The outer room was filled with "observers," particularly young boys. A compulsion to finish the liquor was coupled with desire to space it out until morning. At times observers, participants, even dancers appeared to be bored. The dancing seemed forced, occasionally grim, not unlike what we had observed in ritual form in the context of an earlier cargo cult in another part of the Admiralties. During much of the night there was joking throughout the room, frequently followed by uproarious laughter that would be terminated by the usual shout in unison from all of those who had been laughing. There was the usual joking about a man who had injured himself while fishing, and Mwaka, a one-legged elderly man, was asked to dance. Mwaka pounded his foot and his crutch and all laughed. Most of the talking was done in Pidgin English since visitors from several linguistic groups were present, but several men did speak in English. Kapur called out to his daughter: "Come, darling, come to your father." At this party all such utterances were considered very funny indeed. Toward morning, only the original group felt obliged to go through to the end. There were no fights, no aggressive behavior other than Kapur's, no insults, no loud shouting or obscenity. Two young men were said to be very sick; they vomited and then slept throughout the following day.

Two later drinking parties in Peri village in 1965 and 1966 featured the collective purchase of liquor. The first was a sedate beer party given by a schoolteacher who was from the village itself, at which no signs of inebriate behavior were noted. At the 1966 party in Peri, the return of one of the authors (T.S.) to Peri was celebrated, along with talk about inaugurating the new meetinghouse where the party was held. There was only one bottle of rum, plus an amount of beer not exceeding two bottles per person. The meal was served at a well-set table: rice, canned meat, chicken, and tea. The group included twelve of the present and past councillors and committeemen of the village, all elected officials, most with traditional legitimacy as leaders. Music came from a battery-operated record player owned by one of the hosts. Spectators watched over the low windowsills. All members of the party were married men, ranging in age from thirty-five to sixty years; a few younger men as well as six or eight older men joined the party uninvited after the meal, but no one objected. Some of the unmarried girls of the village were asked to come in to join the dancing but they did not drink or eat. A few children wandered in and out. No one abstained totally from drinking but most of the men took little and did not ask for more. Rapail Manuai, in his mid-fifties, of prominence in village affairs, danced and drank as much as he received from the limited stocks until the party ended. Most of the other councillors just sat smiling and nursing their drinks. Rapail kept challenging them to dance, not to drink; he became noisily insistent and resentful. Two of the younger men who had joined the party unasked, and who drank as much as they could get, did much of the male dancing. No interest was shown by the men at the party in the young women who danced, for dancing and drinking were considered to be male matters (with the recent revival of traditional dancing this has now changed). About 1:00 A.M. most of the observers had left and it seemed that the drinks had long since been finished, but Rapail, Kraman, and Kanawai were still going strong. The kerosene lamp began to run out of fuel and the record player was slowing down. When the lamp expired, the three inebriates refused to go home. Kanawai and Kraman began to "big mouth" in the village square outside the meetinghouse. Rapail stated that he would keep on dancing, then he abruptly started for his nearby house and passed out in the clearing. While they were being taken to their houses, Kanawai and Kraman were shouting curses and obscenities in voices that could be heard through most of the village. Kraman began shouting the name of his brother-in-law Tano, calling for him to come to him, shouting, moaning, and weeping. Tano had married Kraman's sister but had not given him any recent gifts even though Kraman wanted a radio and Tano had just returned from teaching in New Guinea where he could have bought him one. Both Kraman and Kanawai were taken home, restrained by small groups of men. They could be heard shouting until they got to their houses. Such grievances are not easily expressed. For Kraman, his night of "big mouth" provided the occasion to advertise to the village that he felt insufficiently compensated for the marriage of his sister to Tano. For Rapail and Kanawai or the young men at Mokareng we can only speculate on personal, individual motives for inebriation.

It was learned from discussions that followed that there had been one previous drinking party in Peri at which alcohol had been consumed in an affinal exchange. At that party the same three men had become inebriated, going into "big mouth" and requiring restraint. By now, it was well established that in any group there are a few who are "bad drinkers." Despite this expectation of recurrent individualistic drinking patterns, Kanawai and

Kraman had been allowed to crash the party and to drink more than others.

Interpretation

In an insightful presentation based on a review and analysis of a wealth of cross-cultural material on "drunken comportment," Mac-Andrew and Edgerton have demonstrated that such behavior has a kind of "impulsivity that possesses the peculiar ability to maintain a keen sense of the appropriate" (1969:85). In concurring with this view, we hope that the preceding observations and the interpretations that follow can indicate "how it comes about" as a first approximation.

Public inebriation is both a state and a status. Aside from personal motives, the inebriate is selected by personality and situation to act for the group as a whole. The inebriate acts on his own needs, which, though in part personally expressive, also move him to occupy this transient status. He serves the group expectation that there will be some drunkenness at the drinking party, regardless of the abundance or scarcity of alcohol, and that some of the drinkers will manifest certain extreme behaviors that validate the entire proceeding.

In all of the parties that were observed, the drinking behavior and the effects of alcohol, mediated by the emergent expectations of actors and audience, may be summarized briefly. There is the expectation, confirmed in behavior, that each individual will have his own characteristic responses to drinking and that they will recur whenever he drinks. The audience acts as if what occurs has novelty, importance, and meaning to be divined. Some behaviors are considered humorous, but most of the extreme displays by the inebriates, such as "big mouth" behavior, incoherent speech, staggering, and vomiting command serious attention.

Other notions in native belief enter into expectation and response to the use of alcohol. One is that of "strength." Long before deprohibition, the whiskey of the European was commonly referred to as "strong water," something that "fights" within one, "strikes" one's mouth and insides. It has power, like other things that affect or disturb the state of the self. In this there are striking parallels to the "strength" of ginger, pepper, lime, and betel nut, which are used commonly in magic, divination, curing, and sorcery for their effects on the self, particularly that part of it which we would gloss as the "soul." The Admiralty native traditionally conceives of the self in a disarticulated way. Each body function, emotion, sense, or feeling is associated with a part of the body or an organ. Shame is in the forehead, anger in the abdomen, fear in the buttocks, thought and memory in the neck. The soul, manifested by consciousness and breath and distinct from thought, is associated with the eyes, more generally the face. Loss of consciousness, signaled by rolling up the eyes and presaged by dizziness, is taken as the separation of the soul, in all or in part, from the body, although life continues under jeopardy so long as there is wind in the heart-lung organ. So the conclusion of the inebriation process is taken as nonfinal death in the loss of consciousness. While this part of the cycle is seen as a state of loss, the early part seems to be a state of gain, paralleling what is believed to happen in all forms of possession, that is, control by an ego-alien being, force, or substance, which occurs in various special states (illness, for example; see Romanucci-Ross 1969). In this gain-loss cycle the inebriate behavior constitutes something added over and above normal, substituting its control over behavior for that of one's own self.

Such behaviors and their folk interpretations occur in religious cults both in group and individual manifestation. They occur as well in "insanity" and forms of illness where the native will invoke possession or some addition to the self, as explanation. Extreme behaviors include convulsions, staggering, and other motor disorders, compulsive behaviors, sudden dramatic alterations in personality, temporary psychosis, seeming coma, agitation, incoherence, "speaking in tongues" (other languages, other voices, and pseudospeech), inappropriate behavior in form, content, or magnitude, violations of "taboo," assumed license, and other aberrant behaviors. Such behaviors have a communicational function and constitute metastable states (see Schwartz 1962). By "metastable state" we mean one of the various extreme states of the personality or culture of an individual, group, or society. Metastable states are potential within the normal state. The transformation to the metastable state requires a heightening of certain variables such as excitation, intoxication, intensity of belief, or commitment. Such a state signifies to others that the possessed person is not for the moment "himself." It is transient and difficult to maintain, yet it has a stable set of recurrent properties when it does occur, hence, "metastable."

The metastable state seen in the class of extreme behaviors passes through the gain-loss cycle commencing with possession through addition to the self of an immanent powerful or disturbing substance or spirit. This is commonly followed by a state of "soul separation" marked by dizziness, or light-headedness, followed by "soul loss," loss of consciousness, and the terminus of the immanent control.

Native interpretation of inebriation is affected by the notions governing other extreme or unusual behaviors. It is not necessary to the above interpretation that alcohol be thought of in explicitly animate terms, although it verges on this. It is enough that it is thought of as a "strong" psychoactive substance for which its users have specific expectations about its effects. The adept drinks to become possessed by this substance and some attain the status of the inebriate. The alcohol may have certain direct sensorimotor and, perhaps, transient personality effects, but behaviors attributed to inebriation are not limited to these effects. Whatever the direct effects of alcohol are, can be seen only to the extent that they can be separated from the effects keyed to the expectations of users in various cultures.

Just as the inebriate is not "himself" as he shouts curses, challenges, and reproaches, the cultist, for example (Schwartz 1962, 1963, 1973), proclaims that his ideas, his program, are not his own but that he is a mere channel through whom God or the Dead speak. The cultist must manifest the symptoms that validate his "disinterested" claim to a role that is responsive to social demand even though it may serve his own covert needs as well. Without such validation, the collusion between the audience and the communicant may break down. In the drinking party he is virtually possessed by the wealth and the power of his host. He is elevated, animated, then "wasted," but in his temporary otherness he may "big mouth" some claims of his own while his behavior validates the event, the drinking party.

V. Alcohol in Asia

270   Beliefs, Behaviors, and Alcoholic Beverages

Notes on Drinking in Japan

Bufo Yamamuro

Historical

Confucius (550–479 B.C.) said, "Drinking knows no limit, but never be boisterous with drinking." Confucianism encourages moderation but not abstinence. Primarily, this teaching was moral and political philosophy but not religion. Its classical literature was early introduced into Japan through Korea. During the reign of Emperor Ohjin (313–270 B.C.), Prince Ujinowakiiratsuko studied Confucianism under the Korean scholars Ichiki and Wani. Confucian teachings later exerted profound influences on Japanese thought and culture.

Buddha (568–478 B.C.) stressed total abstinence. The last of his five commandments forbade drinking.

1. Never kill living beings.
2. Never steal.
3. Never be lewd.
4. Never tell a lie.
5. Never take strong drink.

These were daily rules for every follower of Buddha. One of the sutras of primitive Buddhism enumerates six sequels of drinking: (1) loss of property, (2) disease, (3) discord and strife, (4) loss of reputation, (5) disturbance of temper, and (6) daily loss in wisdom. Other sutras mention ten disadvantages and thirty-six faults of drinking. Not only personal abstinence but refraining from the sale of strong drink is an essential qualification for Bodhi-sattva (Buddha elects) of Mahāyāna (the Greater Vehicle). Except on rare occasions for medication, Buddha emphatically advocated the strictest principle of total abstinence. Buddhist scriptures, naturally, are full of teachings on the matter. Buddhism was introduced into Japan in A.D. 552 and became the national religion before long.

The native religion of Japan is Shintoism, with a shamanistic background, which later developed into monolatry. Japanese history dates back to 660 B.C. when the Emperor Jimmu, the first emperor of the present dynasty of the imperial family, was enthroned. The prehistoric myths contain many references to *sake,* taken from fermented rice, but this was originally sweet sake without alcohol content. Divine sake is inseparably entwined with

Shinto worship. However, the Miyake Shrine dedicated to Prince Ninigi (grandson and legal successor of the goddess Amaterasu), the national ancestor, and the Tsuma Shrine dedicated to Princess Konohanasakuya, the national mother, are situated in the province of Hyuga (Miyazaki prefecture), the southern island of Kyushu, and both exclusively used *amazake* (sweet sake without any alcohol content) from time immemorial. This ancient custom was followed by the Grand Shrine of Ise and many others. Moreover, sake was used only at the time of festivals.

Sake was etymologically an abbreviation of "sakae" (prosperity) because the merry feeling associated with intoxication reminded drinkers of prosperity. The original form of the Chinese character 酒 representing strong drink, was 酉, which symbolizes the shape of a pot for strong drink. (The prefix 氵 is the emblem of water.)

The origin of alcoholic beverages was *yashiori no sake*, fermented by Prince Susanoono, younger brother of the goddess Amaterasu. He made the eight-headed monster serpent drunk with it, and killed him. Prince Yamatotakeru, son of the Emperor Keiko (A.D. 71–131), again intoxicated Kumaso, the vicious Ainu lord, and killed him.

There are a number of Shinto sake gods, the most conspicuous among them being Okuninushi-no-Mikoto (Ohmiwa Shrine), his son Ohyamakui-no-Mikoto (Matsuo Shrine), and Sukunahikona-no-Kami. These gods belonged to the Izumo race, original inhabitants of southern Japan, which was conquered by the Tenson race, forefathers of the more temperate present imperial household and their followers.

The most primitive method of fermentation was to chew the grains to imitate natural fermentation. Another method was to lead sprouting and saccharifying grains to fermentation. During the reign of the Emperor Ohjin a Chinese named Susuyari became a naturalized subject and taught an excellent method of fermentation. In this way refined sake (a transparent liquid) gradually became popular, taking the place of amazake and raw (unrefined) sake. Rice, leaven, and water were used to produce refined sake. Even in Shinto festivities or ceremonies, refined alcoholic sake became predominant.

After Buddhism became the national religion, prohibition was decreed from time to time. The following dates are on record:

Under Emperor Kohtoku, March, A.D. 646
Under Empress Kensho, July, A.D. 722

Under Emperor Shomu, July, A.D. 732
Under Emperor Shomu, May, A.D. 737
Under Empress Koken, February, A.D. 758
Under Empress Shotoku, July, A.D. 770

These imperial decrees were usually intended to counteract menaces, due to famines or epidemics, by religious and moral effects rather than economically.

Lord Tabito Ohtomo, an outspoken and reactionary decadent, contributed thirteen poems in praise of sake to the noted *Manyo Shu,* a collection of forty-five hundred thirty-one-syllabled Japanese poems published about twelve hundred fifty years ago, of which the following are examples:

> Far better to get drunk and weep
> Than sagaciously speak like a wizard.

> Rather be a pot of sake than a human being
> To be saturated with sake.

> If only merry in this present world
> Never mind being insect or bird in the next.

During the Heian Era (A.D. 794–1184) with the capital in Kyoto, prohibition or temperance was often decreed to guard against luxury, riotous festivities, and extravagant banquets. Denkyo and Kohboh, two outstanding Buddhist leaders, were both staunch advocates of total abstinence.

The Kamakura Era (A.D. 1184–1333), with the seat of authority in Kamakura, marked the start of the feudal age, and Bushido, or knighthood, came into power. Under the influence of Myoe, noted Buddhist saint, the Hohjohs, the feudal rulers, exemplified temperance and thrift, laying foundations for Bushido. The Mongolian invasion was a great national calamity, and Tokiyori Hohjoh prohibited the sale of sake (dated 30 September 1252). It is recorded that 37,274 pots of sake were destroyed in Kamakura alone. After this manner was the spirit of loyalty and patriotism fostered in those days. Eison and Ryokan were distinguished Buddhist social workers and courageously upheld national prohibition. Eisai was the great pioneer of Zen Buddhism. He brought tea seeds from China and universally encouraged tea drinking instead of sake drinking. He composed a volume on the "Tea-Drinking Regimen." Throughout Japan, a stone pillar stands at the entrance of every Zen Buddhist temple with the inscription: *Garlic and wine never to be admitted into the gate.*

The popular Buddhism of Shinran, founder of the Shin sect

intended for the salvation of the masses, tended to "only-believism" and antinomianism. Together with the new Nichiren sect, it loosened the principle of total abstinence.

During the Edo Era (1603–1867), laws to diminish sake production drastically were enforced from time to time to meet floods, famines, and other emergencies. A considerable number of feudal lords established prohibition or encouraged temperance on their estates. Some leading scholars advocated or required total abstinence among their followers.

The Restoration of Meiji (1867) was the dawn of a new international civilization and culture. The new temperance movement prospered among early-day Protestants. On the other hand, Western liquors were imported with the introduction of new drinking customs. Around 1886 the Yokohama Temperance Society, Hokkaido Temperance Society, a Japanese branch of the Woman's Christian Temperance Union (WCTU), and other temperance groups were organized, together with the Hanseikai of the awakened Buddhists. A national organization, the Japan Temperance Alliance, was formed in 1897. A Prohibition Law for Minors was instituted on 1 April 1922. Ever since then the temperance organizations have fought to raise the obligatory abstinence age to twenty-five. The WCTU has supplied teaching materials to all schools regularly for many years and the Salvation Army has endeavored to promote the cause of total abstinence among the masses. The Emperor Hirohito is not only a distinguished biologist but is also internationally known as a staunch total abstainer and nonsmoker.

Drinking Customs

In the present section some of the drinking customs peculiar to Japan will be described briefly.

Toso.   The toso custom was originally introduced from China over a thousand years ago. On New Year's Eve a number of medicines were presented to each native village. These were put in a sack and hung in the wells. On New Year's Day they were brought out and mixed with sake, to be taken for the prevention of disease. If a family member has it, the family should be free from disease. If one family has it, the entire community should be free from disease. The youngest in the family drinks the toso cups first, then the elders in ascending order of age. At the imperial palace an unmarried lady offered the toso cups to the emperor. When people make New Year's calls nowadays they are offered cups of toso. At present, toso is ordinary sake drunk at the New Year season.

Shirozake. White sake is specially prepared and used particularly for the Doll's Festival on March 3. The festival is observed by girls with dolls of the emperor, the empress, ministers of the left and the right, three court ladies, five musicians, a number of footmen, left-hand cherry tree, right-hand mandarin orange, and so forth. Rhombic rice cakes and pellet rice dumplings are offered to the dolls. The celebration of the festival has a history of over one thousand years. It was originally an aristocratic event but gradually became popularized among the common people. Family members and guests take cups of white sake in its celebration.

Moonlight Party. In autumn, when the sky is clear, the moonlight party is held to view the full moon. August 15 and September 13 (lunar calendar) are the dates for moon-viewing banquets for poets and persons of a romantic turn. Autumnal plants, such as pampas grass, *Patrinia scabio-saefolia*, Chinese bell-flowers, etc., are put in a vase, on one side. Boiled potatoes are offered to the moon on the other side. On a wooden stand at the veranda a big liquid measure of sake and white dumplings of boiled flour are placed. Enjoying cups of sake, poems are composed by every participant.

Sansankudo (literally, three-three-nine cups). At the Shinto wedding rite in particular, cups of sake are taken both by the bride and bridegroom to solemnize the ceremony. Three cupfuls are offered to each of the new couple thrice. Usually, three cinnabar-varnished, round and shallow cups are piled up for the purpose.

Sakazuki (cup). Originally, small round and shallow unglazed earthenware cups were used. Even today they are used in Shinto ceremonies and offerings. However, lacquered wooden cups of the same shape are most commonly used nowadays.

Sakana (relishes taken with sake). As accompaniments of sake, various fishes and vegetables are taken. In banquets they precede the serving of the proper meal or rice. Slices of raw fish, sea breams broiled with salt, vinegared dishes (particularly fish), dried cuttlefish, peanuts, bean custard, mashed sweet potato sweetened and mixed with chestnuts, sweet white kidney beans and black peas, vinegared herring roes, boiled and cooked vegetables, and the like, are most frequently provided.

Sakazuki-goto (events of cups). Promises between two parties, marriages, and so forth, are represented by this term.

Kan. Sake is poured into an earthen bottle and heated by

putting it into a kettle of warm water over a fire. Sometimes it is directly boiled in a pot. The most appropriate temperature for drinking is said to be 50° centigrade.

Niiname-sai (harvest festival). On November 23, offerings of the new crop of rice and new rice wine, sake, are made to the emperor and Shinto deities who are imperial ancestors. In the year of enthronement of every emperor, this festival is called *Daijoh-e* and is held on a far larger scale.

Japanese attitudes on drinking are characterized in the following proverbial expressions:

What is the cherry-blossom (national flower) without wine?

Wine is the panacea for all ills.

Good wine makes good blood.

When the wine goes in, the wit goes out.

Firstly man drinks wine, then wine drinks wine, and finally wine drinks man.

Bag of liquor and sack of food. (referring to those who eat the bread of idleness)

The Contemporary Scene

The war brought about radical changes in various aspects of Japanese life. In consequence of wartime scarcity, strong drink and tobacco were rationed. Though a dry and tobacco-free day was observed throughout Japan each month, on the other hand many weak abstainers yielded to drinking as one of the few consolations available in those weary and fearful days. With the gradual postwar return to normal life, the production of alcoholic beverages has been restored almost to the prewar level.

Things Oriental and Occidental now coexist and mingle in Japan. Modern big cities like Tokyo and Osaka have many bars, cafés, cabarets, night clubs, etc., where strong drink is provided, besides the traditional pot-houses or restaurants. Surrounding the hundreds of American and British bases of the security forces, large numbers of beer halls are prospering. Cocktail parties are often held for the reception of Western residents and visitors.

The national consumption of domestic alcoholic beverages in the fiscal year 1952–53 is shown in table 1. In addition 490 liters of whiskey, valued at ¥2,394,000,000, and beer valued at ¥636,000,000, were imported. Total liquor imports amounted to about ¥3,300,000,000. Besides these, a large quantity of tax-free liquors, wines, and beers is brought in by the American and British security forces. Some of this supply is black-marketed for Japanese consumption. Japanese beers meet public approval in Western lands. Their production was to be raised to 1,980,000 koku for the 1952 liquor year (October 1952–September 1953), compared to 1,620,000 koku in the previous year. Their export in 1952 amounted to 14,570,000 liters, valued at ¥1,087,770,000. The distilling of Western liquors (whiskey, brandy, etc.) amounted to 140,771 koku in 1952, including 55,370 koku of whiskey.

TABLE 1.   Consumption of Domestic Alcoholic Beverages in Japan, Fiscal Year April, 1952–March, 1953, by Type and Class of Beverage

Type	Class	Amount (koku[a])
Refined sake	Extra fine	1,175,877
	1st class	342,390
	2nd class	1,439,138
Beer		1,550,592
Synthetic sake	1st class	49,097
	2nd class	536,233
	Miscellaneous	142,124
	Mirin for seasoning	38,518
Shochu (Japanese liquor)		12,921
Fruit wine		8,714

a.   The koku is 1.8039 hectoliters or 47.66 U.S. gallons.

Arrests for illicit brewing or distilling numbered 43,265 cases and 16,443 koku were confiscated in 1952.

Before the war there were 17 dry villages; 106 partially dry villages; about 200 dry factories, mines, railroad temperance unions, and the like; 15 dry steamers; and about 3,800 temperance organizations affiliated with the Japan Temperance Union (formerly the Japan National Temperance League), with a combined membership of well above three hundred thousand. The war drastically undermined and diminished the temperance forces. The American and British occupation brought with them a series of alcohol-related problems. Beer halls, cabarets, night clubs, etc., encircling the bases; violence and crimes by drunken servicemen; the smuggling of Western liquors following the reopening of international traffic; and also illicit manufacture by Korean residents have recently aroused public concern.

As the number of motor vehicles is increasing, traffic accidents are rising sharply. The Tokyo Metropolitan Police Board operates a number of Japanese-made machines for determining blood alcohol by the breath test, but the test is not yet universally adopted in Japan.

Despite recommendations by the World Health Organization, alcoholism is not yet taken up as a public health problem by the authorities and the general public, as when dealing with narcotic addicts. Japanese-made disulfiram is on sale now and is prescribed for the treatment of alcoholism in rehabilitation centers affiliated with the Japan Temperance Union. American films, as *Something to Live For*, have introduced and popularized the ideas of the Alcoholics Anonymous (AA). To meet the urgent need of those who seek advice or help from the Consultation Section of the Japan Temperance Union, a Japanese equivalent of Alcoholics Anonymous was started in September 1953. Close touch is maintained between this Japanese group and the AA group of American servicemen in Tokyo.

Temperance education has been neglected hitherto. As a new move, lantern lectures on alcohol questions have been initiated at high schools, civic centers, churches, factories, women's and young people's groups, etc., by the executive director of the Japan Temperance Union. New pamphlets and handbooks on alcohol problems are also in preparation.

The Japanese National WCTU is endeavoring to have references to alcohol, tobacco, etc., inserted in various secondary-school textbooks. All the temperance forces are striving to have the prohibition age raised from twenty to twenty-five. A majority in Parliament appears to favor the bill personally and it has passed one of the two houses from time to time, but it faces persistent blocking by opposing forces.

The Japanese people has been traditionally tolerant of and lenient toward misdemeanors of drunkards, as irresponsible and innocent. However, the temperance forces are planning to submit a new bill to the Parliament for their severer handling. Another effort under way is to make the financial support of rehabilitation centers for alcoholics a national or public responsibility through new legislation.

Changes in Japanese Drinking Patterns
Margaret J. Sargent

During a century of intensive modernization, social change has affected much of the traditional social system and values of Japan. Drinking patterns—as an integral feature of this complex literate society—seem still to be in a process of reorganization. On the whole, the traditional patterns of drinking can be regarded as culturally integrative: there is a continuation of some of the ritual and social functions of alcohol into modern drinking, as well as a recent incursion of certain additional social functions. At the psychological level, a change is possibly occurring in the form of an increase in the use of alcohol for anxiety reduction (Horton 1943), and this will be investigated in the present study.

In order to expose the changes in drinking during this transitional period, traditional patterns will be contrasted with modern drinking behavior. First, information will be presented from anthropological studies of Japanese village societies, most of which were completed before 1954, to delineate the more traditional patterns of drinking. Recent trends will then be described as suggested by a survey of the drinking patterns and attitudes toward drinking in the general population of a region of western Japan.

Traditional Drinking Patterns

The brief descriptions of drinking patterns contained in anthropological studies yield a fairly consistent picture of the traditional role of drinking as it appeared in village societies early in the 1950s.

The alcoholic beverage most frequently consumed was sake, containing 14 to 16 percent alcohol, made from fermented rice. The cheapest beverage was shōchū, containing on an average 25 percent alcohol, made by distillation from mash left over after making sake, or from sweet potatoes. Cornell and Smith (1956) found doburoku to be popular because of its cheapness and potency; this was an unrefined mash-fermented drink said to be made illicitly by local Koreans. Beer and whiskey were occasionally drunk, especially at bars in the local towns, but were at that time considered rather expensive for general use.

The use of alcohol, always sake, was common in religious ritual, which would frequently be followed by ceremonial drinking. In house-building ceremonies, for example, the officiating carpenter first offered food and sake to the god of the carpenters,

Itsubashira-no-kamisama, and then poured a ceremonial cup of sake for all the men present, and a feast for all followed; "most males are soon maudlin with drink, and there is much laughter, singing and dancing" (Norbeck 1954). Ceremonial drinking took place also—as it still does—at weddings, funerals, banquets, and "congratulatory occasions" such as New Year. Typically, solemn formal behavior would gradually become transformed with the aid of alcohol into informal convivial camaraderie. "Various games and rituals, such as the mutual exchange of wine cups, are brought into play to step up the drinking, which in most areas leads to speedy and hilarious inebriation" (Beardsley, Hall, and Ward 1959:110). Younger women seldom took alcohol, and older women would only very rarely drink to the point of intoxication. Drunkenness in young men was rare and not generally encouraged, but the autumn festival in some villages provided an exception. The young unmarried men *(seinendan)* would carry a portable shrine through the streets; "contributions from a house to house collection are usually sufficient to purchase enough saké to get all the seinendan drunk," which they might do on this occasion without censure. Then, "they may wander . . . about the community in a sodden state with arms about their friends—behavior which is avoided at all other times—until sleep overcomes them" (Norbeck and Norbeck 1956:671).

In adult male drinking parties, etiquette required drunkenness or even "a simulated display of drunkenness" (Dore 1958: 208). Lemert's (1958) description of Salish Indians' apparent inebriation after imbibing extremely little alcohol, drunkenness being the expected behavior, bears some resemblance to the Japanese speedy reaction to small quantities of alcohol. Drunkenness in Japan, however, did not normally continue to the next day and so it did not interfere with other activities. Plath gives a glimpse of the philosophy which prescribes drunkenness: "The ideal self must be capable of entering into relationships of human feeling and intimacy. . . . Ability to melt into the nexus is prized. Drinking parties are an example of how this is manifested. . . . To drink and 'not crumble' *(kuzurenai)* is to reject an opportunity mutually to offer human sympathy" (1964). From the psychological point of view one may view such inebriation as the result of the emphasis on controlled and correct behavior on the one hand, and the availability of volatile emotion on the other, set in a culture having a permissive attitude toward drinking. Release of sexual inhibitions and aggressive behavior while drunk were rare: "Drunkenness . . . does not often result in unpleasantness or quarreling, for almost any foolish behavior under the influence of alcohol can be over-looked" (Cornell and Smith 1956:198). There was permissiveness toward drunkenness and protection of the drunken: "The Japanese man does not anticipate rejection from others because of his drinking and is less likely . . . to feel guilty about his drinking. . . . The Japanese woman takes on the role of ministering and caring for the [drunken] man" (Caudill 1959:216).

In summary, Japanese traditional patterns of drinking, as they appeared in village communities in the early 1950s, indicate the prevalence of heavy drinking and drunkenness in certain confined social groups, mainly adult males and generally excluding women and children, and in certain well-defined situations. The functions of alcohol may be said to include the following: ritual functions in the symbolization of status changes, functions as an offering to ensure the benignity of the gods, and ceremonial and social functions in diminishing social distance and strengthening group bonds. These social functions were of some importance because Japanese society emphasized formality and politeness in personal interaction to such an extent that on some occasions only alcohol could release the inhibition of the expression of affectivity. Fallding considered these integrated drinking patterns to be the only benign type of drinking, in which "alcohol is not needed to generate relationships, but to express the solidarity generated by trust" (1964:718).

Alcohol Consumption and Alcoholism Prevalence

Changes in drinking patterns, which have occurred particularly during the last decade, are indicated by the rise in consumption and production of alcoholic beverages and an apparently increasing alcoholism.

The annual consumption of absolute alcohol of the drinking-age population (aged fifteen years or over) increased from 0.9 U.S. gallons per capita in 1953 to 1.3 gallons in 1963 (Japan, Tax Admin. Agency 1958, 1960, 1964). (The comparable estimate of consumption in 1963 in the United States was 2.15 gallons [Efron and Keller 1964].) The absolute alcohol contained in the alcoholic beverages produced annually in Japan, after decreasing from 29½ million gallons in 1939 to 8½ million gallons in 1947, rose to 87½ million gallons in 1964 (Japan Handbook 1965; Minryoku 1965; Japan, Nat. Tax Off. 1965). (Illicit production, according to government estimates, is included in these data.)

As indicated in figure 1, until 1956 beer and sake were produced in roughly equal quantities, but from 1956 the production of beer soared; by 1964 it reached 468 million gallons compared with sake production of 262 million gallons. In 1964, 82 percent of the general population drank beer, 72 percent sake, 53 percent whiskey, 50 percent grape wine, and 5 percent shōchū (*Asahi Consumers' Survey* 1965).

Alcoholic admissions to state psychiatric hospitals in Tokyo increased from 0.47 percent in 1946 to 5.21 percent in 1957 (Noguchi 1960), but this rise is probably due partly to changes in admission policies and diagnostic procedures. Alcoholics averaged 14.9 percent of psychiatric hospital patients throughout Japan from 1959 to 1961 (Japan, Min. of Justice 1962). Deaths due to cirrhosis of the liver in 1962 were 9.9 per 100,000 in Japan and 11.3 in the United States (*Japan Handbook* 1965), but the proportion of cir-

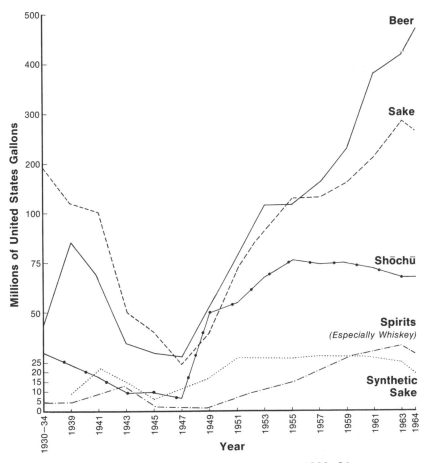

Fig. 1. Production of alcoholic beverages in Japan, 1930–64.

rhosis cases with associated alcoholism is not necessarily the same in the two countries. According to the estimate of Arai (see Moore 1964), the prevalence of alcoholism in the general population of Japan was 3 percent,[1] a rate similar to that in the United States in 1960 (Efron and Keller 1964). Japan, France, and the United States therefore share the three highest reported rates of alcoholism in the world (Popham and Schmidt 1958). The comparison of estimates is limited in scope since they are derived by different methods, at different points in time, and with varying diagnostic approaches. These data, however, like my periodic observations from 1953 to 1966, may be said to support the view (Noguchi 1960; Chafetz 1964) that there has been a recent increase in the prevalence of alcoholism in Japan.

A Survey of Contemporary Drinking Patterns

Method

A survey was made in 1965 of a stratified sample of 200 subjects resident in Nishinomiya (population 323,319), where I was living at that time. Nishinomiya lies between Kobe and Osaka in western Japan and comprises a variety of districts, urban, semiurban, and rural. Three districts, two suburban and one rural, were selected as they seemed typical residential districts for each occupational group, white-collar, trade, and labor; subjects were then picked at random from the electoral registers of the three districts. In the proportions of the sexes, the sample was not statistically different from the population of Nishinomiya (Nishinomiya City Off. 1962); however, the sample was not representative in terms of age-groups as it contained more subjects under thirty and over fifty than the general population of Nishinomiya ($p < .05$). This difference should not affect the comparison of the drinking patterns of different age-groups where the chi-square method of contingency is employed.

Modifications in behavioral patterns have tended, on the whole, to appear first in those sections of the Japanese population which are most influenced by Western customs and attitudes, and probably drinking patterns are similar in this respect. Owing to their education and their greater contact with Westerners, the higher social classes tend to be influenced to a greater extent than the lower, and for this reason the survey deals mainly with the upper and middle social classes. The percentage of subjects in each occupational category was white-collar 55 percent, trade 34 percent, and labor 11 percent. As the sample is predominantly white-collar, its findings relating to the *sarariman* (salarymen) class, which has become such an important phenomenon in postwar Japan, may be of particular interest.

Fourth-year Japanese university students of social psychology, experienced in interviewing techniques, visited the subjects' homes and conducted a standarized twenty-minute interview. Thirty subjects were not available for interview owing to absence or to lack of leisure. The subjects interviewed included ninety-two men and seventy-eight women between nineteen and seventy years of age; on the whole they showed cooperation and interest. No claim is made that the small sample portrays all the varieties of drinking customs found in the different regions of Japan, but there seems equally no reason to assume that the trends found in Nishinomiya are exceptional.

The theory which prompted this survey is that modern Japanese drinking patterns incorporate to a greater extent than traditional patterns the use of alcohol for anxiety reduction. (The term "anxiety reduction" is used interchangeably in this paper with "alleviation of anxiety.") It is assumed that younger subjects portray modern patterns while older subjects retain traditional features of drinking. The hypothesis to be tested is that the use of alcohol to alleviate anxiety is associated with membership of the younger age-groups. The questions in the interview concerning anxiety were phrased thus: "Do you think some people drink because they are anxious? to forget a disappointment? to get rid of angry feelings? to get a 'lift' when they are feeling bored?"

As a measure of drinking, the quantity-frequency index, devised by Straus and Bacon (1953), was used. Subjects were classified, according to the amount of absolute alcohol consumed on an average drinking occasion during the previous year, as drinking a "small" quantity (less than 1.3 ounces absolute alcohol, equivalent to roughly 1⅔ large bottles of beer, or 1¼ tumblers of sake, or 1⅔ doubles of whiskey), a "medium" quantity (1.3 to 3 ounces) or a "large" quantity (3 ounces or more). Drinking occurring more than once per week was classified as frequent, two to four times per month as moderately frequent, once a month or less as infrequent.

Three attitudes were investigated by means of three sets of statements (see table 2): attitudes toward drinking as supportive of social solidarity, toward drunkenness, and toward drinking by women. Five of the statements for the attitude toward drunkenness were taken from Allardt (1957); in addition, a Japanese proverb was included. The subjects' responses of agreement with the statements were weighted as shown in table 2, and added to yield a score for each subject on each of the three attitudes. Weighting of scores was based on two main considerations: (1) A subject's agreement with all the set of statements for any one attitude might be due to a mental set of compliance rather than genuine affirmation, so scores were weighted to yield a total of zero when the subject agreed with every statement. (2) It was desirable that extreme attitudes should be indicated by high total scores, so statements indicative of extreme attitudes were allotted high weights. For each attitude subjects were divided into a high-scoring and a low-scoring group, each of roughly equal size. The associations between attitudes and other characteristics were then measured by the chi-square method.

Results

The hypothesis that the use of alcohol for anxiety reduction is associated with membership of the younger age-groups was supported to the extent that significantly more subjects in their twenties than those aged thirty years and above showed awareness that people use alcohol on account of anxiety ($p < .05$). If the source of the awareness was projection referring to the subjects' own behavior or the observation of their peers' behavior, then the hypothesis was further confirmed. Of the 170 subjects interviewed, 163 were users of alcohol; the nonusers, 2 men and 5 women, had never drunk alcohol. The characteristics of respondents which were related significantly to awareness that people may drink on account of anxiety were: male sex ($p < .01$); age twenty to twenty-nine years ($p < .05$); commencement of drinking before age twenty ($p < .001$); first inebriation before age twenty-two ($p < .001$); recent drinking in places such as bars, cabarets, and stand-up stalls (*sakaba*), where social controls tend to be inoperative ($p < .01$); alteration of behavior or mood by alcohol ($p < .01$); permissive attitude toward drinking by women ($p < .001$). Characteristics not so related were occupation, education, religious affiliation, and attitudes to drunkenness, to misuse of alcohol, and to alcohol as supportive of social solidarity.

The classification of subjects' drinking according to the quantity-frequency index is given in table 1. The index provided a basis of comparison with a very different population, United States college students (Straus and Bacon 1953); the extent of drinking in the female users, American and Japanese, was almost identical, but in men there was significantly more drinking in the Japanese group ($p < .001$). Only 25 percent of the Japanese women drank more than one drink on an occasion or more frequently than once per month. Among the Japanese men 39 percent received the highest quantity-frequency rating; all of these drank frequently, but only seven drank large quantities. This high rating was associated with white-collar occupation ($p<.05$); absence of religious affiliation ($p<.05$); drinking for personal rather than social reasons ($p<.001$) (this association was found also in Iowa subjects [Mulford and Miller 1960]); and the attitude toward alcohol as supportive of social solidarity ($p<.001$). Men with the highest rating admitted less awareness than other subjects of the use of alcohol to alleviate anxiety ($p<.01$).

TABLE 1.   Quantity-Frequency Index of Drinking

Q-F Index[a]	Men		Women	
	Number	Percentage	Number	Percentage
1	14	16	46	63
2	8	9	18	25
3	12	13		
4	18	20		
5	35	39		
Not known	3	3	9	12
Total[b]	90	100	73	100

a.   1 = Drinks infrequently (once a month at the most) and consumes only small amounts (not more than approximately 1.3 oz. of absolute alcohol); 2 = Drinks infrequently and consumes medium or large amounts (more than 1.3 oz. of absolute alcohol); 3 = Drinks more than once a month, but consumes only small amounts; 4 = Drinks two to four times a month and consumes medium or large amounts; 5 = Drinks more than once a week and consumes medium or large amounts.

b.   The total does not include the seven abstainers (two men, five women).

The results of the questions on attitudes are given in table 2.

The alcoholic beverages served to subjects when drinking on recent occasions included beer 127 times, sake 82, whiskey 21, and shōchū 3 times. The beverages generally preferred by the under-forties were beer and whiskey, both originating in the West, while the older subjects preferred the native sake ($p<.001$). White-collar workers' preference for whiskey, though it failed to reach significance in this study, was highly significant in Suminoe's larger Tokyo sample (1962). White-collar occupation was associated with a permissive attitude to drinking by women ($p<.001$)

TABLE 2.   Respondent Attitudes toward Drinking as Supportive of
Social Solidarity, Drunkenness, and Drinking by Women

	Percentage Agree	Weighted Score
I. Drinking as Supportive of Social Solidarity		
1. Drinking certainly improves the way people get on together	89	+1
2. Sake is a broom which sweeps out care (Japanese proverb)	60	+1
3. Sake reveals the inner man (Japanese proverb)	77	+1
4. A few drinks are necessary to break through the formality of some occasions	94	+1
5. Agreement about business and other contracts may be assisted by the use of alcohol	54	+1
6. Drink may cause a man to neglect his work or his family	64	−2
7. Drink causes fighting and other unpleasantness too often	57	−3
II. Drunkenness		
8. Getting drunk enables men to show the friendly feelings they have for each other	63	+1
9. It is important for men to be able to get drunk once in a while in order to relax and talk things out	69	+1
10. A man is none the worse for a good booze occasionally	36	+1
11. Abstinence doesn't always build a treasure house (Japanese proverb)	63	+1
12. Being drunk is shameful	66	−2
13. To get drunk shows a lack of moral stamina	58	−2
III. Drinking by Women		
14. Women should be allowed to drink as much and as often as men	29	+1
15. It is all right for a woman to take a drink or two when visiting	86	+1
16. A drink now and then at home does no harm to a woman	83	+1
17. Drinking is all right for older women, but younger women should abstain	43	−1
18. Women should never take alcohol under any circumstances	13	−2

and also with the attitude to drinking as supportive of social solidarity ($p<.01$).

Subjects were offered a multiple-choice question on the definition of misuse of alcohol as administered by Allardt to 400 residents of Helsinki (1957). The responses of the Japanese sample defined a much wider range of behavior as misuse than the Finnish group ($p<.001$); 25 percent of the Japanese against 7 percent of Allardt's subjects defined as misusers even those who sometimes have a drink or two at parties.

Discussion

The traditional pattern of Japanese drinking seems to have represented a concrete example of the cultural integration theory of drinking as described, for example, by Mangin (1957). The theory may be said to include the following factors: enhancement of the sense of social solidarity; lack of conflict, guilt, or ambivalence; noninterference with performance of social roles. In terms of Lemert's (1962) ascription of costs and values to drinking, the values outweighed the costs.

Yet widespread tensions are thought to have long existed in Japan, and Bellah (1957) describes how, in Tokugawa times (1603–1868), they became socially patterned and institutionalized: a general hypochondriacal concern for health led to a prosperous medicine business; tension relief was offered by the gay quarters; an ultimate meaning behind the central value system was supplied by religion. Although much of the traditional social system is retained today, certain additional factors may contribute to tension (Vogel 1963; Matsumoto 1960; Jansen 1965; De Vos 1963; Abegglen 1958). First, there is the anomie due to the gradual dissolution of established rules. Second, we find the rise of the salarymen, symbols of Japan's *akarui seikatsu* (bright new life), who stop off after work for a drink because their firms demand socializing activity, and also perhaps because the nature of modern work leads to a need to restore a sense of personal participation in society. Lastly, the increase of individual freedom, and coincidental reduction of familial guidance, may add to the responsibility of the individual. Many workers have remarked on the unusual dependency of the Japanese male. "A Japanese, on reaching man's estate, already has the habits of dependence and trustful respect thoroughly ingrained" (Stoetzel 1955). Some *Nisei* (American-born offspring of Japanese immigrants) have found difficulty in adjusting to American society partly owing to inability to overcome dependency needs (Babcock 1963); as individualism increases, this difficulty may occur in Japan also.

Such factors have probably played a part in weakening the traditional social system with its integrated drinking patterns. Yet social change in Japanese institutions has proceeded smoothly by the speedy adoption of new norms of behavior. The changes in drinking may also be said, following the theory of DuToit (1964), to consist in the substitution for traditional patterns of a different, but not necessarily deviant, type of drinking behavior. In young people the new pattern has become the modal behavior, and it seems probable that the traditional patterns will slowly die out. In prewar Japan, permissiveness to drunkenness was confined to a definite area of ritual, ceremonial, and recreational drinking. In effect, in defining the free areas within which drunkenness was accepted, the permissive attitude acted as a social control of excessive drinking outside them. The new mode of drinking, however, fails to define unambiguously the areas in which drunkenness is permitted behavior. Moreover, the dangers of alcohol as a factor in traffic accidents and crime have been emphasized in mass communication media in recent years. Behavior under the influence which contravenes the social code meets with less tolerance than formerly. Shame control, characteristic of traditional-directed cultures (Riesman 1950), is giving way to guilt control. Disapproval of drunkenness is increasing and Japan appears to be gradually adopting the social ambivalence toward alcohol typical of some Western countries (Myerson 1940). Yet in the present transitional stage, Japan seems still to be more permissive of drinking, more protective of the drunken, than almost any other complex society.

Note

1. The date was not stated but presumably Arai's estimate (see Moore 1964) refers to the early 1960s. No estimate of prevalence was available for earlier times, but the general impression given by most writers is that alcoholism was rare (Benedict 1947; Yanagida 1957; Noguchi 1960; but cf. Yamamuro 1958).

Use of Alcohol and Opium by the Meo of Laos

Joseph Westermeyer

At the present time we are in the throes of what is perceived to be a serious problem with drugs. Better understanding of the society-individual-drug triad is needed. It is hoped that this paper will contribute to such understanding.

The Meo are a tribal people who inhabit the mountains of several southeast Asian countries. In Laos they comprise the largest minority group, numbering between one hundred thousand and two hundred thousand people. These mountaineers produce and consume two potentially addictive substances, opium and distilled grain alcohol. My close contact with the Meo over two years disclosed a marked difference between the opium and alcohol patterns of usage. Questions as to the origin and meaning of this difference provided the motivation for the following study.

This paper reports on a sample of Meo resident in Laos during the years 1965 to 1967. I visited fourteen Meo villages. A total of seven months was spent in one village; others were visited for a few days to a few weeks. During these visits, I was generally a house guest in Meo homes. Communication was carried on without a translator in Lao, the lingua franca of the area. Working and social contacts with Meo people led to several close friendships, as well as a wide circle of acquaintances. Frequent invitations into Meo homes provided abundant opportunity for me to observe the patterns of alcohol and opium usage.

Prior to going to Laos, I had completed course work for a master's degree in anthropology; and a main purpose of the sojourn was to obtain data for the thesis (Westermeyer 1968). My employment as a general physician in the Public Health Division of the U.S. Agency for International Development provided me a subsidy and an additional role from which to establish contact with the people and customs. Professional work in a hospital and in village health activities provided the opportunity for me to become acquainted with the addicted users.

Meo people inhabit mountainsides one thousand to two thousand meters above sea level. Climatic conditions are ideal for vigorous opium-poppy growth. Slash-and-burn agriculture yields corn and upland rice. Hunting of small and large forest animals supplements the diet. A few domestic animals are often kept for spirit sacrifice or sale.

The Meo live in politically autonomous villages of one hundred to three hundred people. Each Meo person belongs to one of twelve exogamous patrilineal kin groups. Polygyny is practiced by men able to afford more than one bridewealth. Every man functions as a farmer, hunter, husbandryman, and—when necessary—warrior. Some have additional roles such as village leader, shaman, musician, ironsmith, or silversmith. All adult women are married and attend to domestic chores. A few older women serve as midwives or shamans.

Meo society is strict and tightly integrated. The hierarchy of family-clan-village obligations places each individual at a distinct social locus, with well-known rights and obligations. Vocational choices, especially for young adults, virtually do not exist. Sex roles are simple and explicit: men should be strong, daring, clever, and ambitious for wealth; women should be industrious, loyal, fecund, and maternal. Norms with regard to truth, honesty, and chastity border on puritanical. Rules for the "correct" Meo way cover all areas of behavior and are explicitly defined. Pro-Meo loyalty and pride are strong. Non-Meo neighboring people tend to be disdained.

Despite the many environmental and psychosocial stresses impinging on the Meo, many modes of expression are available to vent thoughts and feelings. Loud marital arguments are permitted. Children can be reprimanded harshly and are free to respond with long, screaming tantrums. Prolonged, involved legal theatrics are indulged in with great zest—often over matters of little apparent import. Structured mourning activity prescribes hours of wailing. Politicking by men and suicide attempts by women provide some limited opportunity for manipulation of one's milieu.

However, emotion and ideas may be expressed in Meo society *only* if they reflect adherence to strict Meo norms and attitudes. Expression of nonconformist attitudes or impulses elicits immediate harsh societal response.

Meo drink alcohol in the form of a strong whiskey distilled from rice or corn mash. Each household makes its own supply. Social imperative strictly regulates when alcohol is drunk, by whom, and in what amount (see table 1). All drinking occurs as a social activity within the nuclear family, extended family, or friendship group. Alcohol usage is closely integrated with other elements of Meo culture: rites of passage, important extra-kin relationships, unpredictable crises, annual celebrations.

Every adult must drink at specific times according to age,

TABLE 1. Alcohol Drinking Events among the Meo

Event	Social Group	Kind of Drinking	Sex	Time of Day
New Year	Household, lineage, friends	Heavy (8+ oz.)	Males and females	Daytime and evening
Wedding	Household, lineage, friends	Heavy (8+ oz.)	Males and females	Daytime and evening
Friendship	Household, friends	Moderate (4–6 oz.)	Males and some females	Evening
Soul day (infant)	Household, lineage	Moderate (4–6 oz.)	Males and some females	Evening
Name day (newborn)	Household	Mild (2–3 oz.)	Males	Evening
Rice harvest	Household, friends	Mild (2–3 oz.)	Males	Evening
Animal sacrifice	Household	Symbolic (1 oz.)	Males	Daytime or evening
Funeral	Household, lineage, friends	Symbolic (1 oz.)	Males	Daytime

sex, and social role. Young adults (teenagers by our standards) and women drink only a fourth to a half the amount drunk by men, and only on the most important occasions. At weddings a bantering drinking contest occurs between the groom and the bride's male relatives. A rigid etiquette governs host-guest drinking: the host offers a toast and drains his glass of whiskey; the guest must then match the host glass for glass.

Symbolic drinking (one fluid ounce of whiskey) or mild drinking (two or three ounces) does not appear to perceptibly alter behavior. Conviviality, lively conversation, and laughter accompany moderate drinking (four to six ounces); participants usually remain seated in the house. Heavy drinking (eight or more ounces) features loud talking, mutual joking, uproarious mirth, and shouting. Motor activity increases, and the celebration may continue out-of-doors. Should someone imbibe to the point of impaired speech, vision, or ambulation, he quietly slips away before his impaired functions attract the notice (and badgering) of his comrades.

Nonsanctioned use of alcohol and the bio-psycho-social "alcoholism" syndromes do not occur among Meo. Enough alcohol is readily available for sporadic binge-drinking, yet it does not occur.

Moreover, even the medicinal use of alcohol common among adjacent ethnic groups is not encountered.

For most Meo the primary importance of opium is its economic usefulness. Each household grows opium to trade for silver and iron—substances integrally woven into Meo ecologic and social systems. As expressed by a Meo adage, "Every home should have opium." At the volition of the individual, opium may also be used as a medicine, for pleasure, or (rarely) to commit suicide.

Many Meo refuse to use opium for fear of becoming "one who enjoys opium." This *nonuse* category comprises 90.2 percent of our sample of 400 Meo villagers aged twenty years and older (see table 2). However, some occasional users very likely report themselves as nonusers either from embarrassment or because infrequent use might be considered more nonuse than occasional use. Since nonusers and occasional users cannot be readily distinguished from one another, the field observer is somewhat dependent on the subject's historical accuracy. A better approximation of nonuse probably would be in the 65 to 80 percent range.

TABLE 2. Prevalence Rates of Opium Use among Meo Aged Twenty Years and Older

Category	Number	Percentage
Nonuse	361	90.2
Occasional	30	7.5
Habitual	7	1.8
Working addicted	2	0.5
Incapacitated addicted	0	.0
Total	400	100.0

Source: Data collected in Xieng Khouang province with the assistance of Xiong Chao.

Of those Meo who do smoke opium, most are *occasional users.* As often as a few times a week or as infrequently as every few years, one or two pipefuls are taken for illness or after a hard spell of work or while the person is relaxing with family or friends. No withdrawal symptoms and no tendency to increase dosage progressively are noted; rather, use tends to wax and wane over time. Occasional users behave and work normally to meet their family and societal obligations. While table 2 reports a 7.5 percent crude rate for occasional use, 20 to 35 percent would be more correct, in my opinion.

Habitual users smoke opium once a day, taking one or two

pipefuls in the evening. Smoking may be interrupted for a few days or even entirely discontinued, without the person's developing evident withdrawal signs. Physically they cannot be readily distinguished as a group, although their opium smoking can be readily observed and is publicly known. Many return to occasional smoking; some continue daily use for years and may in later life begin to smoke more often.

The *working addicted* smoke two to four times during the day. Deprived of their opium for a few days, they develop generalized aching, abdominal cramps, loss of appetite, diaphoresis, and weakness. Shoddy dress, the smell of opium smoke, and cyanosis of the lips and gums readily identify their addiction. While such individuals still perform work and indeed are able to raise their own opium, their ambition and energy are dulled. They rarely taper off or stop smoking, and they manifest extreme concern for their opium cache and smoking equipment. Their extremely low prevalence rate compared to other categories of opium users is shown in table 2. Another survey, in which only addicts were counted, was done in the same area as the first survey. Of the several thousand inhabitants in the area of the second survey, thirty-two persons were addicted to opium smoking; thirty-one of these were working addicts and one was an incapacitated addict (see table 3).

TABLE 3. Meo Opium Addicts by Age and Sex

Age (in years)	Male	Female
Less than 20	1	—
20–29	3	2
30–39	3	2
40–49	6	2
50–59	5	4
60–69	2	1
70 and older	1	—
Total	21	11

Source: Data collected in Xieng Khouang province with the assistance of Xiong Sai.

Incapacitated addicts smoke five to ten times a day and perform little or no work. Preparation of the opium pipe and deep inhalations from it alternate with periods of stupor. Such men, usually in their fifties or sixties, are totally dependent on others for their opium supply. Since smoking requires large amounts of opium as compared to parenteral use or ingestion, large portions of the family's resources may be thus consumed. While an impoverished incapacitated addict may beg for opium, he does not resort to thievery. He can be readily identified by his unkempt appearance, long dirty hair, marked weakness, dull expression, and thin wasted condition; his hands are thin and uncalloused. Withdrawal is prolonged and severe, the person shows inability to eat, insomnia, diarrhea, dehydration, and incessant whining. Table 2 indicates that no incapacitated addicts were encountered in the sample; one fifty-six-year-old man was present in the table 3 survey. I encountered several incapacitated addicts (all elderly men) while I was carrying on my hospital duties.

Patterns of opium usage vary with age and sex. Children may rarely receive small amounts of opium orally for illness. Occasional opium smoking among teenaged males or females infrequently occurs in homes where the parents smoke opium. Young women with children and young men starting families virtually never use it. However, a few young unmarried adults are addicted to opium. Table 3 indicates the predominance of addiction among persons aged forty and older, and the greater percentage of male addicts. Only women not raising children and whose husbands smoke opium use opium regularly.

Discussion

Hypotheses have been sought with two goals in mind: (1) to understand the Meo case, and (2) to shed light on societal aspects of intoxication and addictive behavior. With regard to the latter purpose, it is important to note that this is an intensive, single-culture study. The Meo are a tribal group of Asian mountaineers who sustain themselves by slash-and-burn agriculture and raise opium as a cash crop. Careful examination should necessarily precede application of these conclusions to Andean mountaineers, African tribesmen, urban Westerners, or other groups of people.

Keeping this caveat in mind, I should like to suggest the following:

1. *The choice of an intoxicant and its pattern of use in a culture is not a chance phenomenon but is related to ecologic, psychosocial, and cultural factors.* The present study provides another case to support the contention, already presented by others, that intoxicant use is determined by sociocultural as well as individual factors. We might say, in addition, that a society

adopts that drug use pattern from which it derives social benefit. From the individual's vantage point, a drug use pattern that enhances coping behavior will be favored within a society. Thus one may conceive of a dynamic relationship in which societies "experiment" with certain drugs and usage patterns and alter these over time. Perhaps, also, the drug use can in turn affect the sociocultural milieu.

2. *Alcohol is a cathartic drug implementing behavioral expression of internal states. Opium is a control drug aiding suppression of disruptive impulses.* The effect of alcohol in reducing anxiety and "releasing" the inhibition of various drives has been described (Bunzel 1940; G. M. Carstairs 1954, also in this volume; Redlich and Freedman 1966). Opiates have been noted to cause reduction of anxiety along with "reduction" of primary drives and impulses (Redlich and Freedman 1966; Wikler 1952). Bailey (1967) hypothesizes that the latter mode of action increases the potential for social and personal adjustment among opium addicts in the United States. In the Meo case, expression of thoughts and feelings is permitted, even encouraged, insofar as these reflect the mores of the culture. Should a Meo not be daring in adversity or should he fail to be ambitious for wealth, he is maladaptive to his society. And if being a misfit causes him distress, no one gives audience to his complaints. On the contrary, expression of un-Meo attitudes by "release" of inhibition would only serve to ostracize him. Under such circumstances, opium provides not only a soothing but also a safe retreat via its drive-reduction action.

3. *Opium use may be functional (as well as dysfunctional) for certain individuals and for their society.* Szasz's (1960) notion that mental illness may be considered within a framework of "problems in living" might be profitably applied to opium use. Indeed, intoxication of any kind can be viewed as an alternative behavior in handling the problems encountered in living within a given ecologic, economic, political, or psychosocial milieu. As expressed by Redlich and Freedman (1966), "for some persons existence without the beneficial effects of these (addicting) drugs would be very difficult or impossible." In line with Ruth Benedict (1934) we might append: for some persons under some circumstances in some sociocultural groups.

Society may also benefit from intoxication and addiction. Nativistic movements, widespread violence, revolution, and anomie have disrupted other societies (Lessa and Vogt 1965). However, the Meo adhere steadfastly to their traditional way despite centuries of external influence and oppression (Yih-fu 1962).

Opium use may contribute to an integrated Meo society by allowing certain individuals, stressed by the demands of their monolithic culture, to continue to live in and contribute to Meo society.

4. *Opium use need not be addicting, even in the chronic user.* While these data are not longitudinal, observations suggest that few Meo opium users ever become addicted. Even the habitual once-a-day smoker appears no more impaired physically or socially than the cocktail-before-supper suburbanite.

5. *Physical disability, crime, and social disruption are not inevitable sequelae of opium addiction.* Most Meo opium addicts limit themselves to smoking two or three times a day and are able to work and produce enough opium for their own needs. Only the incapacitated addict cannot raise his opium, and he is too deteriorated to cause harm.

6. *Cross-cultural study of the use of addictive substances requires lengthy field observation and careful use of terminology.* Reports in the literature concerning Meo opium use are conflicting (Halpern 1964; LeBar and Suddard 1960; Srisavasi 1953; G. Young 1961). Moreover, this study fails to agree with many aspects of previous accounts. Careful examination into this discrepancy reveals two general areas of difficulty.

First, terms such as "addiction" are not applied uniformly or in the usual technical sense of the word. Use of opium does not necessarily imply addiction, for example. Clear and explicit use of such terms is necessary to render the data comparable.

Second, prolonged personal observation is required to collect data on use of intoxicating substances. For example, most Meo opium and alcohol consumption occurs at home. Thus, an invitation into the home as a friend is necessary. Use of a translator obstructs this process of friendship making. Informant data must be closely checked against firsthand observations. Observation of intoxicant use might require participation in the use of it, as is true for alcohol use among Meo. If participation is not required, as for Meo opium use, the observer must at least be a trusted guest with whom the host is comfortable. In short, prolonged field work without translators and with that elusive "rapport" is essential.

Daru and Bhang:
Cultural Factors in the Choice of Intoxicant

G. M. Carstairs

The Problem

Throughout the year 1951 the writer of this article was engaged in a field study which involved his living in intimate daily contact with the inhabitants of a large village[1] in the state of Rajasthan, in northern India. In the course of that year, he got to know this community fairly well; and he was struck by one unexpected aspect of the caste system which permeates Hindu society. This was the violent antithesis shown in the community's attitudes toward the two most prevalent forms of intoxication—that caused by drinking *daru*, a potent distilled alcohol derived from the flowers of the mahwa tree (*Bassia latifundia*), and that due to *bhang*, which is the local name for an infusion of the leaves and stems of Indian hemp (*Cannabis indica*) which is readily cultivable in this region. Each had its partisans, and each decried the other faction.

It may be noted, in passing, that these were not the only forms of *nasha*, or intoxication, recognized. Villagers frequently spoke of the nasha caused by drinking cups of sickly-sweet tea infused in milk. Some went so far as to blame the breakdown of traditional piety on this modern indulgence in "English tea." They would also describe the nasha induced by a few puffs from a communally shared cigarette, and of that brought about by an unaccustomed feast of meat. Instances were cited of men who had become addicted to chewing opium; but in recent years this has become so prohibitively expensive as to have dropped out of the picture. It was remembered by the warrior-caste, the Rajputs, one of whom explained that in the old days they would take opium before a battle in order to steady their nerves and to inhibit untimely bowel movements. Another Rajput, of humbler rank, put it more prosaically: "Yes, they'd issue a lump of opium to every man in those days, and glad to get it.—Might as well enjoy it now—may not be here tomorrow."

Here in Rajasthan the Rajput caste held a position of social supremacy. It is they who are the rajahs, the rulers. For centuries their semifeudal authority has governed the state, which was divided into a number of kingdoms, each with a hierarchy of subordinate rulers, down to the village *thakur*, who is a Rajput squire of a few acres. They traditionally justified their wealth and prestige by their willingness to fight in defense of their land and their

religion. On the smallest scale, it was to the thakur and his kinsmen that the ordinary villagers turned for protection against ma-
rauding bands, especially in times of famine or of war.

As fighting men, the Rajputs had certain special prerogatives, notably the right to eat meat and drink alcohol. These privileges, as well as their forefathers' bravery in battle, are commemo-
rated in a rich store of poetry and song. The writer recalls many
evenings spent listening to minstrels reciting epics of war and of
the hunting field, while drummers played and strident women's
voices sang with the refrain: *Pi lo, pi lo manna Raja!* ("Drink on,
drink on, oh King!"). His Rajput hosts were careful to point out on
such occasions that daru should be taken with circumspection,
only in the proper measure (*niyam se*), and with due formality. Yet
for all their protestations, "Oaths are but straw to the fire i' the
blood," and a typical Rajput party tends to become boisterous,
bawdy, and unbridled.

Besides the Rajputs, only the Sudras (the artisan castes) and
the Untouchables—and not all of them—are accustomed to take
meat and alcohol. These lower orders also observe a certain formality in their drinking. Usually they go in a group to the village
grogshop, and there the daru is passed from hand to hand in a
small brass bowl. Each man, before taking his first drink, lets fall a
drop or two and says, "*Jai Mataji!*"—invoking the demon-goddess
Kali in her local embodiment. In so doing, they fortify themselves
with the knowledge that that great goddess, mother and destroyer
in one, relishes a diet of blood and alcohol.

In striking contrast, the members of the other top caste-
group in the village, the Brahmans, unequivocally denounce the
use of daru. It is, they say, utterly inimical to the religious life—
and in matters of religion the Brahmans speak with authority. Certainly no Hindu who has tasted or even touched daru will enter
one of his temples (not even a goddess temple) without first having a purificatory bath and change of clothes. The first requirement of those who begin to devote themselves seriously to religion is always: "Abhor meat and wine." Priests and holy men
insist that a *darulia* (an alcoholic) is beyond the pale of possible
salvation. And yet again and again the writer was able to see
respectable Brahmans and holy Saddhus who were benignly and
conspicuously fuddled with bhang. To his eye, they were drunk as
lords—drunk as Rajputs—and yet they would have been mortally
offended if the comparison had been drawn, because this form of
intoxication they believed to be not only no disgrace, but actually
an enhancement of the spiritual life.

It might have been thought that if one form of intoxicant were condemned, so would be the other. In time, however, the writer was able to learn not only the subjective characteristics which distinguish these two states, but also the important cultural values which are associated with their use, and a solution to the riddle began to emerge.

Different Effects of Daru and Bhang Intoxication

The physiological and psychological effects of the ingestion of alcohol are sufficiently familiar to require no further elaboration. As Ravi Varma (1950) has shown, the stages of inebriation have also been described in ancient Sanskrit texts. He quotes the pre-Medieval writer Susruta as distinguishing three phases: first, elation and conviviality with increase in sexual desire; next, a progressive loss of sense of propriety with overactivity and failing coordination; and finally a comatose, dead-drunk state, "like a felled tree," in which, "though alive, one is as it were dead." As will be shown below, the Rajputs were vividly aware of the "release of sexual and aggressive impulses" which Horton (1943) has shown to be the basic role of alcohol in every community which resorts to its use.

The effect of taking *Cannabis indica* in one or other of its preparations is less familiar to Occidental readers; and yet it is an intoxicant which is second only to alcohol in the volume of its use, the variety of its recipes, and the profusion of its names.[2] Descriptions of its effect show a number of discrepancies, which may be attributed in part to the varying concentration of the drug in different preparations, and also to the fact that it is often taken in conjunction with other drugs. Thus Porot (1942) reports that most North African cannabists are also alcoholics. In the Middle East it is used often in conjunction with an aphrodisiac.

When a cannabis preparation is taken alone and in moderate strength (as is the case with the village bhang drinkers), Porot describes the following sequence of events: (a) a transient euphoria, a rich, lively, internal experience, in which ideas rush through the mind and there is an enormous feeling of superiority, of superhuman clarity of insight; (b) sensory hyperesthesia, and coenesthesias: sights and sounds become unusually vivid and meaningful; (c) distortion of sense of time and space; (d) loss of judgment; (e) exaggeration of affects, both of sympathy and of antipathy; (f) the phase of excitement is succeeded by one of placid ecstasy, known to Moslems as *el kif*, or "blessed repose": the "will to act" becomes annihilated; (g) after some hours of the trancelike state, sleep supervenes.

As a Frenchman, Porot was interested in the cult of cannabism which was created by a circle of writers and painters in Paris during the 1840s: an intellectual vogue which has enriched medical literature with some vivid accounts of the subjective aspects of the intoxication. This reportage was facilitated by the fact that the condition does not interfere with self-awareness, so that the participants had the sensation of being onlookers at the same time as actors in the scene. As Théophile Gautier (1846) wrote: "Je voyais mes camarades à certains instants, mais défigurés, moitié hommes, moitié plantes, avec des airs pensifs d'ibis debout sur une patte d'autruche."

But Gautier, as Guilly (1950) has pointed out in a recent essay on the "Club des Hachischins," was not altogether a reliable witness. His account was frankly embellished, designed to exaggerate the bizarre and the orgiastic elements of the situation; and in so doing he illustrates a finding of his contemporary, Baudelaire, who also was fascinated by the effects of the drug and carried his experiments to extreme lengths. Baudelaire (1860) pointed out that cannabis affected people differently according to their degree of intellectual refinement. He distinguished "spiritual" from merely material or brutish intoxication; and to this one can add that the quality of the intoxication can be influenced by the expectations with which the subject enters into it. For example, Tunisian addicts would smoke their *takrouri* in a quiet room, scented and decorated with flowers and with erotic prints calculated to stimulate hallucinations proper to their self-induced anticipation of paradise.

Frivolous though his interest was, Gautier seems to have tasted enough of the drug to have experienced the state of lethargic ecstasy—in Baudelaire's words, "l'apothéose de l'Homme-Dieu"—which he described as follows: "Je ne sentais plus mon corps; les liens de la matière et de l'esprit étaient déliés; je me mouvais par ma seule volonté dans un milieu qui n'offrait pas de résistance. . . . Rien de matériel ne se mêlait à cette extase; aucun désir terrestre n'en altérait la pureté. . . ."

There have been other European experimenters who have described the effects of cannabism but none who have been outspoken in its praise. Walter de la Mare (1924) wrote that, "Like opium, it induces an extravagant sense of isolation," and he went on to quote the experience of his friend Redwood Anderson, who reported on the effect of taking small doses of the drug. He was able to describe the euphoria, the rush of ideas, and the intense subjective feelings of awareness and heightened significance of all his perceptions; but he was not seduced by this near-ecstasy, rather struggling to resist the weakening of voluntary control and to repudiate these illusions of godlike intuition.

In this he was at one with Baudelaire, who indulged very profoundly in this as in other forms of intoxication and, in the end, like a true Westerner, protested against any drug which would hamper the exercise of free, individual assertion and volition. He wrote: "Je ne comprends pas pourquoi l'homme rationnel et spirituel se sert de moyens artificiels pour arriver à la béatitude poétique, puisque l'enthousiasme et la volonté suffisent pour l'élever à une existence supra-naturelle. Les grands poètes, les philosophes, les prophètes sont des êtres qui, par le pur et libre exercice de leur volonté, parviennent à un état où ils sont à la fois cause et effet, sujet et objet, magnétiseur et somnambule."

It is necessary to refer at length to these subjective experiences because, although to the superficial observer the behavior of the bhang drinker might seem not unlike that of an alcoholic (except that the progress of intoxication is at first delayed, for up to ninety minutes, and then proceeds by rapid stages to a profound stupor), the subject's inner experiences are very different. To quote an early medical investigator, Hesnard (1912): "Ses symptomes en sont bien plus riches pour celui qui l'éprouve que pour l'observateur." This was convincingly demonstrated to the present writer when he was prevailed upon to share in the Brahman group's potations on two occasions. He experienced the time distortion, the tumbling rush of ideas, the intensified significance of sights, sounds, and tastes and, more strongly than anything else, the feeling of existing on two planes at once. His body sat or lay in a state of voluptuous indifference to its surroundings, while consciousness alternated between a timeless trancelike state and a painful struggle to keep awake, to keep on observing, and acting (in this case, to keep on writing down notes on his introspective experiences). It became clear to him, in retrospect, that throughout the intoxication his bias of personality, and perhaps his less conscious fears of surrendering to a dreamlike state, resisted the somatic pull of the drug; and yet he was able to enter sufficiently into the fringe of the real ecstasy to quicken his future appreciation of what the experience meant to those who welcomed and valued it.

Hitherto, it will be noted, the state induced by bhang has been discussed in the terms of reference used by Western observers. The writer's own experience confirmed their clinical accounts, with emphasis on feelings of detachment, of extreme introspection, of the loss of volition coupled with a dreamlike impression of heightened reality. Moreover, the recognition of his own fear and repudiation of the state opened his eyes to two possibilities: (a) that other Western observers might have shared his own reluctance, if not inability, fully to submit to this intoxication; and (b) that to Hindus, with their different cultural heritage and personality bias, the experience might represent something different, at once less frightening and more congenial. It was with this in mind that he reviewed his notes of some hundreds of conversations with villagers, in order to consider what were their associations to daru and to bhang respectively.

It should be pointed out that this discussion concerns the use rather than the abuse of these intoxicants. There were many habitual drinkers of both, and instances of alcoholic delirium were described by several Rajputs, though not witnessed by the writer. The only Brahman who could be called an addict to bhang in the strict sense was also an opium eater, and at seventy-five was one of the oldest men in the village. It is a vexed question as to whether cannabism, when carried to extremes, incites to crimes of violence, as P. O. Wolff (1949), Dhunjibhoy (1930), and Porot (1942) assert, or whether, as Bromberg and Rodgers (1946) and G. B. Wallace (1944) have shown in careful statistical studies, this association is not supported by the facts. The present writer's study of the literature supports the view that crime (even the berserk attacks on the crusaders by the hashish-inspired followers of the Mohammedan Old Man of the Mountains, from which the word assassin is said to be derived) is, like the voluptuous daydreams of the Tunisians, merely one of the ends which cannabism can be made to serve during its brief phase of excitement, and not a necessary consequence of taking the drug. In this village, at any rate, there were no instances of crimes attributable to the drinking of bhang, nor was there any evidence to support the suggestion of Dhunjibhoy, among others, that it gives rise to a characteristic psychosis. It remains open to proof whether such cases are not, as Mayer-Gross (1932) maintains, simply schizophrenic illnesses occurring in a cannabis-taking population.

Villagers' Associations to Daru and Bhang

In the following series of quotations from a number of villagers' conversations, it will be helpful to bear in mind that Rajputs are distinguished by the addition of the title *Singh* (lion) to their name; among the Brahmans, a common second name is *Lal* (red, the auspicious color). For the sake of clarity all Brahman names have been transcribed to conform to this rule.

The first obvious difference to emerge is that while the Brahmans are unanimous in their detestation of daru, the Rajputs do not present a united front in its defense. "Some Rajputs," explained Himat Singh, "those who are worshippers of God, they do not eat meat or drink wine—that is the first thing for them to give up. Wine spoils men's mind: some swear and give abuse, which is inimical to holiness." Such Rajputs, however, are few and far between: "The rest, they eat, drink and remain *must*."[3]

Many Rajputs prided themselves on drinking with discrimination, a fixed measure every day. Thus Nahar Singh: "My father used to drink a fixed quantity of daru, from a small measure, every night. It was his niyam, his rule." A young man called Ragunath Singh was emphatic in asserting the warlike traditions of his caste, and their need for meat and drink: "Panthers and tigers don't eat grass—and that's what Rajputs are like, a carnivorous race." He also, however, stressed that liquor was a dangerous ally: "If you take it to excess it destroys your semen, the good stuff, the strength of your body—but taken in right measure it builds it up."

Gambhir Singh mentioned that his father, a former inspector of police, used to allow himself a generous measure every day: "It helped him in his work, made him fierce and bold, ready to beat people when that was needed."

This stress on restraint, and on small measures, soon tended to be forgotten in the course of an evening of Rajput hospitality, when glass after glass was filled and emptied at a draught. In his cups, Amar Singh used to boast of his ungovernable temper, of men he had killed in the heat of anger, of his sexual prowess with prostitutes. His friend Gordhan Singh chipped in with a description of a typical Rajput celebration: "They sit drinking heartily till they are senseless, and then they talk loudly and make fools of themselves, and spill their food down the front of their shirts, and shout to the dancing girls; and some of them pass out altogether—oh, it's a fine sight to see, it's good fun."

The former ruler of the village and of the surrounding principality expressed conflicting views on daru. On the one hand, he aspired to gain a "spiritual rise" through the practice of prayers and austerities, and this necessitated a strict rationing of his customary indulgence in alcohol. Quite often, however, something would happen to interrupt his abstemious intentions, and on such a day his eloquence in praise of wine was noticeably stimulated: "Red eyes are thought by us Rajputs to be very beautiful. They are the sign of lust. Those who have the good fortune to have red lines in the eyes, they are thought to be very lusty. Rajputs are very lusty, Sahib. It is because of their meat and drink: it makes them so that they have to have their lust, poor fellows." At this point he began to quote verses in praise of wine: "It makes the eyes red, it keeps the pleasure going between the pair, the husband and wife: how shall I praise you enough, oh twice-distilled!" And again: "In time of war, when the drum beats, only opium and daru drive out fear."

On another occasion, the ruler quoted a ribald couplet to the effect that without meat all food is grass, and without daru even Ganges water has no virtue. But this blasphemy alarmed him into a momentary sobriety. He hastily repudiated the verse, but a few minutes later he was exuberantly describing the scene at a wealthy Rajput's wedding party: "They will be sitting drinking far into the night, with dancing girls entertaining them. They will call the dancing girl to sit on their lap, then they will get stirred and take her into a room and bar the doors; and the others will beat upon the door and say, 'Eh, Rao Sahib, we also want to see this girl.' Poor girl, where can she go, all doors are locked! Enjoy till morning, she must do what you want."

The ruler's younger brother was emphatically not one of those Rajputs who renounced their pleasure in alcohol in the interests of religion: "Sahib, I am not interested in these things. These religious matters, usually one begins to be interested in them after the age of fifty."

And before then?

"Before then, Sahib, eat, drink and make merry."

Rajputs not infrequently referred to bhang, but never with strong feelings either of approval or condemnation. It is mentioned as a refreshment given to guests who arrive after a long journey. An elderly retainer called Anop Singh said: "We are not in the habit of drinking bhang, though we'll take it if it comes our way. Sometimes holy men come, and they are great ones for bhang, so you have to join them if they invite you, and have some too." On one occasion the writer found a young Rajput landowner called Vijay Singh profoundly fuddled with a large dose of bhang which had been given to him, without his knowledge, in a spiced sweetmeat: "I didn't know I was eating bhang or I wouldn't have taken it—it's not a thing I like. It makes you very sleepy and turns your throat dry. . . . I don't like it, it makes you quite useless, unable to do anything. Daru is not like that: you get drunk but you can still carry on."

The Brahmans, on the other hand, were quite unanimous in reviling daru and all those who indulged in it. They described it as foul, polluting, carnal, and destructive to that spark of Godhead which every man carries within him. As Shankar Lal put it: "The result of eating meat and drinking liquor is that you get filled with passion, rage—and then what happens? The spirit of God flies out from you."

The ruler's own attempt to reconcile religious devotions with a measure of indulgence in alcohol was rejected with contumely by Mohan Lal, a scholarly teacher. "He is all wrong: he is a bogus lecher. Always busy with wine and women, how can he find his way along this stony and thorny path?"

In their references to the use of bhang, the Brahmans were matter-of-fact rather than lyrical. "It gives good *bhakti*," said Shankar Lal: "You get a very good bhakti with bhang." He went on to define bhakti as the sort of devotional act which consists in emptying the mind of all worldly distractions and thinking only of God. The "arrived" devotee is able to keep his thoughts from straying off onto trivial or lustful topics; in his impersonal trance he becomes oblivious to mundane concerns so that you "could hit him in the face with shoes a hundred times, and he would remain unmoved" (Mohan Lal).

Brahman informants made many references to a nearby pilgrimage center presided over by a very influential priest. Both he and his predecessors were described, with admiration, as being mighty drinkers of bhang and heroic in the depth of their devotional trances. The chief object of worship at this place was an ancient phallic symbol of black stone, representing the god Shiva; and this god in turn was often cited as both a bhang drinker and a paragon of the contemplative life. It is by modeling themselves on his example that religious ascetics practice severe and prolonged austerities, training themselves to withdraw their entire attention from the distractions of the sensible world until they can exist for hours in an oblivious, inward-looking state. The ultimate reward of this asceticism is that the Saddhu is enabled to divest himself of his body (which becomes imperishable, though apparently lifeless) and to pass directly into reunion with the spirit of the universe. (One is reminded of Baudelaire's "l'apothéose de l'Homme-Dieu.") Bhang is highly regarded as conducing toward this condition and is taken regularly by most Saddhus. In the precincts of the great Shiva temple, the writer frequently encountered holy men, dressed in little more than a coating of sacred ash, who staggered about in the early stages of bhang intoxication. If he

addressed them, they would reply only with an elusive smile or
with an exclamation like "Hari, Hari, Hari!"—repeating one of the
names of God. Ordinary village Brahmans, who did not aspire to
such feats of asceticism, made a practice of devoting some minutes
or hours every day to sitting in a state of abstraction and prayer,
and in this exercise they found a modicum of bhang to be most
helpful.

Relevant Themes in Hindu Culture Pattern

Both the Rajput and the Brahman castes, at least in this large
village, belonged to the economically privileged section of the
community. Their male members had all received at least
enough education to make them literate in Hindi, and in an unsystematic way had been instructed in the fundamentals of their
religion and made familiar with the main features of the Ramay-
ana and Mahabharata epics which illustrates those teachings in a
variety of dramatic episodes. Hinduism encompasses so wide a
range of practical and philosophical beliefs, of myths and ritual
ordinances, and contains so many contradictory elements, that
one theologian, after twenty-five years of study, came to the conclusion that there were only two indispensable features in this
religion: reverence of the Brahman, and worship of the cow (G.
Carstairs 1926). These features are epitomized in the formal
greetings exchanged by Rajput and Brahman. The former salutes
the priestly caste with, "I clasp your feet," and the latter replies,
"May you live long and protect the Brahmans and the cows." In
so doing, they acknowledge each other's caste in its respective
status of spiritual and temporal primacy.

The fundamental orthodox Hindu beliefs, as Taylor (1948)
has pointed out in an analysis drawn from study of a community in
an area contiguous with Rajasthan, stem from the concepts of
karma (predestined lot), of the cycle of rebirth, and of dharma
(right conduct), observance of which leads to promotion in one's
next rebirth and ultimately to the goal of all human endeavor,
which is *moksh,* or liberation from the cycle of reincarnation altogether. Socioeconomic relationships are accepted as inevitable, as
is the hierarchic structure of caste. Indeed, "the individual's security in this society comes from his acceptance of his insignificant
part in a vast pre-ordained scheme: he has little anxiety, because
he is not confronted with a variety of choice." Rajputs and Brahmans are alike in knowing that virtue consists in performing the
duties appropriate to that station in life into which one is born,

and in minimizing one's indulgence in sensual and emotional satisfactions of a private nature. Thus Nahar Singh, a Rajput renowned for his religious zeal, said: "Those of us who take religion seriously, but have still not wholly renounced the world, we can do it by taking care not to let our affections become too deeply engaged in things of lesser importance. We should do our work, fulfill all our duties, and be affectionate to our families—but all that should be on the surface of our daily lives. Our real souls, deep down, should not be involved in any of these emotional ties. . . ."

Mohan Lal expressed similar views: "The religious man lives in the world, but apart. He is like a drop of water on a lotus leaf, which moves over its surface but is not absorbed." His caste-fellow Bhuri Lal described the ideal pattern of "nonattachment," leading in the end to release: "Moksh is obtained by purging the self of all carnal appetites and withdrawing from the illusions of this world. A wise man is cool-tempered." Immediately after this, he went on to talk of sexual morality. Sex, he said, should be strictly controlled. It should be regarded as a duty, and used only for the purpose of perpetuating one's male line. He himself had been afflicted with four daughters before his two sons were born, and then, "As soon as my second son was born, I gave up having sex. You say I look young? That's because I have practiced celibacy for years."

This exaltation of asceticism, of self-deprivation, of trying to eliminate one's sensual appetites, is a basic theme. Again and again in Hindu mythology one encounters heroic figures (by no means always virtuous ones) who practice austerities so severe and prolonged that their spiritual power becomes prodigious: the gods themselves beg them to desist and offer to grant anything they ask. Taylor has related this to the absoluteness of paternal authority in the home; the pattern is firmly laid down that one can achieve success and recognition only by self-abnegation and prostration before the all-powerful father figure. A student of Kardiner (1945) might be tempted to carry the analogy still farther back, to the Hindu child's wholly indulgent experience at the suckling stage, during which he actually usurps his father's place, because parents are not supposed to sleep together until the child is weaned. In this context, the *tapassya* which constrains even the gods can be seen as a return to the infant's fantasied omnipotence.

The values discussed thus far are held in common by both castes, with the difference that the Brahmans, being at the pinnacle of the spiritual hierarchy, have a special obligation to lead a pious life. More than ordinary men, they must pay constant attention to the fulfilling of religious duties. Their lives are beset with recurring threats of defilement and their days are punctuated with acts of absolution. Among the many forms of self-denial to which they are accustomed are the avoidance of anger or any other unseemly expression of personal feelings; and abstinence from meat and alcohol is a prime essential. They are rewarded by being regarded, simply by virtue of their birth in this high caste, as already quasi-divine. Ordinary men address them as *Maharaj*, the greeting given to the gods. As one of them put it: "Even now, when people see a man is a Brahman, they pay much respect in comparison to other castes. He is much more closely related to God."

In this region the Rajputs represent the temporal aristocracy, as the Brahmans do the spiritual. Their caste is one of warriors and landlords. Until the social reforms of 1948, their rajahs exercised arbitrary and autocratic rule over the innumerable small principalities into which Rajasthan is divided. They owed allegiance in their turn to the ruler of their state—in the case of this village, to the maharana of Udaipur. By virtue of their role as warriors, the Rajputs were accorded certain privileged relaxations of the orthodox Hindu rules: in particular, those prohibiting the use of force, the taking of life, the eating of meat and drinking of wine. These all represent violations of basic canons of Hindu dharm, and so they are hedged about with restrictions and formalities in order to minimize their evil effects. Violence is a part of their lives, but they are taught to exercise forbearance, to rebuke an offender twice before chastising him. In warfare they obeyed a code of chivalry not unlike that of the medieval knights. Similarly, the meat of only a few animals is counted fit to eat, and then only of the male of the species; and hence, also, the emphasis on restriction and invariable "measure" in drinking daru.

The Rajputs find themselves in a curious position. Their social preeminence is due to their role as defenders of religion, and they are as conservative in belief as they are in politics; and yet their own cherished traditions emphasize their deviation from "right living" in the orthodox Hindu sense. The conflict is heightened by the circumstance that in their caste, even more than in all the others, patriarchal authority is stressed. As the writer has pointed out elsewhere (1953), both sons and younger brothers in Rajput families have to learn to defer in utter subservience to their fathers and elder brothers. Whereas in the Brahman caste this domestic discipline is made tolerable by the fact that it is impersonal, simply a facet of a general obedience to propriety which the elders observe in their turn, among Rajputs it is different. There is a great difference between the status of the head of the family and that of his subordinates. For example, a younger son inherits an estate only one-twentieth the size of that which comes to the first-born. The head of a Rajput family is anything but an impersonal figure. Coached from infancy by a succession of sycophantic retainers, he has an inflated idea of his personal importance, coupled with an often well-founded suspicion that he is surrounded by rivals and enemies. The tensions which arise in such a setting explode from time to time in violent quarrels. Another corollary of the peculiar upbringing of the Rajputs is that they are taught to put great stress on individual bravery and ferocity in the face of danger. The test of real danger is all too seldom met with, but every young Rajput lives with the anxiety that he may not prove adequate to the occasion when it comes. As a result he tends to be boastful, touchy, and readily inclined to assuage his anxieties in the convivial relaxation of a drinking party.

Discussion

In her much-quoted study of patterns of drinking in two South American villages, Bunzel remarks, of such sociological appraisals in general: "It should be borne in mind that each group represents a different problem: it is necessary in each case to find out what role alcohol plays *in that culture*" (1940:386). She was able to demonstrate two widely differing ways of using alcohol. In Chamula there was little aggression or promiscuity or severity of discipline; there, heavy drinking was indulged in from childhood and was attended with no guilt. In Chichicastenango, on the other hand, she saw a strict paternal authority and an insistence on the repression of aggressive and sexual impulses, which found release in the course of occasional drinking sprees; and these were followed by feelings of severe guilt. The Rajput drinking pattern, obviously, has much in common with the latter.

A more general frame of reference has been given by Horton (1943) in his survey of alcohol in primitive societies, which led to his drawing up three basic theorems: (*a*) the drinking of alcohol tends to be accompanied by release of sexual and aggressive impulses; (*b*) the strength of the drinking response in any society tends to vary directly with the level of anxiety in the society; (*c*) the strength of the drinking response tends to vary inversely with the strength of the counteranxiety elicited by painful experiences during and after drinking.

The first of these theorems is abundantly borne out by the behavior of Rajputs in their cups. It is clear also that the presence of socially approved prostitutes and lower-caste servants and dependents enables the carrying out of these impulses in a manner which excites no retribution, and so the third theorem operates in support of their drinking heavily. On the side of restraint is the knowledge that sensual indulgence is an offense against the Hindu code of asceticism; but this code does not weigh heavily on most Rajputs.

On Brahmans, on the other hand, the code weighs very heavily indeed, being associated with their fondest claims to superiority over their fellow men. A Brahman who gets drunk will be outcasted, condemned to associate with the lowest ranks of society. Consequently the threat of this "counteranxiety" is sufficient to make the drinking of alcohol virtually impossible to Brahmans (at least in the village). There is no reason to suppose, however, that they, any more than the Rajputs, are devoid of anxiety. But the differences in emphasis on individual self-assertion (stressed by Rajput upbringing but constrained by their fiercely authoritarian disciplines) and on the unimportance of personal and sensual experiences (stressed in the Brahman code) seem to imply that the anxieties of the Rajputs will be more acute while those of the Brahmans will be more diffuse and more readily sublimated in the religious exercises which play such a large part in their adult lives.

Another consideration is raised by Shalloo's analysis of the way in which Jewish cultural values operate to minimize the incidence of alcoholism in their community. In his view, the Jews develop strong familial and communal ties and stress social conformity and conservatism in mores because they are aware of the critical and often hostile scrutiny of the Gentiles among whom they live. He concludes: "Such an analysis indicates that we are dealing with an 'isolated sacred society' as against a Gentile 'accessible secular society' " (1941:273).

In our Indian example, the Brahmans repesented a "sacred society" but not an isolated one. Far from being alien, they represent the ideal religious aspirations of the masses of ordinary Hindus, those who are obliged to "eat, drink, and keep their passions alive," as Shankar Lal once put it. If the Brahmans are abstemious, it is not through an exaggerated fear of the censure of their fellows. On the contrary, their consciousness of their exalted state often makes them high-handed and inconsiderate in their dealings with those of lower caste; and moreover, they are not abstemious.

If Horton's theorems hold good for alcoholism, must a new set be constructed to account for cannabism?

The answer which the present writer would suggest to the problem posed at the outset of this paper would be on the following lines: there are alternative ways of dealing with sexual and aggressive impulses besides repressing them and then "blowing them off" in abreactive drinking bouts in which the superego is temporarily dissolved in alcohol. The way which the Brahmans have selected consists in a playing down of all interpersonal relationships in obedience to a common, impersonal set of rules of Right Behavior. Not only feelings but also appetites are played down, as impediments to the one supreme end of union with God. Significantly, this goal of sublimated effort is often described in terms appropriate to sexual ecstasy, as is the case with the communications of ascetics and mystics in other parts of the world. Whereas the Rajput in his drinking bout knows that he is taking a holiday from his sober concerns, the Brahman thinks of his intoxication with bhang as a flight not from but toward a more profound contact with reality.

Westerners, like the Rajputs, are committed to a life of action. They are brought up to regard individual achievement as important, and sensual indulgence to be not wholly wrong if it is enjoyed within socially prescribed limits. In spite of the existence among a sophisticated minority of the cult of nonattachment, the principles of yoga are unfamiliar to the West, and the experience of surrendering one's powers of volition is felt to be threatening and distasteful—as European experimenters with hashish (and the writer, with bhang) have found. P. O. Wolff (1949) is, however, too sweeping in suggesting that cannabism is a peculiarly oriental taste. The Rajputs are far from being the only Easterners who dislike it or feel no need of it. Porot has pointed out that Indian hemp could easily be cultivated in the Far East, and yet it is practically unknown to the peoples of China and Japan. La Barre's (1946) account of Chinese personality suggests that that people have little inclination to despise the material pleasures of this world; and the Japanese would be the last, one would suppose, to renounce the active life.

On the basis, presumably, of his own religious convictions, Wolff has implied that the ecstatic intuitions experienced through cannabism, far from having any validity, represent a flouting of "an inviolable moral law." This is the antithesis of cultural relativism. No one is left in doubt where Wolff takes his stand. Were the present writer to emulate this candor, he would have to say that of the two types of intoxication which he witnessed, and in a measure shared, in this Rajasthan village, he had no doubt that that which was indulged in by the Brahmans was the less socially disruptive, less unseemly, and more in harmony with the highest ideals of their race; and yet so alien to his own personal and cultural pattern of ego defenses, that he much preferred the other. It was a case of *video meliora proboque, deteriora sequor.*

Postscript

Since the above article was written, Aldous Huxley (1954) has published an eloquent and perceptive account of the experience of mescalin intoxication, which is shown to resemble that induced by bhang. Huxley was particularly struck by two aspects: in the initial stage, by the primordial vividness of visual impressions, in perceiving ordinarily commonplace objects; and in the later stages, by the feeling of superhuman insight into the nature of things, accompanied by a complete detachment both from his own self and from those of his fellow men. He regards mescalin as a "gratuitous grace" which facilitates the sort of mystical experience which he finds both chastening and rewarding, in much the same way as Brahmans and Saddhus regard bhang as an aid to contemplation. Yet he is unrealistic enough to wish that Americans, and Westerners generally, should take to this drug in preference to alcohol and tobacco. If the thesis of this paper is valid, Westerners have refrained from taking mescalin (which has long been available to them) because its effect does not accord with their desires. Unless there is an unforeseen reversal of their basic values, they are as little likely to follow Huxley's advice as are the Brahmans to abandon bhang in favor of the Rajputs' daru, or vice versa.

Notes

1. The village had twenty-four hundred inhabitants, of whom ninety-three were Rajputs and eighty-five Brahmans.
2. These include: bhang, charas, ganja (India); kif (Algeria); takrouri (Tunisia); kabak (Turkey); hashish-el-kif (Middle East); djoma (Central Africa); dagga (South Africa); liamba (Brazil); grifa (Mexico); marihuana (South and North America). There are, however, many other names descriptive of particular sweetmeats, cakes, drinks, etc., containing the drug.
3. *Must* describes the rage of an elephant which is in heat.

Drinking Patterns and Alcoholism in the Chinese
K. Singer

Brief Review of Literature

The earliest observation, so far as I can trace, is that of Hsu who reporting as a social worker on China before World War II stated that alcoholism as a cause of mental disorder was as rare in China as it appeared in the United States (1955:276). La Barre the anthropologist, from his observations as a naval officer during World War II in Kunming, concluded that "the Chinese are not so voluntarily addicted to excessive use of alcohol as have been some northern European peoples. . . . The fact seems to be that in spite of ample and even copious consumptions of alcohol on defined occasions, its use appears never to become an emotional problem" (1946:376). Lin (1953) in Taiwan found only two alcoholics in a survey of twenty thousand inhabitants and further reported that in seventeen years among the population there had been not more than ten cases of alcoholism (Chafetz 1964).

The most thoughtful account of drinking patterns and related behavior in the Chinese to date is that of Barnett (1955) who studied the Cantonese in New York City. However, his findings among Chinese Americans cannot be extrapolated to the Chinese people as a whole. In a condition like alcoholism where sociocultural factors are usually given pride of place in etiology, generalizations concerning an ethnic group are not justified without reference to social context and milieu. It is obvious that American Chinese have evolved in a different direction from those in their homeland. The former have become in some respects highly acculturated, yet in others remained orthodox and reacted to compression from the dominant cultural group by preserving norms discarded elsewhere. Nevertheless Barnett's observation that the incidence of alcoholism in Chinatown Chinese is low and that alcoholism as a social problem is relatively unimportant is noteworthy as providing support for the influence of sociocultural factors as such in the etiology of alcoholism.

Further evidence for the low incidence of alcoholism in the Chinese overseas is provided by Wedge and Abe (1949) who in considering the racial incidence of mental diseases in Hawaii found no case of alcoholism in a receiving hospital.

Demographic and Social Characteristics

Hong Kong is a colony of the United Kingdom with an estimated population at the end of 1969 of four million thirty-nine thousand.

About 98.5 percent are Chinese and 58 percent of the population are of Hong Kong birth. Most of these and the greater part of the migrant population are Cantonese having originated from the neighboring Kwangtung province of China. Eighty-two percent live in the urban areas which comprise 40 square miles of the total land area of 398½ square miles, making the population density one of the highest in the world.

Economically Hong Kong has grown and prospered in her free port and been able to surmount the stress of a rapid increase in population, owing mainly to influx of refugees from China, from six hundred thousand at the end of the Japanese occupation in 1945. In the last decade rapidly growing industrialization (64 percent of the people are engaged in industry) has replaced the traditional entrepôt trade of the colony which has risen to a place among the twenty-five leading trading countries in the world (*Hong Kong Annual Report* 1969). As a result there has been substantial improvement in housing, education, and recreational, health, and social welfare amenities. The standard of living is high compared to other Asian countries. However, much unequal distribution of wealth remains and pockets of poverty abound.

The main religions are Taoism and Buddhism with Christianity accounting for 10 percent of the population. Pervading the various religions and the social fabric are the religious aspects of Confucianism which is strictly not a religion but an ethical code. It defines behavior that is proper between peoples of various ages, sexes, and degrees of relatedness and between friends and strangers. To the casual observer the Chinese may appear relatively unconcerned about religion or at least concerned more with observance of rites and rituals than with experiential aspects. Certainly they are tolerant in their general outlook and free from bigotry and fanaticism in their religious beliefs. This may stem from Confucian philosophy which emphasizes supremacy of reason and the wisdom of avoiding extremes. At any rate the Chinese combine various religious practices including the Christian without any sense of incongruity.

With increasing affluence and impact of Western culture the people, especially the younger generation, are shedding traditions and assimilating new values.

Drinking Patterns

The observations that follow are based on the author's knowledge of the Chinese community in Hong Kong acquired over a number of years from personal involvement. They are supplemented by examination of published materials and interviews with representative members, with alcoholic patients, and with their relatives and friends.

Traditional Beliefs and Attitudes

The Chinese regard drinking as immoral but do not feel very strongly about it. Drinking finds a place in the four vices or disasters: "womanizing, gambling, drinking, and smoking (narcotics)." Also "the good son does not drink." But there is no real moral code against moderate drinking, little concern with drinking or alcoholism as a problem, and little guilt or hostility attendant upon drinking, provided the rules and procedures are followed.

Traditional beliefs attribute to alcohol the following "ninefold harm": (1) impairment of intellect; (2) impairment of morals; (3) predisposition to physical illness; (4) impairment of sex performance; (5) shortening of life span; (6) impairment of fertility; (7) passing on of inherited defects; (8) increased risk of suicide; and (9) increase of criminality. Alcohol is also traditionally believed to be beneficial, if taken moderately, as follows: (1) relief of rheumatism (alcohol for this purpose being taken mainly by men and especially in winter when it is supposed to be "warming"); (2) increase of blood circulation; (3) increase of blood production (i.e., useful for treating anemia and for this purpose certain wines are routinely taken by women after childbirth); (4) improvement of mental well-being; (5) relief of exhaustion; (6) improvement of digestion; (7) improvement of complexion; (8) improvement of appetite; and (9) expulsion of wind.

Drinking is sanctioned in defined situations. Alcohol is regarded as food and drinking as one phase of eating. It is noteworthy that the Chinese term for banquet is *yum* or "drink." The prime purpose of drinking at banquets is to facilitate social intercourse. Children though not usually allowed to drink take part in these gatherings, are exposed to alcohol, and learn the rules from an early age. Banquets are given for various life events like marriages and births and are attended by a large number of relatives, friends, and acquaintances. At these functions moderate drinking is the rule though copious amounts may be consumed by some. Pressure is put on one to drink but no stigma attaches to the abstinent. One drinks individually at one's own pace, at toasts which may be numerous, and occasionally at drinking games in which large quantities may be consumed. These games are now a dying art and indulged in mainly by the older generation. Popular still is *tsai mui* or "guessing fingers." The object of such games is to make the opponent drink. The victor prides himself on the clarity and expertise needed to win, the loser on his capacity to hold his liquor. Intoxication at banquets leads to expansiveness and verbosity, rarely to physical violence or sexuality.

Regular drinking at meals is an accepted custom, though contrary to the common belief that almost every family indulges in this, only a small minority do so. The average drinker will take a few ounces at each meal. He drinks to attain a sense of well-being and improve his physical health. Drinking also fits in with the ritualistic aspects of eating. Drinking at meals is the prerogative of the head and other adult males of the family. Children and females are usually discouraged from drinking. A small minority will actually encourage all members of the family to indulge. Children are then taught at an early age, exceptionally as early as one. They are given one to two teaspoons of wine at each meal in the belief that it promotes their health. Such a belief is likely to be held in the lower social classes. A few of the upper classes also train boys in their early teens to drink for social reasons. The majority, however, prohibit children from drinking.

A small amount of alcohol is consumed entirely for its medicinal value. An example is port taken after childbirth "to improve the blood."

It is commonly assumed that the use of wine in the numerous ceremonies for various life crises, e.g., rites for the dead, provides yet another important source of alcohol for consumption. In fact the small quantities of wine used are entirely sprinkled on the ground.

The Chinese disapprove of excessive drinking, secret drinking, drinking alone, and intoxication. Aggressive and noisy behavior and public drunkenness are strongly condemned. The last is an extremely rare sight. The alcoholic is regarded not as suffering from a disease but a reprobate.

In conclusion drinking in the Chinese whether at banquets or at ordinary meals is an institutionalized mechanism interweaving intimately the social, ritualistic, and physiological aspects of these functions.

Drinking Behavior

Most adult males drink at some time or other but probably not more than one-tenth drink regularly at meals. Males drink much more frequently and in larger amounts than females, a reflection of the subordinate status of the latter. Apart from a small distinct minority who are taught to drink from early childhood, the age at which the first substantial drink is taken is usually between fifteen and twenty-five. The lower social classes drink more frequently, usually consuming Chinese wine regularly at meals. The upper classes prefer Western beverages and drink mainly at banquets. With increasing affluence and westernization the drinking of Western beverages is on the increase.

The average wine drinker alters his drinking pattern as necessary. His drinking does not obviously impair his work, family social life, or physical or mental health. He rarely develops intoxication and when he does he sleeps it off.

Types of Alcoholic Beverages

Chinese-Type Alcoholic Beverages

These are drunk at meals. Table 1 lists those commonly used. It will be seen that their alcoholic content is generally high, averaging about 50 percent by volume. They are also much cheaper than Western beverages and this is why the lower social classes drink more than the upper, in contrast to the pattern usually found elsewhere.

While all wines are regarded as beneficial for health if taken in moderate quantities, certain wines are particularly favored for their medicinal value. An example is "snake wine." Three types of snakes are used in its manufacture, the Indo-Chinese ratsnake, the cobra, and the banded krait. They are believed to benefit the upper, middle, and lower portions of the body respectively.

Western-Type Alcoholic Beverages

These are preferred because they produce less hangover and are more palatable and more prestigious. They are generally ten times more expensive than Chinese wine.

Brandy and whiskey are the most popular. The former is regarded as having medicinal qualities. Beer is the drink of the poorer classes, regarded as somewhat harmful, "cooling" and "dissipating the blood," and avoided by women. Western wines are not consumed with meals with the exception of port and Martin Rose which are preferred by women for their medicinal value.

Alcoholism

Prevalence

Alcoholism in Hong Kong as in most Asian countries is not at present a matter of prime concern. It appears that though drinking is frequent, alcoholism is uncommon. But it is not as rare as commonly assumed to be the case in the Chinese.

TABLE 1.   Commonly Used Chinese Wines in Hong Kong

Name	Made from	Alcoholic Content (percentage by volume)
General Purpose Wines		
Sheung ching	Rice	30
Sam ching	Rice	42
Sie ching	Rice	53
Fai tiu	Rice	30
Mau toi	Millet	55
Ko leung	Millet	60
Fan chow	Millet	65
Medicinal Wines		
Ng ka pei	Rice wine with herbs preserved	53
"Rose wine"	Rice wine with rose petals preserved	57
"Snake wine"	Rice wine with snakes preserved	36
"Tiger bone wine"	Rice wine with tiger bone preserved	60
"Lizard wine"	Rice wine with lizard preserved	39
"Gelatinous rice wine"	Gelatinous rice and millet	30
Mo kai tsau	Rice wine, usually Sheung ching, with wild pheasant preserved	30
Dong kwai tsau	Rice wine, usually Sheung ching, with chiretta preserved	30
Kwai yuen ki kok tsau	Rice wine, usually Sheung ching, with chiretta, medlar, and feverfew preserved	30

Jellinek's Estimation Formula

As with other countries factual data concerning the extent of the problem are lacking. It has not been possible to form an estimate of the incidence by applying Jellinek's formula because of the lack of figures for deaths from alcoholic cirrhosis of liver in the population as a whole. However, it is known that in the hospital population judging by autopsies and needle biopsies alcoholic cirrhosis is less common than, say, in the United States. Although cirrhosis of liver is common in Hong Kong the overwhelming majority are of the postnecrotic or posthepatic type (J. Gibson 1970). This suggests a low incidence of alcoholic cirrhosis and alcoholism in the general population though one would not quite be justified in applying findings in a hospital population to the general.

First Admissions of Alcoholic Psychosis to a Psychiatric Hospital

First admissions of alcoholic psychosis to Castle Peak Hospital, which as the only psychiatric hospital admits patients from the whole colony, have risen from 8.8 per million male Chinese adults in 1962 to 44.4 in 1970 (table 2). Readmissions averaged 32 percent of total admissions. Total admissions of alcoholic psychosis in 1970 were 21 per million general population and compare with a rate of 55 per million for England and Wales in 1960. These figures cannot be used as indications of the relative size of the problem in these places as among various factors, England and Wales have proportionately many times more beds and a much older population.

TABLE 2.   Admissions of Alcoholic Psychosis to Psychiatric Hospital

Year	First Admission Rate of Alcoholic Psychosis per Million Chinese Male Adults	Proportion of First Admission of Alcoholic Psychosis to All First Admissions (in percentage)
1961	3.5	0.4
1962	8.8	1.2
1963	12.9	1.6
1964	8.3	1.0
1965	11.1	1.2
1966	17.6	1.8
1967	36.0	3.5
1968	30.0	3.4
1969	. 44.0	6.1
1970	44.4	6.1

Of more relevance to the size of the alcohol problem is that the proportion of first admissions of alcoholic psychosis to all first admissions has also risen steadily in Hong Kong from 1.2 percent in 1962 to 6.1 percent in 1970. The latter compares with 1.3 percent for Norway in 1949, 2.5 percent for Finland in 1949, 5.1 percent for the United States in 1950, and 8.6 percent for Sweden in 1949 (Mayer-Gross, Slater, and Roth 1969). These figures are again not strictly comparable as they may reflect different practices in diagnosis and disposal of alcoholic psychosis rather than actual differences in incidence. However, as regards Hong Kong the rise in admissions is unlikely to reflect changes in diagnostic practice or in increased acceptance of treatment on the part of alcoholics relative to other psychiatric patients. In conclusion, although the Hong Kong figures cannot be used even as rough indices of the size of the problem, they do indicate that (a) alcoholic psychosis and by implication alcoholism are not uncommon—contrary to common assumption and (b) there is a rising trend of these conditions in the Chinese in Hong Kong.

Consumption of Alcoholic Beverages

Data (table 3) were obtained (*Hong Kong Trade Statistics*, 1960–69) on import, local manufacture, export,and reexport of the various types of alcoholic beverages. Consumption was estimated by subtracting export and reexport from import and local manufacture. From a knowledge of the alcoholic content of the various beverages, consumption was calculated in terms of imperial gallons of absolute alcohol. The resulting figures were added to form totals for Chinese- and Western-type beverages. From data on adults of drinking-age population (aged twenty or more) obtained from census figures, the average per capita consumption per year in adults was calculated in terms of imperial gallons of absolute alcohol.

TABLE 3.   Consumption of Alcohol in Hong Kong

Year	Total Consumption of Absolute Alcohol from Beverages (1000 imperial gallons)			Per capita Adult Consumption of Absolute Alcohol (in imperial gallons)		
	Western Type	Chinese Type	Total	Western Type	Chinese Type	Total
1960	219,000	N.A.	—	0.13	N.A.	—
1961	243,000	N.A.	—	0.14	N.A.	—
1962	275,000	N.A.	—	0.15	N.A.	—
1963	341,000	1,380,000	1,721,000	0.19	0.74	0.93
1964	362,000	1,544,000	1,906,000	0.19	0.81	1.00
1965	440,000	1,643,000	2,083,000	0.22	0.83	1.05
1966	533,000	1,635,000	2,168,000	0.27	0.80	1.07
1967	493,000	1,432,000	1,925,000	0.23	0.70	0.93
1968	581,000	1,600,000	2,181,000	0.26	0.72	0.98
1969	636,000	1,641,000	2,277,000	0.28	0.71	0.99

Note: N.A. = data not available.

An inspection of the figures gives the following impressions. (1) Consumption of alcohol maintained a steady level from 1963 to 1969, apart from a slight dip in 1967 when there were political disturbances and a depression in the economy. The steady level of consumption indicates a steady number of drinkers since there are no grounds for assuming a simultaneous increase or moderation of drinking levels in the population generally. The steady level of consumption does not, of course, give an indication of the trend of alcoholism during this period since it takes a number of years of drinking to develop the condition. (2) Per capita consumption of Western beverages showed an upward trend, rising from 0.13 gallons in 1960 to 0.28 gallons in 1969. (3) Consumption of Chinese beverages showed a slight downward trend from 1965 to 1969. The trends in (2) and (3) are consistent with the common observation that the traditional Chinese drinkers who consume Chinese wine are decreasing in numbers and are being replaced by a new type of westernized drinkers taking Western beverages. (4) Consumption of Chinese-type beverages averaged four times that of the Western type, indicating that the majority still drink Chinese wine. (5) Total consumption from 1964 to 1969 averaged about 1 imperial gallon of absolute alcohol per adult per year and compares with about 1.6 imperial gallons per adult in the United States in 1953–57 (Pittman and Snyder 1962:324). As Chinese women account for much less of the consumption than women in the States the figures for consumption in male adults in the two places must therefore be closer than those for adults of both sexes. One may therefore surmise that the Chinese male adult drinks only somewhat less than the American.

Calculations for consumption are bedevilled by the problem of illicit supplies of liquor and illegal distilleries. Manufacture of "moonshine" undoubtedly occurs and there is no way of estimating the extent to which it contributes to the amount of alcohol consumed. There is no reason to believe, however, that illicit sources have increased or diminished in recent years and have significantly affected the trend of consumption from licit sources. But because of the presence of illicit sources the statistics for consumption supplied are minimal estimates.

Offenses of Drunkenness

The police do not regard offenses of drunkenness as a significant problem in the community and do not usually categorize them separately from other types of crime. Enquiry showed, however, that crimes of drunkenness constitute only a small proportion of total crime. The number of cases reported for such offenses in 1968 and 1969 was 1.75 percent of all arrests. This compares with a figure of 45 percent for the United States in 1965 for arrests for such offenses (Nat. Inst. of Mental Health 1969). Although many factors other than prevalence of alcoholism must influence police arrests such as the strength of the police force and its policy concerning arrests, nevertheless the figures taken together with other available evidence reinforce the assumption of a low prevalence of alcoholism in the community. An alternative possibility is that the Chinese when intoxicated refrain from disorderly behavior in public and avoid getting arrested.

Possible Reasons for the Low Rate of Alcoholism

There is no wholly satisfactory explanation for the low rate of alcoholism and the question lends itself to extensive speculation. Amid the gamut of assumptions concerning the role and interplay of social, cultural, psychological, economic, and biogenetic factors that cause or prevent alcoholism we may single out for special mention the traditional Chinese sociocultural structure, informed by Confucian philosophy, which proscribes excesses, teaches propriety in interpersonal behavior, and stresses intellectual control rather than emotional display. Such teachings have engendered strong disapproval of intoxication, especially in public, and may be an important factor in the prevention of alcoholism. Other probably significant factors are the restriction of drinking to meals, with possible physiological and psychological implications, and the absence of strong ambivalent feelings about drinking.

It may also be mentioned that the Chinese do not have drinking-centered institutions and groups which enable one to drink regularly and frequently to the point of intoxication or maintain blood levels at heights great enough and long enough to develop alcoholism. Public drinking houses and taverns are conspicuous by their absence. In Hong Kong, under Western influence, bars have appeared but these are patronized almost entirely by Westerners. Nor does liquor play an important role in social gatherings at home or other than at banquets which are relatively few and far between. Tea and not alcohol is served to visitors. People are not asked to drop in for a drink and evenings with friends at home are not spent in drinking. It would thus appear that ample cultural and sociological grounds exist to explain the "low susceptibility" of the Chinese to alcoholism though a genetic explanation can still not be ruled out.

The Chinese Alcoholic

The following is an account of the Chinese alcoholic derived from alcoholics with psychosis admitted to a psychiatric hospital in Hong Kong. They are not necessarily representative of the alcoholic population of Hong Kong as a whole.

The Chinese alcoholic is far more likely to be a male than a female. He would be in his fifth decade on admission, belong to the lower social classes, have little education, and be somewhat superstitious in outlook and general beliefs. He probably started drinking in his third decade taking wine regularly at meals three times a day with his family. Later he would also drink alone and between meals. Under these conditions he would have a fairly constant low concentration of alcohol in the blood which would cause minimal visible symptoms. On the other hand he would develop tolerance and tend to consume larger quantities. He would usually be able to control the quantity consumed but be unable to abstain for a single day. He would refrain from drinking excessively in social gatherings or at work and be able to keep his job. He would rarely get severely intoxicated and in view of the apparent lack of any indication of his addictive status he would be taken by surprise at the first occurrence of a physical or mental complication of his alcoholism. Although it is a matter of common observation that the Chinese drinker rarely gets violent when intoxicated, many of the alcoholics admitted to a psychiatric hospital have a history of violence associated with drunkenness.

The main reasons the Chinese alcoholic would give for drinking would be hedonistic and social. Secondary reasons would be to relieve physical and mental exhaustion. He would regard the habit as masculine. He would not appear to belong to any clear-cut prealcoholic personality type or show marked psychological or psychiatric deviation. Some psychological vulnerability may however be assumed and it cannot be overlooked that alcohol brightens his usually dull and often impoverished existence. He would be unlikely to have experimented with sedatives or narcotics though he would have a higher likelihood of having done so than the general population. He would regard narcotic consumption as grossly immoral and with highly detrimental effects on the physical and mental condition. This is a picture of the usual and traditional type of Chinese alcoholic. He resembles the French wine drinker. The modern Chinese drinker belongs to a smaller but steadily enlarging group. He consumes Western beverages and belongs to the upper social classes. Probably an increasing proportion in this group is composed of younger people and women.

The Narcotic versus the Alcohol Problem

In contrast to alcoholism narcotic consumption is a major problem in Hong Kong. This conforms to the pattern in other Asian countries and is the reverse of that in the West. Various formulations have been advanced to account for this inverse relationship. These are usually based on generalizations which derive drinking and drug taking from the psychic needs of the individual. It has been asserted, for example, that the high prevalence of narcotic consumption in the East is due to cultural sanction of the passive and peaceful traits they enhance (Wikler and Rasor 1953). Similarly the high prevalence of alcoholism in the West is accounted for by cultural sanction of active and aggressive traits promoted by alcohol. The increasing prevalence of drinking in Hong Kong with westernization is consistent with the hypothesis. Nevertheless it has not been found that the East and the West do in fact sanction the traits mentioned to the exclusion of their opposites. If Chinese culture sanctions the passive and peaceful so does the Judeo-Christian as witness the eight beatitudes. On the other hand, activity, competitiveness, and success are as much sought after and promoted by the Chinese as by the Westerner.

More significant perhaps for the development of the narcotic-alcoholic prevalence pattern in Hong Kong are the historical events which have led to easy availability of narcotics for a prolonged period for large numbers of the population. Where a proportion of the population has a high degree of psychological vulnerability, given a situation where an addicting drug which provides a crutch is available, addiction will occur; and given a situation where two drugs are equally available, addiction to the more powerfully addicting drug will become a problem of the greater magnitude. Hong Kong for a considerable time after it was ceded to the British in 1841 served as a center for the opium trade both with China and towards the end of the nineteenth century with the United States. Opium was easily available and its consumption by a large proportion of the population became a practice sanctified by tradition. It would be strange indeed if such a situation failed to lead to a high prevalence of narcotic consumption. Periodic efforts at restrictions since the 1880s were made but its use went unabated. It was not till 1959 that stringent efforts were carried out to enforce the law against consumption.

The historical view does not preclude the relevance of personality factors in the genesis of the Eastern pattern of addiction. The existence of diverse assumptions and speculations in the literature regarding their role, even within the same race and culture, caution against generalizing about their significance.

Treatment and Legislation

Because alcoholism is not considered a major problem in Hong Kong no specific program exists for dealing with its prevention or treatment. Facilities for treatment and rehabilitation of cases have developed within existing government mental health services in its hospitals and outpatient clinics. These have been able to cope with the problem. Treatment in general hospitals is limited to withdrawal with little subsequent rehabilitation. The number treated by private practitioners is unknown but probably small. No legislation exists for compulsory commitment for treatment on grounds of alcoholism, except to a psychiatric hospital on grounds of mental disorder.

An Alcoholics Anonymous and an Al Anon family group meet once weekly. Members are mostly middle-class British, engaged in business or government-employed. Meetings are conducted in English and attended by a few Chinese bilinguals. There is need for such groups conducted in Chinese for the Chinese, as group therapy has been found useful in the rehabilitation of Chinese alcoholics admitted to a psychiatric hospital.

As regards legal control, alcoholic liquors are one of the few groups of imported commodities subject to duty in this free port. Duties are also levied on locally manufactured alcoholic beverages. The rate of duty is low ranging from U.S. $0.26 per gallon on Hong Kong brewed beer to U.S. $12 per gallon for liquors and spirits of non-Commonwealth origin. All firms engaged in import, export, and manufacture or sale of dutiable commodities must be licensed.

Premises serving alcohol are required to be licensed but are not limited in their service to any period of the day. Legislation, effective in February 1971, restricted the serving of liquors to and employment of those aged eighteen and above at these premises.

Conclusion and Summary

A common assumption from the literature is that the Chinese drink, often in large amounts, but rarely suffer from alcoholism. Such an assumption with its implications for etiology is based on an inadequate number of studies on small populations of expatriate Chinese and none on Chinese in their native setting. It was therefore thought useful to examine the drinking patterns and problems of alcohol in the Chinese people of Hong Kong.

The Chinese in Hong Kong traditionally drink at meals and banquets and not without food. Drinking is incidental to eating and drinking-centered institutions and groups are absent. The main aims of drinking are to promote conviviality and improve health. Moderate drinking is sanctioned on defined occasions, drunkenness especially in public strongly disapproved.

First admissions of alcoholic psychosis to a psychiatric hospital have risen steadily from 8.8 per million male adults in 1962 to 44.4 in 1970 and from 1.2 percent of total first admissions in 1962 to 6.1 percent in 1970. These figures suggest that (a) alcoholic psychosis and by implication alcoholism are not as rare in the Chinese as was formerly believed, and (b) there is a rising trend of these conditions in Hong Kong.

Consumption is calculated to be about 1.0 imperial gallon of absolute alcohol per adult (aged twenty or more) per year during 1963–69. Consumption of Chinese beverages is four times that of western in terms of alcoholic content. Trends in the consumption of Chinese and western beverages indicate that the traditional Chinese drinker who consumes Chinese wine at meals, belongs to the lower social classes, and resembles the French wine drinker, is gradually being replaced by the new type of westernized drinker who takes western beverages, usually spirits, and belongs to the upper classes. Probably an increasing proportion of the latter type is composed of younger people and women.

The greater magnitude of the narcotic as compared with the alcohol problem in Hong Kong, a pattern similar to that in other Asian countries and the reverse of that in the western, is regarded as due not so much to cultural characteristics as commonly supposed, but to the easy availability of narcotics. In Hong Kong opium smoking became widespread and traditional because this powerfully addicting drug was available to large numbers of people over a long period until recently. The eastern pattern of addiction can therefore be understood viewed from an historical perspective.

Treatment and legislation are on the whole adequate to cope with the problem. There is need for Alcoholics Anonymous and Al Anon family groups conducted in Chinese. The alcohol problem is at present not a major one. In view, however, of evidence suggesting a rising trend of alcoholic psychosis and by implication alcoholism in the years 1962–70, the situation needs to be kept under review.

VI. Africans and Alcohol

Alcohol as a Contributing Factor in Social Disorganization: The South African Bantu in the Nineteenth Century

Bertram Hutchinson

The knowledge and use of alcoholic beverages is common to many, if not to most, primitive societies, although their alcoholic content (and hence their physiological effect) varies widely. Their consumption, however, is invariably subject to certain social conventions equally diverse in their severity whose function is that of retaining within definite limits the degree of permissible intoxication and the liberty of behavior which is socially tolerated. These limits are normally determined, in a given society, by the light of the fundamentals of its organization, so that while advanced states of drunkenness may be tolerated, or in some circumstances even required, secular or religious offenses which might endanger social equilibrium are not generally excused merely on the grounds that the misconduct arose from the effects of alcohol.

The social control of the consumption of alcoholic beverages is first made effective at the personal level, control being manifested not only in the explicit sanctions which discourage drinking beyond what is socially approved but also, more significantly, in the subconscious restraints which society (by virtue of the values which the individual absorbs during childhood and youth) exercises tacitly. For although during alcoholic intoxication certain inhibitions of a more superficial nature may certainly be released, other forms of behavior remain inhibited—the nature of these ultimate prohibitions being to some extent common to all societies. In consequence, while the individual is more or less free to enjoy alcohol for the temporary euphoria which it offers him, yet society in normal circumstances is protected from the danger of disorganization which would otherwise follow uninhibited behavior, as it is also protected against the effective loss of its members following alcoholic addiction. But even within the setting of these restraints the consumption of alcohol, unlike the consumption of other narcotics such as betel, coca, and tobacco, is nevertheless not allowed to remain an entirely personal matter. Perhaps because the intoxicating effect of alcohol is more dangerous to society, "solitary" drinking in these societies is normally extremely rare: indeed, in most of them the drinking of alcoholic beverages is emphatically a group diversion.

Social control is therefore also manifested in the association of these beverages mainly with social, rather than individual, life. When alcohol is regarded as essentially a means of promoting conviviality, the principal setting for its consumption is found in formal and informal meetings of kinsmen and friends; and it is clear that companionable drinking facilitates society's exercise of control in ways that would be impossible if man drank alone. Moreover, this social interpretation of alcohol's function offers the not wholly secondary advantage that the use of alcohol can be recruited as a positive agent of social stability. Thus we find a third stage in the socialization of alcohol manifested in its association with secular and religious ceremonial. The symbolic use of alcoholic liquors with which we are familiar in the history of our own society, from the ritual libation of Hellenic religion to the rites of the Christian church and the drinking of toasts, is also widespread in primitive society. It is at this level that alcohol, in being linked to ritual, suffers the final metamorphosis, and from being a simple source of personal indulgence becomes a factor (albeit, perhaps, a minor one) in the maintenance of the social status quo.

These considerations, it must be added, are applicable only in conditions of social stability. Where this stability is lacking, as in periods of rapid acculturation, control of the use of alcohol, as of other forms of social control, is likely to become weakened. It is our purpose in this note to show how, among the Bantu tribes of Southern Africa, alcohol became a significant source of social disorganization, instead of being, as before, an aid to or a neutral factor in social cohesion.

The traditional importance of beer and beer drinking in Bantu culture is so familiar that it is unnecessary to make more than a general reference to it. Solitary drinking appears to have been extremely rare, although group and ritual consumption of beer took place frequently. Indeed, the convivial beer drink played a central part in the cementing of old and the creation of new friendships, and in reinforcing the ties which linked kinsmen together. Such everyday conviviality, while it had important social functions, had no ritual meaning. Nevertheless, the conduct of the beer drink was strictly regulated. Although brewing was itself a woman's task, women were excluded from beer drinks, or were permitted to take part only in such as were held separately from the men. The carrying of weapons was forbidden, and intoxication was not held to justify violent or offensive behavior, continued respect for age, status, and authority being insisted upon. The beer drink gave refinement to daily life, and a man anticipated with pleasure the opportunity which marriage would give him of offering this hospitality to his relatives and friends.

The importance of beer in the daily life of the community had its parallel on more formal occasions. Beer was offered, for example, as a recompense to members of work teams, to potential relatives-in-law at the conclusion of marriage arrangements, and on similar occasions. Ceremonies such as marriage or funeral feasts were scenes of abundance, their success being largely measured by the quantity and the strength of the beer offered to the guests. The investment of beer drinking with symbolic value is seen even more clearly, not only in its use as a form of tribute or taxation offered to the chief, but also in its ritual function in initiation ceremonies, harvest festivals, and religious propitiatory rites. At almost all times of its consumption, therefore, beer had a significance beyond that of mere personal indulgence, and Bantu traditional culture illustrated rather strikingly how alcohol may be made subservient to the strengthening, rather than the weakening, of group cohesion.

II

The coming of Europeans to southern Africa severely disturbed this equilibrium by changing the manner in which beer was produced and consumed, and by introducing wine and ardent spirits hitherto unknown to the Bantu people, and to whose unfamiliar potency they fell victim. There is little reason to doubt that the introduction of the new liquors was primary both in time and in the severity of its consequences for Bantu society. Nevertheless, these alcoholic beverages of European origin did not begin seriously to affect the Bantu tribes until the middle of the nineteenth century— or about two centuries after the first Europeans had settled in the Cape. On the other hand, by the beginning of the nineteenth century in the western Cape and elsewhere the colored population (that is, persons of mixed racial origin) were already suffering severely (e.g., Fawcett 1836). But while missionary reports from Bantu regions rarely mention the matter in the first half of the nineteenth century, we know that throughout this period European traders were introducing brandy, together with other less harmful trade goods, to the Bantu people (Hutchinson 1956). The missionaries themselves foresaw the consequences of this trade, and in an attempt to avert them established among the tribes during the years 1830–50 a number of trading stations where European goods, with the exception of alcoholic liquors, could be purchased by tribesmen who wanted them (Great Britain 1851; Hutchinson 1957). It is clear to us now that these attempts to isolate the Bantu people from a major and growing feature of the South African economy were almost certain to fail. For not only was the country, under European rule, producing yearly large quantities of both wine and distilled liquors, but these products, being of an extremely poor quality, were largely unmarketable in Europe. The Cape producers were consequently obliged to seek a means of disposing of their goods in the domestic market, small though this was. As a result, it became customary on many European farms by the middle of the century for laborers to be given as part of their wages "tots" of wine five or six times a day (cf. Walker 1957), and by 1885 a missionary from the Berea district of the Cape wrote, "The neighbouring farmers, who are the only employers of labour in the neighbourhood, produce a very cheap wine, which will hardly pay for carriage to Cape Town. They, therefore, endeavour to dispose of it in one way or another to our people, and are thankful for every penny gained by the sale of it, or are saved by giving it instead of tea or coffee to those who are at work for them. In these times of scarcity, the latter feel the need of something before they go out to the fields, and are often taken unawares by the effects of drinking on an empty stomach" (United Brethren 1885:583).

Meanwhile, although the sale of European liquor within the reserves had been legally prohibited, widespread smuggling rapidly made this regulation ineffective. Brandy and other liquors were readily obtained from canteens set up on the boundaries of native areas, and many of the Bantu people, including women and children, not uncommonly traded profitably in this way (Cape of Good Hope, House of Assembly Papers 1883). In some parts of the country the results were disastrous. In the Tamacha district, it was reported, men, women, and children became "degraded and demoralised by their inordinate appetite for strong drink," and many died from the deleterious effects of alcohol, or committed criminal offenses which had their origin in drunkenness (Cape of Good Hope, *Blue Book* 1880:173). In the district in which the Moravian mission at Goshen, Kaffraria, was established drinking became "to a terrible extent a national vice among the whole tribe" (United Brethren 1885:67); and among the Tembu of the Wodehouse division in 1874 "a passion for intoxicating liquors (was) spreading slowly but surely . . . a large trade (being) illicitly carried on in the wildest and most abominable adulteration of Cape spirits" (Cape of Good Hope, *Blue Book* 1874, 1875, 1884).

There is little reason to doubt that these developments and

others like them fostered the social disorganization which other forces had already begun; and even the political organization of certain tribes was affected where the chief or the members of his council were frequently or, as happened among the Tembu, were habitually drunk. Speaking of conditions in this tribe in the year 1883, a European special magistrate stated in evidence to the Cape Native Laws and Customs Commission, "When I was in Emigrant Tembuland, where brandy was smuggled, I would sometimes send for the chief, and he would be drunk, and remain so for a week. When at last he came, he would be in a 'boozy' and muddled condition, his headmen being in the same condition. Wherever this fellow went he wanted brandy. The consequence was that nothing could be done in the location, where all depends upon the headmen" (Cape of Good Hope, House of Assembly Papers 1883:par. 5,096). In such circumstances the business of the tribe was necessarily brought to a standstill, for reasons which weakened if they did not entirely disable the prestige of the chieftainship. This disorder was naturally and increasingly reflected in personal behavior among the tribe generally. While it is true that some groups suffered more than others, nevertheless wherever the place of the traditionally regulated beer drink was taken by irregular drinking parties the conduct, especially the sexual conduct, of the participants became, in terms of the tribe's traditional values, quite outrageous. "Our wives go to the canteen and drink," complained one Bantu witness before the same commission. "They throw away their clothes and are naked. They are becoming lost to all sense of decency" (Cape of Good Hope, House of Assembly Papers 1883:pars. 4,322–24). Children were said to be learning to drink from their mothers. The desire for alcohol was sometimes so compelling that Bantu families sold all their assets in order to obtain it and, thus reduced to indigence, suffered further degradation when they were deserted by their menfolk who were obliged subsequently to seek paid employment in the cities. In 1893 there were in Victoria West considerable numbers of both men and women living in conditions of extreme poverty and degradation which a missionary witness before the Cape Labor Commission attributed, perhaps with some pardonable exaggeration, to the prevalence of drunkenness among them (Cape of Good Hope, House of Assembly Papers 1894).

How widespread such conditions were in the rural areas of the country is difficult to discover. There is no doubt, on the other hand, that matters eventually reached such a critical stage that there arose among the Bantu people themselves an opposition to the unregulated supply of the new beverages that became increasingly articulate, especially among the older generation. Bantu witnesses before the Native Laws and Customs Commission of 1883 were unanimous in their desire to see canteen owners expelled from native areas. Even tribesmen who were themselves eager to obtain alcohol were sometimes aware of its undesirable consequences and were ready to support some form of government control (Cape of Good Hope, House of Assembly Papers 1883). A group of tribal councillors thought it necessary to ask a missionary to urge in the appropriate quarters the desirability of some form of control of the sale of brandy in the native reserves because "they did not wish to drink in the presence of their wives and children." Men who wished to drink, they added, could ride to the nearest town—a procedure which, they foresaw, would have the dual advantage of isolating their womenfolk from the new liquors, and of preventing men appearing drunk in the tribal setting (Cape of Good Hope, House of Assembly Papers 1883). Indeed, it appears that in some districts (as in the King Williams Town division in 1875) a temporary diminution in the incidence of drunkenness occurred through the force of Bantu public opinion alone (Cape of Good Hope, *Blue Book* 1875).

But for a number of reasons it proved difficult for the administration to put such controls into operation, however desirable they appeared in theory. The South African wine-producing interests especially were opposed to control, for as we have seen the cheap supply of wine and spirits to canteens and the free issue of wine to native laborers was a convenient means of disposing of their surplus produce for which they found no market abroad. If prohibition were introduced, said one wine farmer in evidence to the Cape Labor Commission, "then you can take a pick-axe and commence uprooting vines" (Cape of Good Hope, Labour Commission 1893). Moreover, in the conditions existing in South Africa during the nineteenth century any control was easily evaded, for demand was heavy and the sources of supply very numerous. The prospect of greater and more accessible supplies of liquor was, indeed, an incentive which drew many young Bantu tribesmen away to the cities and the minefields: by 1876 there was a large African population living in the vicinity of the Kimberley diamond fields because liquor as well as employment could be easily obtained in the locality (Great Britain, Parliamentary Papers 1876). In Port Elizabeth a few years later weekend "orgies" had become customary among the Bantu population living there, and at such times "nude, drunken, frantic Kafirs fight, yell and franti-

cally gesticulate until the scene is disgraceful in the extreme"
(Cape of Good Hope, Select Committee 1883:par. 144). And although in this city the authorities subsequently undertook the
control of all alcoholic liquor, the result appears to have been
negligible: ten years later, in 1893, the resident magistrate there
described conditions among Bantu migrants in the following
terms. The Bantu migrants, he said in evidence, "mix Kaffir beer
with honey, and then it is more maddening than brandy. I think it
drives them mad. You know what they are when in that state.
They will think nothing of four or five of them beating one to
death. I had a case of six setting on one man. They did not kill, but
injured him. . . . Out of seventy inquests held last year (1892),
thirty were from drink, and one was directly killed by it. The
deceased drank off a breakfast cup of brandy and fell down dead. I
suppose the brandy was adulterated so we could not touch it.
They put tobacco and bluestone into it. The Kaffir does not like it
if it is not adulterated and does not cut like a saw all the way down
his throat" (Cape of Good Hope, House of Assembly Papers 1894:
pars. 20,800–20,805).

It was also reported during the same period that in Cape
Town workers leaving home in a chilly dawn went first to the
canteens for a glass of brandy. Many remained there for the rest of
the day and at last emerged intoxicated. The loss of labor resulting
from this habit became so great that European employers sought a
legal restriction on canteen opening hours in the hope that absenteeism might be thereby reduced (Cape of Good Hope, Labour
Comm. 1893).

The Boer War at the turn of the century appears to have
brought about a temporary decrease in the incidence of drunkenness among migrant Bantu, but with the return of peace former
habits were resumed. Local administrative officers making their
annual reports (later published in the Cape of Good Hope *Blue
Book on Native Affairs,* 1904) once more strongly urged the need
for new legislation to check African consumption of alcoholic liquor. A Liquor Licensing Act was already in existence by this
time, but it had been only moderately successful even in the limited localities where it had been applied. The loopholes in the
legislation were such that an African who resided in a "restricted"
area could obtain unlimited supplies of liquor from adjoining districts where the sale was unrestricted. In the Cape registered
voters, being specifically exempted from the provisions of the Licensing Act, served as middlemen supplying liquor to the African
population (Cape of Good Hope, *Blue Book* 1904).

Such attempts to control the liquor traffic, however, did much to undermine the status of the relatively harmless traditional beer drink among both rural and urban Bantu. In the European farming areas where many Bantu were employed the beer drink, often regarded by the whites as "nothing less than a drinking bout" (Cape of Good Hope, *Blue Book* 1903:11), was censured as it had been in the cities largely because it interfered with a reliable supply of labor. While it proved a difficult matter to control directly a custom so deeply embedded in the traditional life of the Bantu people, other factors (such as the persistent tendency for Europeans to confuse the regulated traditional beer drink with the disorderly drinking of liquors of European origin) were leading to the same conclusion. Although, as we know, the brewing of beer was traditionally a family matter, by the end of the nineteenth century shopkeepers were selling ready-prepared sprouted or malted grain for brewing, and in so doing began a process which ultimately brought about the separation of brewing from the domestic setting it had hitherto occupied. Hence, by 1908 commercial beer drinks were organized, which "guests" could attend on the payment of a fixed sum (Cape of Good Hope, *Report on Natives* 1908). In this way the beer drink changed its character from a convivial meeting of relatives and friends to a heterogeneous gathering of people who had in common perhaps only a liking for beer and the ability to pay for it. Personal behavior at such meetings was not easily controlled since, having paid to come, everybody present sought his money's worth in beer and enjoyment. In Natal the commercial beer drink was the setting in which the old traditional ways of regulating sexual behavior were defied, for, although beer drinks were not formerly attended by both sexes together, it rapidly became common for young men and women to spend their evenings together drinking beer in a hut from which older people were excluded (Natal 1909). By 1914 such parties had become commonly noisy and violent since (again contrary to tradition) weapons were now taken to these diversions, fighting occurred, women and girls were assaulted. A Bantu councillor from the Transkeian territories describing these meetings said, "Nowadays, when a man went to a beer-drink . . . he took his sticks with him. A spectator at a beer-drink would probably observe the young men standing in groups here and there, and perhaps a little distance apart there would be a young fellow and a girl. If these young men in the group observed that the girl was in love with the young fellow, they would pick a quarrel with (him), and then a fight would follow. There were some people who dispersed their beer-drinks at sunset, but evils occurred in the dark, for some one would start a disturbance and everybody would join in and there would be quite an affray" (Transkeian Territories Gen. Council 1914:109). But while such developments as these were becoming widespread, in many tribes social control still remained sufficiently potent to prevent the most violent outbreaks of drunkenness and the irregular behavior which accompanied them. It was in the cities and the mining compounds that the effects of liquor were most profound, and towards which the various efforts at legal control were chiefly directed.

In 1897 the Transvaal Mining Industry Commission sent to South African mining companies a questionnaire on labor conditions and related matters. Of the seventy-four mine managers from whom replies were received, all stated that alcoholic liquor continued to be sold to their Bantu employees despite the legislation designed to prevent it. Moreover, added a majority, the deleterious effects of this trade were such that for considerable periods many of their workers were incapable of carrying out their functions (Transvaal, Mining Ind. Comm. 1897). Eating houses and trading establishments made a large part of their profit from the sale of liquor. It was stated in evidence that of the ten such establishments existing in 1897 on the boundaries of the East Rand Proprietary Mines alone, all depended so heavily on the liquor trade that its prohibition would force them to close down (Transvaal, Mining Ind. Comm. 1897). In 1899 from 12 to 14 percent of the African employees in the Crown Reef compound in Johannesburg were said to be absent because of intoxication, and the "number quite drink sodden was very great" (Great Britain, Parliamentary Papers 1904). The general manager of another mine on the Witwatersrand, describing conditions there during the weekends, said, "On Sunday night our compound was a simple hell, to put it even mildly. Liquor was being sold all over the place yesterday. Hundreds of boys could be seen sitting and drinking in groups everywhere. Two police were once seen and nothing was attempted by them in any way. The whole thing ended in a serious row in the compound, and the compound police were badly mauled" (Transvaal Chamber of Mines 1898:135). On the diamond diggings the situation was similar. In 1898 there were in the Barkly West division thirty-five canteens whose sales of alcoholic liquor to Bantu migrants were such, according to the civil commissioner, as to reduce them to "drink-sodden, hopeless wrecks of humanity" (Cape of Good Hope, *Blue Book* 1898:13).

The degree to which the liquor traffic rapidly became associated with prostitution is noteworthy, for this association had significant consequences for the traditional forms of Bantu social organization. In the mine compounds themselves the problem was largely avoided by a total prohibition of women within the areas reserved for male Bantu workers. Elsewhere, however, such restrictions did not apply, with the result that during and after the last quarter of the nineteenth century prostitution became a normal accompaniment in the cities and the labor centers to the provision of liquor. Many mineworkers, at the expiration of their contract, no longer returned to their families in the rural areas, but preferred to stay in a beer-house in the company of a temporary concubine. A similar position was noted in Natal, where men returning from working in the mines were "speedily relieved of their earnings, and, after an orgy of a week or ten days' duration, re-engage themselves for another term of service and go off without even visiting their homes" (Natal 1909). In the city of Durban itself a system of temporary "five-day passes" for Bantu women was established, officially in order that they might visit their relatives in the city, but rapidly modified by the women as a convenient means of bringing beer into the urban area. During the year 1907 some forty thousand women came into Durban in this way, and many of them remained there as prostitutes or concubines as long as they escaped detection. Describing the conditions in which these women lived in his evidence to the Transvaal Liquor Commission of 1910, the Durban chief magistrate said, "in the majority of cases they lodged under all sorts of unfavourable conditions, in 'risksha sheds, back kitchens, compounds and the like, under no adequate control. During the time they were in the town they were provided by their male relatives and others with all kinds of luxuries, meat, sweets, sugar, etc. The demoralization of the women and girls was going on at a very great pace; the allurements of the town also were so great that as soon as a fresh brew could be made, women would come back again under any pretext that could be invented, and, in many cases, this resulted in women staying in town altogether and taking to a loose life" (Transvaal, Liquor Comm. 1910). There is also other evidence that throughout South Africa at this time indigent Europeans played a large part in the illicit liquor trade, employing European women and children as agents—the white women not uncommonly being prostitutes with a clientele among the African population (Union of S. Africa, Comm. of Assaults on Women 1913).

Some ten years after the interval of the First World War the general position had changed very little, the unpublished evidence of the Native Economic Commission (1932) and the conclusions of the South African Institute of Race Relations leaving little doubt that prostitution continued to be closely allied with the liquor traffic. In a study made at the same period in the Rooiyard slums of Johannesburg, Ellen Hellmann comments, "The Native beer customer after drinking his fill, will make advances to the women around him; nor will he fail to find a woman who, for 2/6, will accede to his request" (1934:58). Indeed, this writer continues, many single Africans or those whose wives remained in the country formed temporary alliances with these women: widows, deserted wives, young girls, tired of working, or the merely dissolute who, married or single, earned a livelihood passing from one man to another as circumstances dictated. To facilitate the provision of liquor in combination with prostitution commercial dance halls were established (*Illicit Liquor Problem* 1935). Children and adolescents drank heavily at location entertainments, as at other times, and it became not uncommon for pupils to come to school in a state of semi-intoxication (*Illicit Liquor Problem* 1935); while teachers themselves were known to drink excessively and to be intoxicated in class (Hellmann 1940).

In an attempt to bring order into the liquor trade among the African population many local urban authorities established municipal beer-halls, where the brewing and sale of beer took place under close supervision. Administratively this system had some success, although Africans themselves objected to it on the grounds that the beer was expensive and that the amenities of the halls were so limited that to go there was like "drinking in a cage" (Union of S. Africa, Ec. Comm. 1932:par. 761). Moreover, private brewing still went on, even though illegal, and Monica Hunter (1936) states that in the thirties in an East London location she observed brewing taking place in a large number of homes in preparation for weekend festivities. But in place of the atmosphere of convivial relaxation which traditionally had surrounded the consumption of beer, the need for secrecy now drove men to solitary drinking, or to drinking with one or two friends, in a closed room or secluded backyard. Beer was now rarely provided free. Indeed, beer brewing had come to be regarded as a means of augmenting a family income, or of providing economic independence for single, widowed, and deserted women (Hellmann 1934).

Meanwhile the liquor laws became one of the principal causes of criminal offense in South Africa. The number of persons, African and European, convicted of liquor offenses in the Union rose from about ten thousand in 1913 to nearly eighty-three thousand in 1936 (Union of S. Africa *Official Yearbooks* n.d.). Of these offenses the majority occurred in the cities, especially on the Witwatersrand (which alone accounted for 81 percent of all liquor offenses in 1935) and drunkenness was significantly more common among the African population there than in other urban areas. Intoxication was frequently followed by violence, the incidence of physical assault growing as the cities themselves expanded. "Johannesburg is a place for business: that is why you see people killing one another," an African councillor from the Transkei remarked with some bitterness (Transkei 1935:176). And in the general dissolution of traditional standards of behavior among the Bantu living in the cities, it was not difficult for the police to find Africans ready to be employed as informers on their fellows; and these informers themselves, as they became known to the suppliers and consumers of liquor and hence no longer of use to the police, drifted into crime. The liquor traffic, it may be said, together with the often brutal police activity which accompanied it (Union of S. Africa, Police Comm. 1937), brought or helped to bring the new system of European law into contempt among the Bantu people. Lawbreakers were shielded, crime continued, and with final and perhaps unconscious irony beer resumed its ritual function—as thanksgiving offering after release from prison (M. Hunter 1936).

III

We suggested that the social control of personal behavior during the consumption of alcoholic liquors was exercised by society in three ways: through the subconscious inhibitions implanted in childhood; by the requirement that drinking take place in company and not alone; and by the linking of alcoholic beverages with ritual observances. In the traditional life of the Bantu people all three means of control were exercised. Moreover, since beer was the only alcoholic beverage with which they were familiar, to control its use was to control all the circumstances in which, traditionally, alcohol could be consumed. The advent of the Europeans weakened the old regulations that guided beer drinking, and led to the rapid introduction of novel drinks which it lay outside the competence of tradition to control.

A variety of other factors, not directly connected with alcohol, also weakened the traditional use of beer. These were factors which attacked the fundamental sources of authority in the tribe, and which consequently led to the disintegration of sectors of social organization which were far more crucial than the beer drink, although this suffered as well. Just as behavior in other sectors of social life was becoming increasingly individualized as the processes of culture-contact continued, so beer itself was gradually transformed into a means of merely personal enjoyment. The social dangers which former controls had sought to repel began to manifest themselves, in this new situation, in the form of personal violence, transgressions of the sexual code, and disregard of authority. Where this happened, social disorganization was accelerated.

But although the disruption of the traditional use of beer was important and widespread (although not universal), the events which followed the introduction of new European liquors were far more potent in their social effect. Because of their novelty these were neither associated with ritual nor with the group drinking which had been so characteristic a feature of Bantu life. Since these forms of control were lacking it followed that only one remained operative—that exercised by the inhibitions imposed in upbringing. Had Bantu society in other respects remained stable it is quite possible that the new liquors would have been brought under social control earlier by this means, and through their gradual adaptation to the other forms of regulation. Unfortunately, disequilibrium had been created already by other and more powerful factors, with the result that, especially among the Bantu urban and mining populations that grew up, the inhibitions traditionally imposed were severely weakened. The new liquors were therefore used as a means of personal indulgence, untrammelled by group or ritual associations, and decreasingly inhibited by values imparted in childhood. The conditions in which the liquors were obtained also did much to encourage their being looked upon as a matter of merely personal and individual concern. They were paid for from individual earnings, obtained through devious and often illegal means, and consumed either in isolation or in a group intent, not on conviviality, but on the personal enjoyment of its individual members, while the state of separation from tribal influences and of relative personal anonymity in which the urban Bantu lived left unchecked disorderly behavior which traditionally would not have been tolerated. Liquor, in becoming associated with unrestrained intoxication, followed by violence, theft, and imprisonment, and with prostitution, became a significant and positive factor in social disorganization, and not merely its symptom.

The European community in South Africa became aware, like any society, of the necessity of controlling the use of alcohol.

The control they sought to impose, however, attempted no more than to deny access to the new liquors—a shortsighted policy which ignored the equally important necessity of linking control with a general system of social values. Such a prohibition, since it did not emerge from the use of alcohol in a community or a ritual context, nor from a set of personal values, had little meaning for the Bantu. It was consequently evaded whenever possible, and the effective social regulation of the consumption of liquor was postponed until such time as a new value system more relevant to the changing social environment emerged from the Bantu people themselves.

Drinking and Attitudes toward Drinking in a Muslim Community

J. Midgley

The contributions of the anthropologist and sociologist to the scientific study of alcohol addiction have, in the main, been confined to cross-cultural comparisons. They have amassed a considerable amount of data not only on drinking patterns in preliterate societies, but on drinking and attitudes toward drinking in a number of ethnic and religious minorities in Western societies. Work on the Eskimo Aleuts (G. Berreman 1956) and the North American Salish Indians (Lemert 1958), for instance, has gone hand in hand with studies of Irish American (Bales 1962) and Jewish American (Snyder 1958) subcultural drinking patterns. Studies of modern Western societies such as Italy (Lolli et al. 1958) and France (Sadoun, Lolli, and Silverman 1965) as well as more comprehensive cross-cultural surveys have also been made (Child et al. 1965).

From these studies certain sociologically oriented theories have emerged. Horton's "level of anxiety" hypothesis (1943) and the current stress on the role of ambivalence (Ullman 1958) in group attitudes toward alcohol consumption are examples of the generalizations that have been derived from such comparative research. Although this work has been both extensive and of value to the core of systematic knowledge that has been built up over the years, it is deficient in certain aspects. Chafetz and Demone, in a review of the available cross-cultural evidence, experience something of this when they write: "When we come to our last nondrinking culture, the Moslem, we were surprised by the lack of published information available. . . . Moslem religion prohibits the use of wine and thus offers investigators a rich field of study, to date sadly neglected" (1962:97). They continue their survey with various snippets of information derived from a somewhat dated Indian medical journal, Bales's well-known crosscultural analysis, and *Time* magazine. Of these analyses they conclude: "Unfortunately these have to remain isolated observations and the material from stories and tales unchecked, for there does not exist for comparison any systematic study of the Moslem drinking patterns, similar to studies of Irish, Italians and Jewish" (1962:99).

It is indeed surprising that to date no research on drinking or attitudes in a Muslim society has been undertaken. That sociologists have not concerned themselves with the fact that five hundred million Muslims—one-sixth of the world's population (Gallagher 1968)—are prevented from taking alcohol by their religion seems a gross oversight.

In Islam the prohibition of alcohol is only one aspect of the religious taboo (*haraam*) on a number of foodstuffs and practices. These include eating pork or any meat not slaughtered by Islamic rite, gambling, the use of narcotics, and, of course, the consumption of alcoholic beverages.

Numerous references to haraam substances occur in the suras (chapters of books) of the Koran: for example, this text from *Sura Baqara:*

> They question thee about strong drink and games of chance. Say: In both is great sin, and [some] utility for men; but the sin of them is greater than their usefulness. [Pickthall 1953:52]

Although the religious prescription is clearly and unequivocably expressed in the Koran, the world's Muslims live not only in predominantly Muslim countries such as the Arab states, Turkey, Pakistan, Malaya, and Indonesia but in Western or Christian societies, where restrictions of this nature do not exist. To talk therefore of universal conformity to the Koranic injunction would, to say the least, be naive. Nor has prohibition always been enforced or historically observed.

It is partly as a response to this challenge that the present work has been written. It seeks to report on drinking and attitudes toward drink in a Muslim community in Cape Town and to serve, perhaps, as a stimulus for further, more extensive research in other Muslim societies.

The Muslims of Cape Town

Islam was introduced to southern Africa in 1667, some fifteen years after the Dutch, realizing the need for their ships to take on fresh supplies, established a refreshment station at what became known as the Cape of Good Hope. The refreshment station, however, soon became a colony. The Dutch East India Company granted land to a number of its servants known as the Free Burghers, who farmed on the outskirts of the settlement. In an attempt to compensate for the shortage of labor (clashes between the settlers and the indigenous Hottentot frequently occurred) the Dutch imported slaves, chiefly from Indonesia and Malaya. The first Muslim slaves arrived in 1667. Their numbers were further augmented through the introduction of the "free blacks," a group of Indonesian clerks, and other free servants of high-ranking Dutch officials. Yet others were exiles from Indonesia, rebels who for their subversive activities were permanently dispatched to foreign lands such as the Cape Colony. To this group of primarily Indonesian Muslims came others of the same faith—Arabs and Indian traders and Turkish coreligionists sent from the Ottoman Empire to consolidate the faith of the local Muslims.

From this handful the Muslim population of Cape Town has increased in size to number about seventy-five thousand today (Rep. of S. Africa 1966). The vast majority draw their ancestry from the slaves imported from Indonesia and Malaya by the colonial Dutch. In spite of much intermarriage they have retained their Islamic religion, although not, as many believe, their racial identity. They are nevertheless still locally known as the "Malays" or "Cape Malays" (Du Plessis 1944). A far smaller proportion of the Muslims of Cape Town came originally from India and Pakistan and unlike the Cape Malays, who have lost their original languages, still speak the Indian dialects (Brand 1968). They have also, generally, remained culturally distinct from the Malays. Since they form such a small proportion of the total Muslim population—about six thousand persons—they have not been included in the samples drawn for the purposes of this study.

For generations the Muslims have resided in tightly knit communities in the vicinity of their forty or so mosques, governed by strong community controls. In more recent years, through the natural expansion of the city, these areas have become overcrowded and some have moved to mass housing schemes more distant from the city center. Others have been compelled to leave their houses (and some of the traditional areas around the urban core) as a result of these having been reserved for white occupation in terms of South African race legislation.

Both groups of Muslims are orthodox Sunnis who have strictly observed the tenets of Islam. Many manage to go on the pilgrimage, the hadj, to Mecca, and some train in the Holy City or at the theological seminaries at Cairo or in Pakistan and return to serve the community as priests (imams). By means of *madressas*, afternoon religious classes conducted by the mosques, the children are further schooled in the rituals and principles of their faith. Although they are a minority group not only to the white but to the other nonwhite peoples of Cape Town, the Muslims have retained their identity in the face of Western and Christian influences.

The predominantly Christian population of the metropolitan area of Cape Town was just under eight hundred and six thousand at the time of the 1960 and the most recent census (Rep. of S. Africa 1966). This number included three hundred four thousand "whites" (the direct descendants of the European settlers), seventy-five thousand African or Bantu people, and a large group of mulatto Christians, known locally as the "Cape Colored."

Unlike the Muslims, the Cape Coloreds, who number about three hundred fifty thousand, have little community integration and less religious fervor. Because so many of their numbers have in recent years come to the city from the rural areas, there is widespread poverty among them and concomitant social conditions prevail. Overcrowding, higher crime rates than in any other population group, high infant mortality, and a severe alcoholism rate typify these conditions.

In a sample survey study of the prevalence of psychiatric disorder (Gillis 1968) and drinking among the Cape Colored people, Gillis, Lewis, and Slabbert (1965) found that 4.7 percent of five hundred respondents were "addicted to alcohol," that a further 3.6 percent were "preaddictive drinkers,"[1] and that only 21.1 percent of the men abstained.

The fact that the Cape as a wine-growing district produces many inexpensive wines that pervade the market contributes further to this problem, for the colored people are chiefly wine drinkers. That the Muslims have been generally able to resist the influences of both their drinking colored neighbors and fairly consistent advertising by the local manufacturers is largely attributable to their religion and the strong social controls in their community.

Thus, while the Muslims generally subscribe to the Islamic prohibition on the use of alcohol, we need to ask what methods or techniques they use to enforce such prohibitive attitudes. How have they managed to resist drink, so widespread among the people with whom they are in daily contact? What are their attitudes toward drink and other drinkers—particularly toward the heavy and addicted drinkers? These are the questions the study reported here sought to answer.

Method

It was decided to draw a sample of Muslim households and to interview equal numbers of men and women. For this purpose an interview schedule containing questions on drinking habits, personal data, and an attitude scale was devised.

The first part of the questionnaire made reference to drinking habits. Respondents were shown a card listing beverages such as tea, coffee, and soft drinks as well as beer, wine, and distilled spirits. They were asked which of these they drank and with what frequency. The interviewers, who were undergraduates in social work at the University of Cape Town, were carefully briefed before interviewing began and were instructed not to indicate that Muslims were being singled out for study.

The respondents were then asked which of these beverages they had tasted even if they did not drink them at all. They were also asked to say whether these beverages had a pleasant or unpleasant taste. All this was done so as to put the respondent at ease and not to give the initial impression that the interviewers were making a study of what for some might have been a "touchy" subject. The fact that drinking is an emotive topic for the orthodox Muslim and even to the less religious somewhat hampered our study. Not wishing to alienate any or to harm the goodwill encountered in the community, we proceeded to ask our questions with care and tact. Even more caution was required when interviewing those who admitted drinking, for not all expressed the confident attitude of one who blatantly violates norms he has actively rejected.

The respondents were also asked to say which of the beverages on the card were "good" to drink and which were "bad" to drink, and they were also asked (if it applied) to say why they did not drink alcoholic substances.

The second part of the interview schedule was a personal data questionnaire in which routine questions such as age, sex, marital status, education, and occupation were asked. Information about religious activities was obtained in the same way. Subjects were questioned on mosque attendance at madressa during childhood and on the religious affiliations of their best friends.

The interview schedule also contained an eleven-item Thurstone-type scale designed to measure the individual's attitude toward drinking. It included items (at the negative pole) such as "Drinking is a waste of time and money," and (at the positive pole) "Drinking serves a good purpose in the community." More to the center of the attitude continuum were items such as "I would not drink but do not object to others drinking." Respondents were shown a card on which the scale items, in large print, were clearly displayed and they were asked simply to indicate the items with which they agreed.

The scale was validated by correlating ratings, obtained by interview, of the attitudes of a group of 30 persons with their scores on the scale. A coefficient ($r=.72$) sufficiently high to allow the researchers to apply the scale to the population was found. When used in the survey, further support for the general validity of this scale was obtained. The difference between the mean scores of nondrinkers and drinkers ($t=5.9$) was found to be significant at $p<.01$ (n=106).

The questionnaire and scales were then applied to samples of Cape Malay Muslims in two selected areas where they were (a) found to predominate and (b) found to be in the minority.

The first area, called Bo-Kaap by the inhabitants (literally "above the Cape," since it is situated on the slopes of the mountain above the city center), is more commonly known, particularly among the whites, as the Malay Quarter. This term is applicable, for here the local Muslims have for generations maintained a family-centered and religiously orthodox existence. They are by far in the majority and there are at least six mosques in the area. Above all, a sense of community and other strong cohesive factors have preserved their identity and religion.

In the second area, a municipally owned housing resettlement scheme, the Muslims are outnumbered seven to one by the mulatto Christians. They have, however, built a mosque and have organized madressas and other religious activities. In this area the researchers were fortunate in having a comprehensive sampling frame at their disposal. The municipal authority which administers the estate has records of, for instance, the incomes, religious affiliations, and family sizes of their tenants and from such data sampling could be undertaken.

In all, a sample of 117 households was drawn. These were mostly of working-class background where the head was employed in a semiskilled or skilled job. In 59 cases a man in the household was interviewed and in 58, a woman.

Limitations of the Study

It would have been of interest to obtain information about the extent of intoxication, the reactions of family members and neighbors to drinking behavior, and about manifestations of feelings of guilt and anxiety on the part of any drinker. However, the strongly institutionalized taboo on alcohol use in the community makes it a difficult subject on which to undertake research and some of those who admitted drinking expressed anxiety when questioned about their drinking practices. Some were evasive and contradictory and since our interviewers were (due to lack of financial resources) volunteer undergraduate social work students, it was thought advisable to restrict the study to one of an epidemiological nature in which statistical correlates rather than a depth analysis of individual cases were sought.

In the light of the strong prohibitive attitudes toward alcohol in the community, it would also have proved interesting to analyze at greater depth the emotional and psychological problems of the drinking Muslim, but this could not be done with our resources.

Findings

The impression that the Cape Muslims generally adhere to their religious proscription on alcohol use was supported by our findings: 12 percent of those interviewed reported drinking. This is fairly consistent with previous findings.

Gillis, Lewis, and Slabbert (1965) included interviews with Malay Muslims residentially interspersed, as many are, among the colored people. Of the 94 Malays interviewed, 13 percent reported drinking, while 1 percent were diagnosed as "addictive drinkers." No further analysis was made. As Gillis, Lewis, and Slabbert point out, "Sampling was not done specifically in the Malay Quarter of Cape Town, all the Malay respondents being encountered in mixed or predominantly colored residential areas. It is possible that less drinking may occur amongst them where they live in their own communities, but this will need further investigation" (1965:62). The present findings are, thus, consistent with those of Gillis and his co-workers.

In an earlier study (Midgley 1967) of conformity and determinants of conformity to religious norms among the Cape Malay Muslims, I had examined the incidence of drinking in the group. The study was not designed specifically to investigate drinking patterns or to measure attitudes toward drink but, rather, to examine correlates of religious conformity. The findings relating to drinking behavior formed only a small incidental part of the main study. Nevertheless in a sample of 191 persons 10 percent reported drinking and those who drank were generally poor conformers to religious norms.

There are also historical records of beer drinking among Muslims of nineteenth-century Cape Town, although it is felt that these refer erroneously to the consumption of alcoholic beverages. The beer mentioned in these reports is in all probability nonalcoholic ginger beer still brewed today in many Muslim households (Du Plessis 1944).

The present study also sought correlates and factors which might offer insight into the breakdown of the community controls enforcing general prohibitive attitudes.

Factors Related to the Occurrence of Drinking

Of the 14 who reported drinking, 12 were regular drinkers (drinking at least once a week, usually on weekends); 4 were daily drinkers. The rest drank less frequently.

A further 11 indicated that they had "tasted" alcoholic beverages, mostly beer, out of curiosity. Thus, only 21 percent of the sample admitted some experience of alcohol. The study had, therefore, succeeded in isolating the drinkers—or at least those who admitted drinking. Applying the information obtained in the personal data questionnaire it was possible to seek correlates of drinking behavior—to isolate those factors which appear to be associated with drinking in a Muslim community.

The drinkers were all men. This was an expected finding, since women play a generally more submissive and a traditional housekeeping role and have, until recently, been comparatively isolated from potential sources of deviance—in this case, liquor advertising and contact with non-Muslims. There was, conversely, no discernible pattern of age. We had rather expected the occurrence of drinking to be more frequent among the younger age-groups who are by far the most exposed to secular non-Muslim forces in the community. No such pattern emerged. Drinking, it seems, is not widespread and when it occurs, it is found among all age-groups.

Similarly no educational or occupational patterns emerged. Practically all those interviewed were of lower working-class backgrounds with unskilled, semiskilled, or skilled blue-collar occupations. Within this group, however, no occupationally linked drinking pattern could be found.

There was, however, an interesting ecological relationship. Sampling, as was pointed out earlier, was undertaken in two areas: in the older established traditional Malay Quarter area and in the new housing resettlement scheme. Drinking was far more prevalent in the latter area and occurred with greater frequency than was expected. For the purposes of the chi-square test the sample was divided into the "drinkers" and the "nondrinkers," those who reported only having tasted alcohol being excluded: of the 14 drinkers, 2 lived in the Malay Quarter and 12 in the resettlement housing, compared with 49 and 43, respectively, of the nondrinkers (chi-square = 13.8, $p < .01$).

One factor that might be used to explain this finding is that the Muslims of the housing scheme are in the minority. In the old Malay Quarter they predominate. But it is surely not only a matter of numbers—the Muslims of the housing scheme are interspersed among the Christian majority while the residential arrangements in the quarter are such that a greater sense of "community" is possible. This homogeneity has much relevance for the learning of norms and their reinforcement.

Further, the constant religious activity in the quarter with its six mosques in a compacted area must have an effect on conformist behavior. People in the housing scheme being well spread out do not live in the shadow of the mosque, as it were.

The question of living in a predominantly Christian neighborhood led us to investigate the relevance of exposure to non-Muslim influences. If a person is exposed, at a personal friendship level, to people who drink, does this influence his attitudes and behavior? A relationship between having intimate Christian friends and the occurrence of drinking was found: 9 of the 14 drinkers and 14 of the 92 nondrinkers had Christian friends (chi square = 25.6, $p < .01$).

An important facet of the upbringing of the Muslim child is his attendance at the madressa or Muslim religious school. In Cape Town, Muslim children attend secular schools with their Christian counterparts and then in the afternoons spend a further hour or two at the madressas which are usually held at the mosques. There they learn the elements of Arabic, the basic tenets of their faith, and to recite the Koran. Usually the Muslim child begins to attend the madressa at about the age of six and will continue to do so until he attains adult status. Many, however, continue to attend the evening classes for working adults. The role of the madressa in shaping and reinforcing attitudes is a powerful one, especially when operating over a period of ten to fifteen years. Quite a number of those interviewed indicated that they had been attending for periods of twenty years or more.

As expected, the madressa plays an important role when it comes to alcohol use. The drinkers were generally poor madressa attenders. The mean number of years attended by the drinkers (about 5) and the nondrinkers (about 10) were significantly different ($t=3.09$, $p<.01$).

Similarly the drinkers were poor mosque attenders: among those whose mosque attendance was known, only 1 of 10 drinkers attended weekly, compared with 17 of 23 nondrinking men (chi square = 15.74, $p<.01$). It is not customary for Malay women to attend mosque except on some of the holy days, and regular mosque attendance is therefore an essentially male characteristic.

Attitudes toward Drinking

On the attitude scale, the possible scores ranged from a minimum of 10 (strongly negative and unfavorable) to 100 units (strongly favorable). The nondrinkers scored a mean of 37.6 units, demonstrating a generally unfavorable attitude toward drinking. A low standard deviation of 6.6 units showed that the attitudes of the nondrinkers clustered fairly tightly about their mean score. The drinkers had a more favorable attitude: 67.5 units.

We also administered the scale to a group of 42 colored people at a religious service and found a mean score of 50.3 units—generally neutral in terms of the attitude scale continuum. Their standard deviation, however, showed that there was far less consensus about their attitude as a group than among the Muslims.

Our initial impression that the Muslims of the Cape have a generally unfavorable attitude toward drink was thus supported. In spite of living in a Western drinking culture, in the close vicinity of the country's wine-growing districts, the Muslims have retained their religiously derived negative attitude.

Attempts to find correlates of this attitude were not very successful. There was little spread along the attitude continuum. Using various measures of association, no significant relationship between attitude scores and age, sex, place of residence, and even friendship patterns could be found. The only factor that correlated significantly, and negatively, with attitude toward drink was length of madressa attendance. Those persons who had experienced less secondary socialization through the madressa system, those who had had less opportunity to learn the norms and have them reinforced, were less likely to express rigidly negative attitudes toward drinking. Correlating attitude scale scores and number of years of madressa attendance, a coefficient of $-.34$ $(p<.01)$ was found.

Note

1. Noting that alcoholism research was hampered by lack of a formal definition of these terms, Gillis et al. devised an operational definition based on answers given to a validated questionnaire on drinking habits and symptoms of alcoholism. The questionnaire was satisfactorily pretested on a known group of forty-four alcoholics at, for instance, a hospital for alcoholics and a state alcoholic rehabilitation center.

Beer as a Locus of Value among the West African Kofyar
Robert McC. Netting

Introduction

The recent growth of interest among anthropologists in primitive drinking has been expressed in accounts of single societies, the assembly and classification of cross-cultural data, and the statistical treatment of such information in order to test hypotheses. Investigators characteristically note the interaction of psychological and cultural variables (Washburne 1961) in analyzing the behavioral effects of alcohol. There has, however, been some tendency to revise earlier formulations relating the degree of drunkenness in a society to the level of anxiety or fear among individual members (Horton 1943) in favor of explanations based on the correlation of sobriety with corporate or formal social organization (Field 1962). The field studies of Sangree (1962) and Heath (1958) stress the functional networks in which alcohol is involved and the social norms and sanctions which condition the responses of individuals in the drinking situation. Less emphasis is placed on the release of aggressive and sexual responses than on the positive aspects of facilitating rapport and social solidarity. It has been suggested that in societies where drinking is an integral part of the culture and only minimally a response to the needs of the individual, the rate of alcoholism will be low (Simmons 1960). I propose to examine a case in which drinking customs are not only well established and consistent with the rest of the culture but in which the alcoholic beverage has become a focus of group interest and the center of a highly ramified functional network. To the extent to which the social values of drinking have proliferated, the potentially disruptive types of behavior have been channeled and controlled. Not only is alcohol addiction absent but the social and personal costs of drunkenness have been significantly limited; there is no drinking problem.

The Kofyar

The Kofyar are sedentary subsistence farmers occupying a territory of some two hundred square miles of hills and plain fringes along the southern escarpment of the Jos Plateau in northern Nigeria. They are one of the numerous isolated peoples known collectively as hill pagans (Gunn 1953). The Kofyar have little political centralization and do not claim a tribal identity beyond village areas such as Mirriam, Dimmuk, and Kwalla (Ames 1934). They are organized in localized patrilineal lineages with virilocal residence. Compounds inhabited typically by single elementary families are dispersed, each surrounded by its own intensively cultivated farm of sorghum, millet, and beans. The Kofyar received only minor influences from the Jukun empire and were never brought under Hausa-Fulani domination. European contact began in 1909 and sections of the hills were not brought under effective control until the 1930s. In recent years, missions and schools have been established in the plain villages along with markets serviced by dry season roads. Though farming is now being expanded to include cash crops, the Kofyar are still largely self-sufficient and lacking in occupational specialization.

The Role of Beer in the Functional Network

The Kofyar make, drink, talk, and think about beer. It is a focus of cultural concern and activity in much the same way as are cows in African pastoral societies. I shall review the complex of Kofyar cultural elements which are integrated around beer and offer some suggestions on the development of values ascribed to it. The cultural emphasis on beer and the lack of negative associations with drinking will be related to the nature of the beverage and to the social sanctions surrounding its use.

    If we choose to regard social relationships as a series of flows, both material and symbolic, from one individual to another, we can see the overt manifestation and acknowledgment of the most important of these flows among the Kofyar in the giving of beer. Among equals, the presenting of beer is a mark of esteem and affection. A jar will be saved for a close friend, and institutionalized friendship among male contemporaries is by means of a named drinking society. Beer is given during courtship by a man to a woman, and the public exchange of beer is typical of lovers in the licit extramarital relationship. Friends or lovers frequently drink together simultaneously from the same calabash. Occasions which involve the entire community are difficult to imagine apart from beer. To celebrate the harvest, beer is made by individuals or by popular subscription and distributed freely. It is, as they say, "just for drinking," and it signifies village satisfaction at the successful completion of the farming year. Major entertainment dances such as the great flute chorus, *koem*, require a large supply of beer. A man who exemplifies the warrior virtues by killing an enemy or bringing down dangerous game on the hunt is honored by a beer feast and the coveted right to drink from a special reserved fermenting jar at funerals for the rest of his life.

Socially valued roles may be singled out by a present of beer. A newly married man or one who has just paid his taxes is entitled to a jar from whomever brews that day. A nursing mother is entitled to take extra beer home with her in a gourd bottle. The even more important political and magico-religious functions of the chief and the diviner merit permanent recognition. Whoever brews beer to sell must set aside a portion, called *mwos miskagam*, the beer of the chief, for the village head. Even when a traditional chief has been deposed as official government representative and tax collector, he insists on maintaining his prerogatives in regard to beer. Following British conquest, a major source of friction on the local level has been the disputes between government chiefs who claim beer as a reward for administrative labors and hereditary priest-chiefs who say that their knowledge of certain ceremonies intimately connected with the earth entitles them to the traditional tribute. One version of the events leading to tribal war and the killing of an assistant district officer in 1930 was that a quarrel arose between the government messenger and the headman over rights to the chiefly beer. Today the outstanding evidence of intravillage factionalism and failure of political cohesion is the decision by a clan segment to withhold its accustomed gift of beer to the chief. Diviners, that is, men whose special knowledge of oracles has been validated by a large beer feast, are also given beer wherever they go.

The Kofyar not only award beer to those who perform important civic services, but they also exact it from those who break social rules. The fine for not taking part in communal work, threatened violence, disrespect for a fellow clansman, abuse, or minor theft is beer. The most severe punishment meted out to a man by his community is exclusion from all occasions for beer drinking. It is the equivalent of social ostracism. Beer flows thus define both the socially valued and the socially censured roles.

In economic situations, beer is the most widely used reciprocal for services. Part of the bride-prices and later supplementary gifts to the bride's relatives may be in beer. The majority of all voluntary labor is repaid in beer. Hoeing and harvesting, stone corral building, the preparation of building mud, and the gathering of thatching grass are all occasions on which a beer party can mobilize large work groups without reference to kinship or neighborhood affiliation. Though rights in land are concentrated on the individual, a system of leases allows redistribution of arable soil according to need. Rent is invariably paid partly in beer. With the current shift to cash cropping and extensive migrant cultivation in a newly opened area, the beer party makes possible cooperation on a large scale among strangers. The fact that no cash is required is of definite advantage to the beginning farmer. Brewing is also a major source of ready cash. A man can get tax money or a woman buy cloth and animals by making beer and selling it, a process which requires only six days. Even if grain must be bought, there is a small but reasonably certain profit to be made. Unlike most agricultural enterprises, the value of labor devoted to brewing may thus be quickly extracted. Where brewing has recently become an organized business in the large compounds of certain chiefs, wives can support themselves and their children by the proceeds, plus forming a sizable labor pool for the chief's farming.

If "malt does more than Milton can/to justify God's ways to man," the Kofyar certainly believe that man's way to god is with beer in hand. Along with blood sacrifices, it is the invariable offering in curing rites, on magical shrines, and to the ancestors. Pains are taken to convince spirits that it is really beer and not gruel which they are receiving. It is blown and poured on the graves of lineage members, and in addition, jars are broken on completion of a grave cairn in the last of four traditional funerary ceremonies. The ancestors, both men and women, gain status in the afterworld by dispensing this beer. Large quantities are brewed by relatives of the dead for giving to both patri and matri kin at the time of the *maap* funeral rites. The village earth ceremonies which occur at irregular intervals to restore fertility and repair natural calamities revolve around the pouring of libations on the ground. The brew house is at the innermost extremity of the hut cluster and is regarded as the most sacred spot in the ancestral compound of each lineage. Any stealing from the brew house or quarreling in front of it could bring supernatural punishment and necessitate a costly cleansing rite. The circumlocution used in referring to harming someone by witchcraft is "to dig up the fermenting jar in the brew house and carry it off." Such desecration could not be imagined by normal people, just as they would not think of indulging in witchcraft.

This wealth of functional associations of beer is not rare as indicated by Washburne's (1961) summary descriptions of other African societies. Perhaps most striking among the Kofyar, however, is the unique conceptual position which beer occupies. When walking through a village, a large part of greetings and small talk concern the presence of beer, recent beer parties, or apologies for the absence of beer. The only words in the Kofyar language for short periods of time are based on the brewing cycle. A week of six days is *shimwos*, "the time of beer." Markets are scheduled to coincide with this time span. Each of the six days is named, and appointments are made in terms of them, e.g., "I will meet you on *Jim*" (the second day of malt grinding and thus five days from the present). Selfishness and magnanimity are almost always phrased in terms of withholding or giving beer to guests. Aggression, quarrels, and interpersonal hostility of all sorts appear at beer parties and ostensibly concern the preparation or sharing of the beer. Folklore is full of references to beer: a spurned hare gets revenge by pushing a woman into boiling beer; a greedy bird tries to steal extra grain for brewing and is caught; God is an important farmer who gives beer in exchange for labor and dispenses it at councils. The culture hero fixed the site of some hill villages by stopping at each to brew, and on the top of the highest peak in the country he left behind a great fermenting jar.

Beer is both the symbol and the essence of the good life to the Kofyar. A hot day when there is no beer ready and no brewing is expected for some time is an occasion for universal commiseration. Though the old days of feuding war were exciting, no story of them concludes without mention of the increased supplies of beer which people now have because of the larger farms possible during peace time. Though people use their new income from cash crops in part to buy bicycles and cloth and to pay bride-price, they always speak first of the migrant farms as a place where beer is cheap and abundant. Whereas the European folktale puts gold at the end of the rainbow, and Ali Baba finds jewels in a cave, the Kofyar story tells of Crownbird opening a magic ancestral stone and finding a jar of beer inside.

Benefits and Cost of Drinking

Why is it that beer is so rich in associations and takes part in such a wide variety of activities? Perhaps we may arrive at some tentative answers by examining the values which beer has for the individual and his society and the way in which the dysfunctional elements, the social costs which may accompany drinking, are systematically limited. Kofyar beer is tasty, nutritious, and only weakly alcoholic. The thick, frothy brew is preferred when fermentation has eliminated much of its original sweetness but not advanced to the point of making it sour. The flavor may be rendered more desirable by its contrast with the prevailing bland diet of cereal porridge. Certainly most grain farmers since prehistoric times have turned part of their production into a fermented drink. In one Kofyar village for which I have figures, an average of 83.5 pounds of millet is produced annually for each household member. Millet is seldom consumed except as beer, and the entire amount converted into beverage would yield just over forty gallons a year per person. Additional brewing is usually done with millet or sorghum purchased in the market.

There is little doubt that beer is a valuable addition to the local diet. The loss of energy resulting from the conversion of grain to beer is fairly small, and nutritionists speak about the "biological ennoblement" by which fermentation produces ascorbic acid, B-vitamins, and microbial proteins (Platt and Webb 1946; Platt 1955). When consumption of fruit and meat is irregular, these food values become especially important. The Kofyar regard their beer as a superior food.[1] They say that if there were enough beer, a man could live on nothing else, though I know of no local cases where this is actually done. On days when drink is plentiful, however, the evening meal is often omitted. Where beer is scarce as with some of the poorer hill villages adjoining Kofyar, porridge is given to work parties. The Kofyar themselves substitute beans and palm oil for beer in rewarding work parties of adolescent boys. Since Moslem and Protestant Christian converts do not drink for religious reasons, the Kofyar are quite aware that beer is not a physiological necessity, yet they attach an affective quality to beer that is not apparent in regard to other more basic foods.

Certainly the Kofyar value the mild euphoria, the sense of happy relaxation which accompanies drinking. Yet there appears to be no particular premium placed on increasing either the proportion of alcohol in the brew or the speed of its consumption. The alcohol content of the beer has not been measured, but I would estimate that it averages 3 to 5 percent. Judging from its effects on myself and others, it would seem rather less potent than the Tiriki brew described by Sangree (1962). Distilled liquor is as yet unknown in Kofyar, European beer is a luxury drink enjoyed at rare intervals by teachers and chiefs, and palm wine is only now being introduced. There are perceptible differences in beer strength in various parts of Kofyar, but, although the techniques of increasing alcohol content are known, they have not diffused. Women marrying into a village where beer is brewed more weakly adopt the local pattern regardless of their previous methods. The alcohol content does not appear to be the crucial determinant of beer's value. The Kofyar could probably get more alcohol into their bloodstreams if they increased the speed of drinking. At a drinking party, groups of five to eight people sit together in huts or in shaded spots and pour beer into calabashes from a jar holding about five quarts. The actual drinking may be quite rapid but there are often waits of an hour or more between jars. Regardless of whether the beverage is being sold or given away, it is doled out slowly. The guests have ample time for conversation and the host can conserve his supply in order to get the most social mileage out of it. Because of the wide distribution of beer and the size of the average brewing facilities, a single compound can usually make only enough for a single day, and drinking bouts extending through several days are rare. It is my impression that an adult drinks on the average of one to two quarts at a beer party. Though the frequency of opportunities for drinking varies according to season, I would estimate that Kofyar men have beer approximately twice a week while women and children who make fewer trips to market and other villages probably drink less than once a week. In one village of fifty-five compounds, there was an average of eleven brewings per month during ten months for which I have adequate records.

The individual satisfactions derived from drinking beer form the basis for its economic value. The announcement of brewing is always welcome; the demand for the finished product is uniformly high. Moreover, beer enters easily into an economic network. It may be carried to nearby markets to be sold. It is infinitely divisible, both in brewing when grain and workers may come from many households or a single one, and in consumption, where it may be sold in small or large quantities or shared in varying degrees. A jar bought by the usual group of five costs each participant twopence. In the relatively undifferentiated society of subsistence farmers, everyone has access to the materials and techniques necessary for brewing. Intensive terrace farming and manuring maintains high productivity so that almost every household has a supply of grain from which to make beer. Under these conditions, beer fits well into a society where the political hierarchy is rudimentary, differences in wealth are small, and the family unit is self-sufficient. The means of its production prevent any monopoly of brewing. It is marketable but cannot be stored for any length of time. Since beer is the preeminent sign of hospitality, wealthy men are expected to distribute it liberally to friends and guests. Beer is a completely consumable good, and used in this way, it prevents accumulation and acts as a leveler.

Besides meshing easily with the structure of traditional society, beer is proving adaptable to the changing needs of a new economy. It allows rapid conversion of agricultural produce or labor into cash. Within the local community, the price of beer is fixed by common agreement and sellers all charge the same amount for a jar of standard size. In the large, impersonal plains markets which are of recent origin, price varies according to the changing cost of raw materials and is arrived at by bargaining. As the cultivated area of Kofyar expands by addition of distant bush lands without change in tools or farming methods, the beer party proves to be a traditional and yet highly effective way for securing communal participation in agricultural work. It eliminates the need for wage labor at the early stages of cash cropping and gives the prospective entrepreneur an opportunity to raise small amounts of capital. Beer as a valued good is both compatible with the forms of an individualistic, egalitarian society and readily usable as a means for the achievement of economic objectives under the fluid conditions of social change.

Perhaps the most striking illustration of the encouraging of some effects of drinking while strictly sanctioning others is seen in group beer parties. The Kofyar value beer as a social lubricant, but not as an explosive. Drinking is understood to be a social act. An individual may have a jar hidden away in his own hut, but when he is ready to drink, he discreetly calls friends or family to share it with him. Drinking is not exclusive. Men and women mingle freely at the compound of beer and sit to drink in mixed groups. Children may be fed beer before they are weaned. The young probably do not consume as much as their elders, but this is due to their lack of money, their home duties, and their lesser participation in work parties rather than to any ambivalence about their right to drink or the effects of alcohol on them.

Approved behavior in the drinking group is that which heightens social interchange, and negatively sanctioned activities are those which threaten group cohesion. It is the drinking situation rather than the alcohol per se which affects individual behavior. For example, beer drinks are culturally defined as occasions on which people may talk with animation and freedom. The period when the group has assembled and before the brew has been passed out is characterized by desultory conversation and a general atmosphere of quiet expectancy. As the first calabashes go around, there is a spontaneous bubbling up of chatter and laughter. This takes place before many participants have even tasted the beer, and there is no later heightening of interchange as people begin actually to absorb some alcohol. The drinking of beer appears to be generally connected with increased activity, and such group enjoyments as singing and dancing cannot be imagined apart from it. The beer party also acts as a proper occasion for the discharge of interpersonal tensions in vociferous argument. Large and small areas of friction are exposed for public review and comment in an atmosphere that encourages emotional catharsis. Strict limits are, however, maintained by the practice of submitting quarrels to older men for arbitration and prohibiting physical violence. A clear line is drawn by the Kofyar between verbal aggression which may be expressed freely and potentially dangerous acts. An argument is immediately halted by bystanders if a man touches his knife or if a scuffle results in drawing blood, no matter how small the scratch. A series of later hearings fixes blame and decrees fines paid by the guilty party to the offended person and often to the entire group in whose presence the quarrel took place. There is never a suggestion that a man is not responsible for his behavior because he has been drinking. Again it happens that some of the fiercest arguments may occur at the place of beer before anyone has drunk.

The convivial atmosphere of the beer drink is certainly conducive to sexual approaches, and this is recognized by the Kofyar. As the situation is culturally defined, humorously bawdy talk, the use of a courting language based on innuendo, and such acts as a man sitting across the legs of a woman are all thought to be appropriate. Women do not come to beer parties alone, however, and if they are to stay all night, a husband, father, or brother should also be present. Lovers have a legitimate, regularized relationship, but covert, promiscuous behavior which might be socially disruptive is generally avoided.

Interaction in terms of conversation, dancing, verbal conflict, and sexual suggestion are all encouraged in so far as they do not lead to hostile acts. Behavior around the beer jar is of the type which moderate quantities of alcohol may stimulate, but it seems often to be generalized from past experiences of the drinking situation rather than resulting directly from the chemical action of the alcohol itself. The Kofyar are not markedly constrained or reticent in ordinary social intercourse nor are they physically isolated from each other. The interaction level may be affected directly or indirectly by alcohol but is not dependent upon it (cf. Heath 1958). Certainly different people have varying tolerances for alcohol and no system of social sanctions can successfully block all potentially disruptive behavior. Yet even the reaction to the rare evidence of drunkenness is usually one of mild amusement rather than anxiety or censure. A man who customarily shouts and roars on his way home from a beer party is regarded as ludicrous rather than disgraceful. It is funny but not scandalous for a person to carelessly uncover his genitals while drinking. Drunkenness is referred to as *mwos tu*, "beer kills," just as "hunger kills" and "sleep kills" refer to natural states of hunger and tiredness. I never saw a person intoxicated enough to lose motor control to the point of staggering or to become sick. In Horton's terms (1943:266), the Kofyar are characterized by slight insobriety in which alcohol is used regularly but with restraint. Stupor is neither the desired goal nor the usual outcome of Kofyar drinking. The drowsiness and eventual sleep that overtake many at the end of a long evening's imbibing are due to a full belly and delayed bedtime as much as to alcohol intake, and no one sees anything wrong with it. The only admonitions dealing with beer drinking have to do with the dangers of remaining away from home rather than with drunkenness. Kofyar men tell each other that they should not stay drinking at night for fear a thief will take their livestock. Women are given supernatural warnings to leave beer parties early in order to prepare the evening meal for their husbands.

There are certainly situations of considerable fear and anxiety in Kofyar society, but beer is not a significant factor in their resolution. Personal problems cannot be solved by private escape because drinking is never done alone. When individuals are overtaken by disease or the group is threatened by some natural disaster, recourse is had to divination, confession, magical rites, and religious observances. It is noteworthy that in these situations as well as in the highly charged atmosphere of witchcraft accusations, drinking has no place, and these are among the very few social gatherings where beer is not consumed.

Conclusion

I have attempted to indicate the way in which the value of beer for the Kofyar depends on factors other than its ability to intoxicate. In each case the value is increased by a limitation of potential costs based on the nature of the beverage and the social definition of the drinking situation. Sanctions to a large degree grow from within the context of drinking rather than from being internalized as feelings of ambivalence or guilt. The Kofyar crave beer as much for its food qualities of taste and nutrition as for the psychological effects of alcohol. The low alcohol content and the deliberate pace of drinking allow the achievement of these ends without intoxication. The nature of beer and home brewing is such that its value may be utilized in a modern economic network while remaining compatible with the forms of an unstratified, unspecialized society. Social interchange in conversation, recreation, argument, and sexual approach is encouraged in the drinking party but is not dependent on alcohol consumption. The emphasis on drinking only in inclusive groups, avoiding physical violence, and checking sexual promiscuity severely restricts the development of personal drinking pathologies and socially disruptive behavior. Beer is thus physically desirable, economically useful, and socially beneficial. It is as a general and unequivocal good that beer can take part in the great variety of social, political, economic, religious, and conceptual relationships detailed in the earlier sections of this paper. As beer becomes increasingly an instrumental entity and a medium which lends itself to the expression of social relationships, the derived values assume a greater importance than the primarily personal satisfactions. The distribution of beer in many ways parallels the flow of money in commercial societies, and beer like money has become through time less dependent on such value as may inhere in its substance and increasingly an accepted symbol of social values and a currency of interpersonal relations. Thus the amount of silver in a dollar or of alcohol in beer are matters of secondary concern. As the functional network of the beer complex expands, the possibilities of using alcohol for private psychological ends are minimized. Beer's value to the individual as nourishment and anxiety reducer is reinforced and ultimately outweighed by a wealth of social values associated with it and by the general absence of personal and societal costs incurred in its use.

Note

1. The same attitude has been noted among the Jukun (Meek 1931) where beer is purchased and consumed in the household as an essential item of daily diet. Regarding beer as primarily a food is characteristic of relatively sober groups where the anxiety-reducing function of alcohol is minimal (Horton 1943).

Problem-Drinking and the Integration of Alcohol in Rural Buganda
Michael C. Robbins

There have been a large number of cross-cultural studies of alcohol use (cf. Heath 1974a). A salient hypothesis to emerge from the evidence accumulated thus far is that when alcohol is well integrated into the sociocultural system its positive social and physiological functions will tend to outweigh its role as a means of assuaging personal psychological problems. This paper summarizes the results of an anthropological study of alcohol use designed to examine this hypothesis in a rural parish in the Buganda region of Uganda. It focuses on the differential functions of a well-integrated, traditional beverage, *mwenge*, a banana beer, and a less integrated, recently developed distillate of it, *nguli*. Together the two constitute the most important locally produced (and consumed) alcoholic beverages in the parish. The empirical hypothesis to be tested is that those persons who mainly drink *nguli* drink more for psychological problem-solving reasons, or personal effects, and less for social and physiological reasons than those who mainly drink *mwenge*.

The Sociocultural Integration Hypothesis

Several studies have shown that drinking can provide, at least for some persons and groups, a means of coping with personal problems, frustrations, and anxieties (e.g., Barry 1968; Jessor, Carman, and Grossman 1968; Jessor et al. 1968). Whether or not alcohol is used in this way, however, depends upon the manner in which drinking is learned, the meanings attached to it, and the extent to which it is an institutionalized part of family and social life, and dietary and religious customs.

In general, it has been found that irrespective of the type of beverage (e.g., fermented or distilled) or the amount consumed, when alcohol is well integrated into the sociocultural system (i.e., positively regarded as a necessary and appropriate component of a wide variety of activities and accepted from an early age), little or no emphasis is placed on its "escape-providing" qualities or psychological problem-solving, personal effects. Instead its positive social value in facilitating convivial social interaction, its cultural value in sacred, ceremonial observances, and physiological value as a healthful enhancement of the diet will assure prime importance. For example, among Italians (Lolli et al. 1958; Jessor et al. 1970), Jews (Snyder 1958), rural Greeks (Blum and Blum 1964) and Austrians (Honigmann 1963, also in this volume), Nahuatl Indians of Mexico (Madsen and Madsen 1969, also in this volume), Andean Indians in Peru (Mangin 1957), and the Kofyar of Nigeria (Netting 1964, also in this volume), research suggests that when drinking is (1) the prescriptive norm, (2) an important expression of social relationships, religious observances, and other customary activities, (3) learned early and in domestic settings, (4) a frequent accompaniment of meals and thought to be of nutritional and medicinal value, and (5) where consumption patterns are regulated and controlled by custom in a known, agreed upon, and consistent manner, its use for personal psychological effects will be minimized. Netting, for instance, has concluded on the basis of his study of the Kofyar, that "as beer becomes increasingly an instrumental entity and a medium which lends itself to the expression of social relationships, the derived values assume a greater importance than the primarily personal satisfactions" (1964:383, also in this volume: 361).

On the other hand, among Irish (Bales 1962), Mexican mestizos (Madsen and Madsen 1969, also in this volume), and many groups of Americans of varying ethnic background including Irish-Americans (Ullman 1960), Italian-American youth (Jessor et al. 1970), and several native North Americans (Dozier 1966; Hamer 1965; G. Berreman 1956), research suggests that when drinking (1) is a source of social and emotional concern, (2) occurs in an ambivalent or nonscriptive normative environment, (3) has been recently introduced, (4) is not interwoven with family, social, or religious institutions, (5) is not a part of meals, (6) is learned later in life, (7) occurs mainly outside of the family in secular situations, (8) is associated with status transformations from adolescence to adulthood, and (9) is thought to be a personal disinhibitor of socially undesirable sexual and aggressive behavior (and as a consequence often is; cf. MacAndrew and Edgerton 1969), alcohol will be used primarily for its personal psychological effects. There is also evidence to show that when alcohol *is* defined for its personal effects it tends to be associated with heavier, deviant drinking and higher rates of alcoholism than when it is defined more for its social and physiological effects (cf. Mulford and Miller 1960; Larsen and Abu-Laban 1968).

In brief, cross-cultural studies suggest that similar behavior such as drinking can play quite different roles, and be conducted for quite different reasons depending upon how it is embedded in the sociocultural system. As Abu-Laban and Larsen surmise:

> The prescriptive normative background, presumably because of an abundance of guidelines which define appropriate drinking behavior, tends to result in an emphasis on the use of alcohol for social rather than personal reasons. The prescriptive norms evidently disapprove drinking for personal effects. . . . Considering the non-scriptive normative background, it seems that permissiveness and anomie regarding the consumption of alcoholic beverages combine to influence the development of a personal-effects definition of alcohol. [1968:41]

Scope of the Present Study

Population and Research Methods

Research was conducted among the Baganda of Uganda for a total of fourteen months between 1967 and 1972. The Baganda are an ethnographically well-known, interlacustrine Bantu population formerly organized into a highly centralized state. Numbering more than a million persons, they are socioeconomically diverse and the predominant inhabitants of the rural and urban areas surrounding the northwestern shore of Lake Victoria. Most Baganda are peasant cultivators of an extensive variety of food staples and cash crops: in particular, plantains, sweet potatoes, beans, cassava, coffee, tea, and cotton.

Fieldwork was conducted in a rural parish (*muluka*) we shall call "Lusozi," located seven miles from Masaka, a town of about five thousand persons. Lusozi includes six villages (*byalo*), each of which has a chief responsible to the parish chief. The parish contains about two thousand persons. Field research methods involved participant-observation of drinking groups and beverage manufacture, key-informant interviews of brewers, distillers, and drinkers, and a social survey of drinking attitudes and practices administered in luganda to a random sample of seventy-six adults (over fourteen years of age) in 1969. Survey items included questions on quantity and frequency of drinking; attitudes toward, and perceptions of, various beverages; reasons for drinking; and socioeconomic background information on each respondent (e.g., age, sex, number of years of schooling, etc.).

The Beverages

Although today the rural Baganda drink several other alcoholic beverages of both traditional and modern origin (e.g., Uganda *waragi*, European beer, pineapple wine, etc.), and a few have even come to prefer them, the two most popular locally produced, regularly available, inexpensive, and widely consumed are *omwenge omuganda* and *enguli* (cf. Robbins and Pollnac 1969). The Baganda have been making *mwenge* since long before contact with the Arabs in the 1840s and Europeans in the 1860s. However, the exact date of origin is obscure. *Mwenge* is made from male plantains (*Musa sapientum*) called *mbidde*. Several varieties are distinguished. The process, in brief, is as follows. Bunches of *mbidde* are cut and then placed in a deep circular pit (*kinnya*) dug in the garden (about five feet in diameter by four feet in depth). They are surrounded by plantain leaves which line the pit and then are covered with earth. To aid ripening a smoldering fire may be started among the plantain leaves. After four days of ripening and fermenting the earth is removed, they are taken out, peeled, and placed in a large (nine feet in diameter by two feet in depth) depression (*lutyatya*) near the pit, which has been lined with long strips of plantain trunk stalk.

The *lutyatya* is waterproof and a hard grass *lusenke* (*Imperata* sp.) is mixed in with the *mbidde*. This is then trampled for several hours (depending on the quantity) and the juice (*mberenge*) is squeezed out. Water is added. Trampling (*kusogola*) is the work of men. Women are forbidden because, as informants say, the work is too difficult and they fear contamination if a woman begins menstruating. Magical rites and taboos are enacted to insure good weather throughout the duration of the process (e.g., certain signs are marked on the ground, visitors are not greeted, etc.). The trampling is exhausting, and requires considerable skill. When completed the *mberenge* is diluted with water forming *mubisi*, and it is placed in a large canoe-shaped vessel (*lyato*). Sorghum (*Sorghum vulgare*) which has been ground to a flour and roasted is mixed in to expedite fermentation and, as the Baganda say, to reduce the sweetness. The *lyato* is then covered with banana leaves and allowed to stand another day. The liquid is then filtered through grass into large gourds (*ebita*) and is ready for drinking.

During manufacture women, children, neighbors, and relatives look on, and often assist, in cutting, digging, peeling, bringing water, etc., but essentially it is adult male work. Table 1 shows that of four samples of *mwenge* analyzed, the average amount of alcohol by volume is 5.57 percent. Seldom is less than ten gallons made at one time. It is then consumed and/or sold at about six to seven cents per quart. About 25 percent of all adult male household heads brew *mwenge* at least once a year. In Lusozi most *mwenge* (and *nguli*) comes from three parish brewers, who make it about every other week, and from several nearby markets, trade centers, and the town of Masaka.

TABLE 1.   Alcohol Content of Beverages

	Percentage of Alcohol	
	Nguli	Mwenge
Sample 1	32.79	3.85
Sample 2	42.71	6.40
Sample 3	38.57	6.40
Sample 4	64.82	5.63
Sample 5	38.96	
Mean	43.57	5.57
S.D.[a]	12.4	1.2
C.V.[b]	28.45%	21.5%

a. S.D. = standard deviation

b. Coefficient of variation $= \left(\dfrac{100 \times \text{S.D.}}{\text{Mean}} \right)$

Nguli (also called local *waragi*) is a "gin" distilled from *mwenge*. The exact date when distillation was learned and employed in this region is unclear, but informants think no more than fifty years ago. Some believe it was introduced by Nubians after World War I. *Nguli* is manufactured from *kidongo* which in turn is made by allowing *mwenge* to ferment in the *lyato* for another day with more sorghum, sugar, and water added. It is then placed in five- or ten-gallon drums and "cooked." After about two hours of boiling, the alcohol and water evaporate and the vapor flows through a copper tube attached to the top of the drum. A lower length of the tubing is placed in a basin of cold water and as the vapors pass through the cooled portion of the tubing they condense to form a liquid.

Nguli is made by both men and women but is illegal. Fines for distilling range from fifteen to fifty dollars. Special manufacturing licenses can be obtained, but are very expensive for the average rural person (upward of fifty dollars). And this only permits the maker to sell to government distilleries at fixed (and low) prices, not to consumers. Most distillers (who are often brewers) prefer to risk arrest and fine. Since the law is enforced only on complaint, and officials are easily bribed (often with *nguli*), this is seldom a problem. However, because it is illegal, it is difficult to collect precise data on the number of distillers. Distilling is also dangerous because drums can explode causing serious injury or death. One distiller mentioned that in twelve years he had experienced three explosions with serious burns. Table 1 shows that of five samples analyzed the average amount of alcohol by volume is 43.57 percent.

Due to the dangerous and illegal nature of the manufacturing process, distillers tend to work alone. *Nguli* sells for about sixty-five cents per quart. It is normally consumed "straight" but can be mixed with other beverages when these are available (e.g., carbonated sweet sodas and pineapple wine). Distilling is profitable and provides a helpful cash settlement for producers. However, it does require some initial capital to purchase equipment, *mwenge*, sugar, firewood, and charcoal, and to pay fines and extend credit to regular customers. It is also a competitive business.

Sociocultural Integration of Alcohol in Buganda

It is postulated that *mwenge* is a more socioculturally integrated alcoholic beverage than *nguli* for the following reasons.

1. *Less ambiguity surrounds the nature and production of* mwenge *than* nguli. *Mwenge* manufacture is prescribed, positively sanctioned, and customary guidelines exist regulating how, and by whom, it is to be made. Considerable cooperation and public interest is evident during (and after) production. *Nguli* manufacture, on the other hand, is of recent vintage, and is a solo, clandestine activity, dangerous and illegal. While many people desire the product, many others do not. Likewise, while some think that *nguli* should be legal, others disagree. *Nguli* is not only

more intoxicating than *mwenge*, but also more unpredictably intoxicating and people are aware of this. Our analysis tends to support this. The coefficient of variation (c.v.) in the amount of alcohol per sample of *nguli* is 28.4 percent whereas for *mwenge* it is only 21.5 percent (see table 1).

2. Mwenge *is perceived to be a common, healthful drink, while* nguli *is perceived to be an economical, potent intoxicant.* Baganda consider *mwenge* to be their "national" (ethnic) drink and it is often referred to simply as "muganda." It is drunk before, during, and after meals and believed to be very nutritious. This is not true of *nguli*.

Informants mentioned the following reasons why they liked *mwenge* in response to an open-ended question (in this order of frequency): (1) contains vitamins; (2) gives strength; (3) everyone else drinks it; (4) settles the stomach; (5) sweet taste; (6) the national drink; (7) doesn't make you drunk or disturb you; (8) makes you feel happy without "hangovers"; (9) readily available.

By comparison they mentioned they like *nguli* in this order: (1) strong enough to get drunk on; (2) a more economical way to get drunk; (3) like the taste; (4) gives strength; (5) makes you less shy; (6) makes you happier.

A comparison of perceptions of *mwenge* and *nguli* was made using a set of bipolar adjectives and a Likert-scaling technique.[1] The results in table 2 reveal that people tend to perceive *nguli* as more masculine, more for younger people, more exciting, stronger, and slightly less healthful than *mwenge*.

TABLE 2.   Perceptions of *Mwenge* and *Nguli* ($n = 60$)

		Mwenge		*Nguli*	
		Mean	S.D.	Mean	S.D.
Very feminine	= 1	3.079	0.965	4.258	1.055*
Very masculine	= 5				
Very boring	= 1	3.063	1.097	4.129	1.274*
Very exciting	= 5				
Old people	= 1	2.238	0.845	3.048	0.688*
Young people	= 5				
Gives sickness	= 1	3.206	0.892	3.145	1.084
Gives health	= 5				
Very weak	= 1	2.952	1.006	4.371	0.944*
Very strong	= 5				

*$p < .001$, t-test (2-tailed).

Considered together then, the data suggest that *mwenge* is perceived as a more common drink, more healthful, and only mildly exhilarating. *Nguli* is seen to be a cheap and strong intoxicant, more exciting, masculine, for younger people, and of less physiological benefit.

3. Mwenge *is consumed by a broader spectrum of the population in a more socially regulated manner than* nguli. *Mwenge* is enjoyed by almost all drinkers and respondents claim they prefer it over *nguli* by a ratio of three to one. Little or no emotional concern is expressed if children drink small quantities. Slightly fermented *mubisi* is given freely to anyone. Public drunkenness and uninhibited drunken comportment, however, are strongly condemned. Baganda clearly recognize that too much *mwenge* can lead to socially disruptive behavior. Numerous proverbs warn that "you can't resist what beer makes you do"; "beer provides an excuse for saying bad things"; "the chicken of a drunkard is always on the verge of death"; "even an old person can be excited by beer"; etc.

Mild intoxication is common and participants appear to talk more, in more animated fashion, and laugh, joke, boast, and engage in more bouts of speech making when drinking than at other times. When drinkers become inebriated they either wander home or are led away by companions. Since drinking settings are the homes and shops of other parish residents, norms regarding hospitality and polite, host-guest relationships are in effect. Householders, bar owners, and/or elders are always present and they insure that loud and aggressive verbalizations and fighting seldom occur. Likewise, few overt exhibitions of sexual behavior take place. Although men claim they desire women more when they are drinking, the formal and public ambience confines this to little more than covert cross-sex joking and flirting. A luganda proverb asserts that "few can drink *mwenge* without dancing" and *mwenge* is considered to be a necessary stimulant for musical and dance performances. Musicians are provided with all they can hold and it is believed that women must be given *mwenge* in order to coax them to dance. This was witnessed on several occasions. In one instance women refused to dance throughout the duration of a village party lasting fourteen hours because they felt slighted over not having received enough beer.

On the contrary, *nguli* is drunk somewhat furtively around the fringes of social settings (or in isolation) and in the absence of social protocol and controls. Intoxicating quantities are consumed in rapid fashion. It is almost always purchased, seldom offered freely as refreshment, and is supposed to be restricted to adults over seventeen years of age. In fact, teenagers as young as fourteen drink it surreptitiously (provided they have the money), and one *nguli* distiller living near a secondary school depends almost exclusively on students for her business. *Nguli* drinkers tend to display more indiscreet behavior, often staggering, shouting, and vomiting. The only incidents of verbal and physical abuse we witnessed in the parish involved someone who had been drinking *nguli*. Villagers believe it has greater disinhibiting qualities than *mwenge*, makes people forget their manners, act crazy (*edalu*), and become sexually aggressive and promiscuous. A few freely translated excerpts from a popular luganda phonograph record by Sempeke entitled "Enguli" express some of these sentiments:

> Enguli makes people suffer
> When you drink it you feel like dancing
> Even if you're a man you're noticed
> It makes your eyes red
> It makes you stagger
>
> When you drink you must eat well
> You must buy intestines and tomatoes
>
> Enguli makes people crazy
> Because of Enguli "Black" [personal name]
> Walked in a queer way
> "Ssewali" [personal name] was beaten by a whip
>   because he was drunk
> It made him walk in a queer way

Many people are aware therefore that *nguli* is associated with uninhibited, disruptive behavior, and some believe its use should be circumscribed.

4. Mwenge *forms an integral part of more cultural activities and social relationships than* nguli. *Mwenge* has had a much longer history and inter alia more opportunity to become incorporated into preexisting cultural institutions than *nguli*. As well as being considered a healthful dietary supplement and medicine prescribed for certain ailments and fevers, *mwenge* is a customary sacrament in numerous traditional rituals and ceremonies. Libations of *mwenge* are used to consecrate new home and garden sites, houses, and canoes. It is also a requisite offering to placate and propitiate ancestral ghosts, spirits, and gods.

Mwenge also plays a significant customary role in ceremonies such as birth and naming, twin ceremonies, marriages, lineage and clan succession ceremonies, funerals, and public celebrations. Marriage arrangements, for example, are jurally confirmed by the prospective bride's father and brother accepting and drinking a presentation of *mwenge* offered by the would-be groom. Large quantities of *mwenge* also constitute a customary portion of the bride-price. A man continues to make gifts of *mwenge* to his father-in-law and brothers-in-law (*Bakodomi*) throughout the duration of his marriage.

Mwenge also flows freely at wedding feasts and celebrations and is presented to *Bakodomi* at the birth of a child. The placenta (or "second child"), which is thought to contain the clan spirit, is buried with food and *mwenge* near plantains. It is believed that the spirit will be absorbed into the plantains, subsequently consumed as food and drink, and thereby be retained. At naming ceremonies the umbilical cord, which has been preserved, is floated in a mixture of *mwenge* and water to divine whether or not the child is the legitimate offspring of the father.

To celebrate the end of wars, warriors used to assemble before the king (*kabaka*) to drink *mwenge*. Each one who had performed bravely was allowed a ceremonial drink. Those who had not were refused and thereby publicly shamed. At death, the king's entrails were cleansed in *mwenge* and water, and the liquid, thought to embody the king, was consumed by his widows. In fact, at all funerals *mwenge* is a required provision to console the bereaved. A man also gives a customary gift of *mwenge* to the person who escorts his wife home from mortuary ceremonies of her deceased kin (and from other journeys).

Mwenge must also be present at feasts and legal and political events. It is used to pay tribute to chiefs and landlords and for fines to redress grievances in the parish courts. Chiefs and landlords also host feasts where beer and food is distributed to commoners and tenants. One informant told Mair, for example, that "the essential qualities of a good chief (are) . . . beer, meat and politeness" (1934:183).

Finally, a luganda proverb expresses the fact that "friendship thrives on beer." It is an expected refreshment to honor visitors and is said to "warm" kinship. Sharing *mwenge* together not only symbolizes friendship but constitutes the medium for the development and expression of ritually bonded drinking partnerships among adult males (*abekinywi*). Drinking partners are the closest of friends.[2] *Abekinywi* always drink together and share *mwenge* whenever they have it. If one partner is not present a special gourd is set aside in the event he might eventually arrive and/or to imply he is there in spirit. *Abekinywi* are usually neighbors and unrelated. Relationships have been known to last a lifetime. They associate together regularly, lend and borrow money, tools, and other goods (often without asking), are close confidants, and help adjudicate each other's domestic disputes. They also protect and defend one another against malevolent gossip or abuse, and speak for, and boast about each other, especially at drinking parties. While *abekinywi* share other drinks as well, the core of these intimate relationships emanates from and is regularly reinforced by reciprocal exchanges of *mwenge*.

By contrast, *nguli* is an exclusively secular beverage which is consumed in a utilitarian manner. Although occasionally present, and taken by some as a supplement, it plays no prominent role in any of the ritual or ceremonial contexts mentioned above. While it can be used as an analgesic to relieve pain, cold, and flu symptoms and to help people sleep at night, it is not considered to be beneficial to health nor a form of nourishment. Some men also believe it makes them more potent and gives them more strength (*amaanyi*). They often take a small dose (two or three ounces) before they expect to have sexual relations. Since there is widespread anxiety among males about their sexual performance (cf. Orley 1970) *nguli* may help relieve tension and alleviate fears of failure. The main concern of Baganda men is ejaculation before the woman reaches a climax. It is even more desirable to delay ejaculation until the woman has attained several climaxes. A man able to do this is said to have strength (*amaanyi*). One unable to do so is derogated as "weak" (*munafu*) or a "chicken" (*enkoko*) based on the observation that chickens copulate for brief durations. Since human and animal research presented and reviewed by Farkas and Rosen (1976) suggests that alcohol *can* delay ejaculation and depress ejaculatory responses and low doses of alcohol also tend to facilitate penile tumescence rates (higher doses decrease it), there may be some basis in fact for this practice.

Integration and the Uses of Alcohol in Buganda

It is clear that *mwenge* is comparatively more integrated than *nguli*. According to the sociocultural integration hypothesis we would expect therefore that those who mainly drink *nguli* will do so more for personal psychological effects and less for positive social and physiological reasons than those who mainly drink *mwenge*.

Sample

To test this hypothesis two subsamples from the total sample of respondents to the drinking survey were selected on the basis of their reported drinking preferences and practices. The first group, designated the "*mwenge* drinkers" (n = 20), is composed of: (1) those who prefer *mwenge* as their favorite beverage, drink it more than any other beverage, and do not drink any *nguli* (n = 15); and (2) those who, although they do not prefer *mwenge* as their favorite beverage, drink more *mwenge* than any other beverage, more than once a month, and do not drink any *nguli* (n = 5).

The other group, designated the "*nguli* drinkers" (n = 21), is composed of : (1) those who prefer *nguli* as their favorite beverage, drink more *nguli* than any other beverage (n = 13); and (2) those who, although they do not prefer *nguli* as their favorite beverage, drink more *nguli* than any other beverage, more than once a month, and their favorite beverage is not *mwenge* (n = 8).[3]

Table 3 contains information on the sex, age, and educational backgrounds of the respondents in each group. Although the *nguli* group contains more females, this difference is not statistically significant ($\chi^2_c{}^* = .253$, $p > .05$, two-tailed test). Likewise, although the *nguli* group appears to have had more years of formal schooling, this difference is also not statistically significant ($t = .244$, $p > .05$, two-tailed test). The *nguli* group is, however, significantly younger than the *mwenge* group ($t = 2.11$, $p < .05$, two-tailed test).

TABLE 3. Sample Characteristics (n = 41)

	Mwenge (n = 20)		Nguli (n = 21)		Total	
	Mean	S.D.	Mean	S.D.	Mean	S.D.
Age	38.15	15.02	28.86	13.08	33.39	14.66
Education	5.75	4.83	6.09	4.07	5.9	4.41
Sex (percent male)	65%		52%		58.5%	

Consumption Patterns

Table 4 presents information on the monthly consumption of the major beverage of each group. These figures are based on the frequency of drinking in a 7-day week over a 4-week month (28 days). The monthly frequency is multiplied by the quantity consumed on each occasion (in ounces). This product is then weighted by the average amount of alcohol by volume in that beverage (see table 1). For example, if a respondent stated that he/she drank 16 ounces of *mwenge* every day the amount of alcohol consumed per month is calculated as: 16 ounces × 28 days × .0557 = 24.9536 or about 25 ounces of alcohol per month. Dividing this product by 28 gives the estimated amount of alcohol ingested per day as .89 ounce. It should be recognized that there are numerous errors involved in arriving at these values (e.g., retrospective distortion, imprecise frequency, and quantity estimates, etc.) and caution should be exercised in accepting them as absolute quantities. Since we suspect no more than random error, however, we feel justified in using them for comparing the *relative* intake of each group.

TABLE 4.   Relation of Beverage Group to Quantity and Frequency of Drinking

	Mwenge	Nguli
Number of respondents who drink		
daily	7	6
4–5 days per week	3	0
2–3 days per week	2	6
weekly	8	4
less than weekly	0	5
Mean number of days/month	15.45	11.83
S.D.	10.75	10.94
C.V.	69.58%	92.52%
Average number of ounces of alcohol per person		
per month	33.94	55.21
per day	1.21	1.97

The results in table 4 show that although *mwenge* drinkers tend to drink more days per month than *nguli* drinkers, this difference is not statistically significant ($t = 1.07$, $p > .05$, two-tailed); likewise, grouping drinking periods into ordinal categories (daily, weekly, etc.) reveals no difference ($D = .238$, $p > .05$, Kolmogorov-Smirnov two-sample test, two-tailed). Furthermore, while it appears that *nguli* drinkers consume more alcohol per month than *mwenge* drinkers, this difference too is not statistically significant ($U = 243$ corrected, $z = .862$, $p > .05$, Mann-Whitney U-test).[4] There appear then to be few if any differences between the two groups in their monthly quantity and frequency of consumption.

Drinking Functions

In order to examine the postulated differences in motivations for drinking between the two groups, information was collected using an attenuated translated version of the Jessor Drinking Functions

Scale (Jessor, Carman, and Grossman 1968). Previous cross-cultural research (Jessor, Carman, and Grossman 1968; Jessor et al. 1968; Jessor et al. 1970) has demonstrated that positive (yes) responses to these items, when a respondent is asked why he/she drinks, provide reliable and valid measures of three main drinking functions: (1) *psychological effects:* motives and attitudes linking drinking to unresolved psychological problems and an escape or relief from problems and inadequacies (e.g., "worry less about what others think of you"); (2) *physiological effects:* motives and attitudes linking drinking to physical pain, aches, fatigue, and a remedy for or relief from them (e.g., "it settles your stomach"); (3) *social effects:* motives and attitudes that link drinking to activities of a social, festive nature or to meet group obligations and pressures (e.g., "it is something to do on special occasions").

In the present study six psychological effects and three social and three physiological items were used. The data were analyzed in two ways (cf. Jessor, Carman, and Grossman 1968). The first considers the number of positive responses a person makes to the items in each of the three functional categories. The second considers the proportion of positive responses made in a category to the total number of responses made in all categories. The latter measure evaluates the differential importance of drinking attributed by a person to that category. Thus, for example, if only three positive responses to all twelve questions are mentioned but two are personal effects, the score (66.6 percent) will be higher in the personal effects category than someone who mentions four personal effects reasons out of ten (40 percent) of the possible twelve.

Results

The results in table 5 reveal that, as expected, *nguli* drinkers mention more personal effects reasons for drinking than *mwenge* drinkers ($t = 1.79, p < .05$, one-tailed). They also show that *nguli* drinkers drink proportionately more for personal effects reasons than for other reasons than do *mwenge* drinkers ($t = 1.69, p < .05$, one-tailed). It can also be seen in table 5 that, as expected, *mwenge* drinkers mention more physiological reasons for drinking than *nguli* drinkers ($t = 1.86$, p $< .05$, one-tailed). They also mention proportionally more physiological reasons than do *nguli* drinkers ($t = 2.47, p < .01$, one-tailed). However, the two groups do *not* differ significantly in either the number of social reasons mentioned ($t = .74, p > .05$, one-tailed) or in the proportion of social to other reasons mentioned ($t = .38, p > .05$, one-tailed).

TABLE 5. Relationship of Beverage Choice to Drinking Functions

Reasons	Mwenge		Nguli		Significance Level
	Mean	S.D.	Mean	S.D.	
Psychological					
number	3.85	1.46	4.62	1.28	$p < .05$
proportion	55.26	15.67	63.9	17.06	$p < .05$
Physiological					
number	2.0	.97	1.43	.98	$p < .05$
proportion	27.0	15.26	16.98	10.39	$p < .01$
Social					
number	1.35	.93	1.57	.98	n.s.
proportion	17.64	12.19	19.03	11.25	n.s.

In general, these results provide modest but consistent support for the sociocultural integration hypothesis on two of the three measures. *Nguli* drinkers tend to drink more for personal psychological reasons than *mwenge* drinkers. *Mwenge* drinkers tend to drink more for physiological reasons. No significant difference was found between the groups in social reasons for drinking.

Discussion and Conclusion

While this pilot study does not claim to be conclusive, pending further research with larger samples and more precise measurements of these and other variables, it does support those who have contended that sociocultural factors are importantly involved in explaining the functions of alcohol use. It especially buttresses those who have argued that whether or not alcohol is used primarily as a means of assuaging psychological problems depends at least in part on the culturally constituted meanings attached to it and the extent to which it is embedded in the sociocultural system. In the present study *mwenge* was found to be a more integrated beverage than *nguli*. And, as predicted, a sample of *mwenge* drinkers drink less for personal psychological effects than a comparable sample of *nguli* drinkers. These results obtain, in spite of the fact that both groups of drinkers are all members of the same rural community and ethnicity, do not differ significantly in consumption patterns, and are substantially the same in sex and educational background.

It *is* true, however, that *nguli* drinkers are somewhat younger in age than *mwenge* drinkers, and this suggests a plausible alternative interpretation of the results—namely, that younger

rural persons are in general drinking more for personal effects reasons, perhaps because they are experiencing more disjunction, frustrations, and dissatisfactions as a result of sociocultural changes occurring in Buganda (cf. Robbins and Pollnac 1969). Further, as reported above (table 2), *nguli* is perceived to be a drink for younger people. Therefore it could be proposed that the relationships discovered between the consumption of differentially integrated beverages and personal effects drinking are in fact masking, or are an artifact of, a more important relationship between age and personal effects drinking. While attractive, this argument tends to be compromised by the following facts. First, there is neither a significant relationship between age and number of personal effects reasons for drinking ($r = -.17$, n.s.), nor between age and proportion of personal to total number of reasons cited for drinking ($r = -.07$, n.s.) when both samples are combined. Second, if the alternative interpretation were true, one would also expect a positive relationship between personal effects drinking and education (years of schooling) since younger people are also more educated. The correlation, for example, between age and education is $r = -.41$ ($p < .01$, two-tailed).

However, as has already been shown, there is no significant difference in educational levels between *mwenge* and *nguli* drinkers (see table 4) and there is neither a significant relationship between education and number of personal effects reasons ($r = -.05$, n.s., one-tailed), nor between education and percent of personal/total reasons cited for drinking ($r = -.07$, n.s., one-tailed) for both samples combined. Significant relationships would probably be expected between these variables if the alternative hypothesis were true. Thus it appears that the relationship between relative beverage integration and personal effects drinking is not an artifact of age. All of this is not to say, however, that "age" is not somehow involved. In fact an even more persuasive explanation can be derived from the sociocultural integration hypothesis itself. Perhaps it is that younger people are inclined to drink more for personal effects reasons *because* they tend to drink more *nguli*. Younger persons are more attracted to *nguli* because it is a cheap, modern, potent beverage. As a consequence they learn to drink in their secular contexts, outside the sphere of customary regulations, and in the absence of directives. This in turn may predispose them to drink more for personal effects reasons (cf. Larsen and Abu-Laban 1968).

It is possible that age is also implicated in the relationship between beverage type and physiological functions. *Mwenge* drinkers, because they are older, may have more physiological complaints and therefore use alcohol as an available, culturally defined remedy (cf. Jessor, Carman, and Grossman 1968). Indeed, the relationship between age and number of physiological reasons mentioned for drinking for both samples combined is positive and significant ($r = .34$, $p < .025$, one-tailed), as in the relationship between age and the proportion of physiological to total number of reasons mentioned ($r = .45$, $p < .005$, one-tailed). These results do not appear to be an artifact of education. There is neither a significant relationship between education and number of physiological reasons ($r = -.24$, n.s., one-tailed) nor between education and proportion of physiological to total reasons ($r = -.16$, n.s., one-tailed).

No explanation can be offered at this time for the lack of differences between the two beverage groups in social reasons for drinking. Both seem to drink for social reasons to about the same extent. More work is called for, however, to delineate more decisively the complex web of interrelationships among these (and other) cultural, biosocial, and psychological variables.

In sum it is proposed that when viewed in concert this study, and other research already cited, support the sociocultural integration hypothesis. Additional research along similar lines would be desirable to assess the various implications that follow from it. Certainly one of the most compelling of these is that a knowledge of sociocultural factors can be employed to both predict and explain variations in motives for drinking. By examining the manner in which alcohol is integrated into a sociocultural system it may be possible to detect sources of problem drinking and therefore anticipate where remedial steps could be taken. Changing the way drinking is institutionalized and socialized may, in other words, be one way of alleviating the undesirable elements associated with it.

Notes

1. This procedure is also known as the semantic differential technique (Pelto 1970:109–10). People were asked in luganda, for example, for each polar adjective pair:

	very weak	weak	neither	strong	very strong
Is *mwenge*	1	2	3	4	5

The same was done for *nguli*.

2. The singular term *omwenkinywe* is similar to the word used to address a blood-pact friend *munyaniwe*. Both terms may be derived from the infinite form of the verb "to drink" (*kunywa*). Beattie (1958) mentions this as a possibility with respect to the culturally and linguistically similar Banyoro. In fact, the region (*Ssaza*) in which our work was conducted (*Buddu*) was until about 1800 a part of Bunyoro (Kiwanuka 1972).

3. Excluded from consideration here are: (1) those who drink neither *mwenge* nor *nguli* (n = 5); (2) those who prefer some beverage other than *mwenge* or *nguli* but drink both *mwenge* and *nguli* in about equal amounts (n = 9); and (3) those who prefer *mwenge* but drink as much or more *nguli* (n = 21).

4. Non-parametric statistics are most appropriate for analyzing these data because of the approximate nature of the quantity and frequency reports of drinking (e.g., "a bottle of *nguli* once a week," etc.). There is also no significant difference between the *nguli* and *mwenge* groups in number of ounces of alcohol consumed a month if the parametric Student's t-test is used ($t = 1.28$, $p > .05$). There is enormous variation around the means of both groups (*nguli* S.D. = 61.91; *mwenge* S.D. = 42.07).

VII. Alcohol Use in Euro-American Societies

Alcoholics Anonymous as a Crisis Cult

William Madsen

Throughout history deprived members of society have frequently banded together in movements aiming to improve their lot or to seek "justice" as they perceive it. This phenomenon is prevalent in contemporary American society, with Indians, blacks, and Chicanos among others forming such movements. In a manner of speaking, Alcoholics Anonymous (AA) may also be viewed as a minority movement, one that seeks a better way for its members in a society that has been largely indifferent or openly hostile to the alcoholic person. Unlike most minority members, however, many alcoholic persons suffer their deprivations as a private ordeal, only coming to realize that they are part of a like group after their first contact with AA. The active alcoholic person's anguish may be harder to bear than that of most other persecuted groups, for he is rarely able to share it meaningfully with fellow sufferers. After affiliation with AA, however, the alcoholic person discovers that he is not a unique phenomenon and that there are others like him who are not only willing to help but have shared his feelings of helplessness, alienation, and terror. Within AA, the strong union among members produced by a common history of emotional and social deprivation has led to the belief that only one alcoholic person can understand another—similar to the feeling in the black movement that the black experience cannot be communicated to whites.

A spiritual or supernatural tone in such movements is not uncommon. The more hopeless a situation seems, the more frequently will the sufferer seek help from "a power greater than himself."[1] As Bronislaw Malinowski (1948) has pointed out, one function of a belief in the supernatural is to give the believer the feeling that he can gain control in a situation that otherwise seems uncontrollable. Many minority movements in seemingly hopeless situations have therefore sought aid and sanction from the supernatural. Such movements have in the past frequently represented a last desperate effort by conquered aborigines to negate the destructive power of their conquerors. Famous examples of these are the ghost dance of the American Indians (Mooney 1896) and the cargo cults of Melanesia (e.g., Belshaw 1950; Worsley 1957). In the same manner, however, deprived and alienated members of powerful and complex societies have been offered a means to power and justice by such saviors as Buddha and Christ. Anthro-

pologists have coined a variety of labels for such religiously in-
spired minority movements. These include: "messianic movements" (Barber 1941), "nativistic movements" (Linton 1943),
"revitalization movements" (A. Wallace 1956), and "crisis cults"
(La Barre 1971).

Typical of such crisis cults is the emergence of a leader who
gained the strength and confidence to rise above his own helplessness through a vision. Such was the origin of the ghost dance and
each of the cargo cults. AA also began with a vision by one of its
cofounders, Bill W. In retrospect, Bill acknowledged that his vision may in part have been preconditioned by his awareness of
Jung's statement that seemingly hopeless cases of alcoholism are
occasionally rehabilitated following a transcending religious experience. Nonetheless, Bill's rehabilitation began with his vision
while he was an alcoholic patient in a New York City hospital in
1934. In the absolute depths of alcoholic despair, Bill first experienced a type of anguish which Assagioli (1971) has called the
"crisis preceding a spiritual awakening." The religious experience
took place and Bill suddenly felt himself freed of the alcoholic
drive (*Alcoholics Anonymous* 1957).

Origins of AA

Bill's vision could be defined as a fairly typical conversion experience. Whatever the psychological dynamics involved, Bill was
given a source of power greater than alcohol. He also felt the deep
need to carry his message of hope to other alcoholic persons. He
shared his story with a fellow alcoholic, Dr. Bob in Akron, Ohio,
and out of the relationship between the two men grew the first AA
group. From those original two members, AA has grown to an
estimated five hundred thousand today.

With very few exceptions, each alcoholic person has joined
AA because of an individual crisis. (There are a few people in AA
who are not alcoholic, but who find in the fellowship an ad hoc
religion that helps them live useful, humane lives.) The movement itself is the product of a grave social crisis: the failure of
other therapies to handle the alcohol abuse problem adequately.
As one young alcoholic person explained it to me: "AA represents
a revolt against the imperialistic claims of the psychotherapists to
our minds and problems. They are good at taking our money and
writing quaint books about us. But they can't help us, and they
certainly don't cure us."

Our failure to adequately treat alcoholism must reflect some
basic misconceptions in those sciences that deal with human be-

havior. Unlike science, Alcoholics Anonymous is a form of folk psychotherapy, relying solely on the empirical evidence of its members' shared experience. It makes no claims to scientific validity, nor does it use scientific concepts or scientific methods. Yet, AA has rehabilitated more alcoholic people than the combined efforts of medicine, psychology, and psychiatry (Maxwell 1967).

The scientific approach to alcoholism has been hampered in part by the extreme specialization in the sciences today. Increasingly scientists are trained to understand one small aspect of the human animal, and then, all too frequently, they try to explain all of behavior by that reference point. This approach has led to a wealth of monocausal explanations of alcoholism—a fantasyland of conflicting interpretations. Too many professionals in alcoholism, when their position was questioned, used to retreat into a verbal ballet of logic to protect their stance. The result is a literature on alcoholism that frequently appears more mystical than scientific (Opler 1959; Watson 1972; Madsen 1974b).

Fortunately, the atmosphere is changing. Some specialists in the field are beginning to be more sophisticated in their conceptions of human behavior. They are now more likely to favor multicausal explanations rather than the simplistic monocausalities of the various dogmatists. Those with adequate training and experience realize that alcoholism embraces biological, psychological, and cultural aspects (e.g., F. Alexander 1963; J. Berreman 1950; Catanzaro 1967; Fox 1967; Jellinek 1960; Landis and Bolles 1950; Mann 1958; Moore 1960; Myers and Veale 1971). Although many of these postulate the eventual discovery of a biological origin for the disease, they realize that, at the present level of our knowledge, alcoholism can only be treated successfully by a many-sided approach. Their interpretation thus agrees with that of Alcoholics Anonymous. However, AA gives the alcoholic person something the therapists cannot offer: the support of a group within which the alcoholic individual can feel normal while learning to live without alcohol.

The social bonding of AA is especially appealing to the primary alcoholic person[2] who invariably from early childhood has lived a life of loneliness fed by a sense of inadequacy. The personality of the primary alcoholic person resembles that of the anxiety-neurotic, and the two may share some biological correlates (Pitts and Ferris 1969). For most primary alcoholic people, the first exposure to alcohol is a peak experience (Maslow 1961, 1964, 1965, 1971) when, for the first time in their lives, they finally have a feeling of adequacy and a new sense of power (Adler 1931; McClelland et al. 1972) that allows them to finally interact freely with others. However, primary alcoholic people rapidly lose their tolerance for alcohol; a compulsion to drink increases, and within a few years, they are totally alienated, powerless, and confused.

Secondary alcoholic persons suffer these effects only after the onset of the disease, which may follow twenty or more years of social drinking. The delta alcoholic person also usually functions well in society until his tolerance for ethanol is destroyed. When any of these persons approaches AA, however, he suffers from acute alienation and a sense of being different and totally alone with his problem.

The relief experienced upon affiliation with AA is enormous. The alcoholic person finds that he is merely a "normal" member of the group rather than an idiosyncratic misfit in society. Most of the descriptions of the initial AA contact reflect the relief felt in this discovery. One person said, "I'd always been a stranger on earth, yearning to find someone who understood me. When I found AA, it felt like coming home to a loving family I'd never known."

Having joined AA, the newcomer is no longer alone, and that very fact begins to engender self-respect, something he has sought for a very long time. His total experience in AA works to reinforce a positive image. The very alcoholism that had alienated him from society becomes the bond linking him to this loving primary group. Thus, his alcoholism is metamorphosed from a destructive force to perhaps the most positive identity he has ever had.

Total abstinence is the basis of success in AA. While some highly contrived and, I think, inadequate research (Madsen 1974*b*) is trying to demonstrate that there is no compulsion in alcoholism (e.g., Sobell, Sobell, and Christelman 1972; Gottheil et al. 1972), the AA member "knows" that "one drink is too many and a thousand are not enough." Despite the opposition of some professionals in alcoholism, I find the AA position obviously valid: The safest way to avoid alcoholic intoxication is to avoid alcohol.

The switch from uncontrolled alcoholism to total abstinence is drastic, and the alcoholic person is struck dramatically by the qualitative difference in his life before and after AA affiliation. In many ways this before-and-after contrast parallels the experience of religious converts. Many AAers describe their drinking years as a period when they were controlled by destructive forces they could not identify. One AAer explained to me: "Back when I drank, I felt like a puppet worked by an unknown master who hated my guts. Every worthwhile thing I tried he blocked by yanking on those lousy strings and getting me drunk." Other AAers visualize their drinking years as a period when an internal evil nature, aided by alcohol, frequently dominated their real and good nature.

The realization that he can live without alcohol comes as an enormous relief to the alcoholic person. As one primary alcoholic individual said: "Every drinking bout was like a game of Russian roulette, but I never really wanted to die or go mad. When I met AA and found that one can break away from drinking, I experienced rapture. It was too gorgeous to describe. I was free!" The double elation of a new freedom combined with the satisfaction of the group bonding usually produces a period of euphoria, which AA calls a "pink cloud." On his pink cloud, the newcomer is safe from alcoholic temptation. However, the euphoria will eventually dissolve and the "AA honeymoon" will end. The newcomer must be indoctrinated with the AA principles before this happens or he will slip and be off on another drunken binge.

Reliance on Sponsor

The strongest insurance against such a slip is to tightly integrate the newcomer into the group. As a basic step, he is urged to rely heavily on his sponsor—someone in the group whose sobriety is fairly long-term and who establishes a special relationship with the newcomer. The new member is also encouraged to attend meetings frequently, to read the literature, and to socialize with AAers. He may also spend much time in so-called "dime therapy"—talking on the telephone with other AAers when he feels anxious. If the indoctrination is successful, when a crisis comes, he turns to AA rather than to a bottle for help. That help is always available without cost in AA.

The ever available help and understanding increase the alcoholic person's sense of loyalty to AA. As a result, he finds himself living up to AA's expectations of him rather than yielding to his own recurrent need for alcohol. His affiliation also helps him resist the usual social pressures to drink. At the same time, AA's own folk psychotherapy remolds the entire value structure of the alcoholic person through the influence of his sponsor, and the effect of attending AA meetings and following AA's recommended steps to sobriety. The core of the person's being becomes the fact of his alcoholism and his need to avoid alcohol. Every decision for the rest of his life will be affected by this guidepost.

In terms that must confuse the psychologist, AA also tells the alcoholic person to get rid of his ego while improving his self-concept. In the jargon of AA, "ego" refers to the totally far-fetched fantasies of self-worth and future promise that grip most alcoholic people between periods of total self-denigration. The alcoholic person is urged to realize his own limitations and set up appropriate goals, rather than to strive for the unapproachable ideals of total perfection. The blow of this so-called "ego-destruction" is softened by the overt signs of approval from his group as he progressively recognizes his fantasies for what they are and develops a more realistic image of his abilities and talents. Further, through group support, he not only comes to accept his potential realistically, but he also develops a positive self-acceptance. With this new image he finds reasonable goals that he can strive for without submitting to excessive stress. He learns to seek serenity in his being and in his activities.

However, primary alcoholism is by any definition a stress disease (Salye 1956) and its sufferers will forever experience periods of anxiety and despair. The psychophysical syndrome of anxiety in the primary alcoholic person is easily triggered, and he then enters the psychic hell he once relived by using alcohol. AA teaches him to hold onto his sobriety through these stressful periods with the knowledge that things will get better. It is at such times that the love, intensity, and tension-relieving laughter of an AA meeting are most effective.

If despite these measures the alcoholic person slips back into drinking, he resigns from AA, but is always welcomed back when he again seeks sobriety. If he maintains his sobriety, he is rewarded by ever increasing prestige. Within AA he finds an integrated value system and the personalized caring relations that typify a folk society (Kroeber 1948). While his sobriety and self-confidence grow, he also learns to cope with the stresses of the larger society in which he must live. As his time in the program increases, he finds that the rewards for a mature and responsible life, which AA calls a "good sobriety," far outweigh those of a "bad sobriety"—which is seen as staying sober but failing to achieve personal growth.

The sober alcoholic person securely in the AA mode becomes dedicated to a continual growth, which he takes "one step at a time" while trying to live "one day at a time," free from the shame of an unchangeable past and the fear of an unpredictable future. For those who "make it" in the program, life can be productive and fulfilling.

388   Beliefs, Behaviors, and Alcoholic Beverages

Notes

1. The second of the twelve steps of AA states that "we came to believe that a power greater than ourselves could restore us to sanity."
2. Ruth Fox (1967) defined a primary alcoholic person as one who experiences an immediate dependence on alcohol from the first exposure to it. The delta alcoholic person, on the other hand, adapts to his dependence on alcohol and is able to control the amount he drinks.

The "Crisis Cult" as a Voluntary Association: An Interactional Approach to Alcoholics Anonymous

Patricia O. Sadler

In a recent paper Madsen (1974a, also in this volume) has indicated that the "crisis cult" concept is useful for understanding some aspects of Alcoholics Anonymous (hereafter, AA). "Crisis cult" typically is used in a specialized way in the anthropological literature, and Madsen demonstrates an awareness of this usage, defining crisis cults as spiritually toned movements, frequently the "last desperate effort by conquered aborigines to negate the destructive power of their conquerors" (1974a:27, also in this volume: 382).

It is my contention that Madsen's reference to AA as a crisis cult constitutes the overextension of a useful term. The purpose of this article is to point out limitations of the crisis cult approach and to suggest a broader anthropological perspective for the study of AA. The scheme that will be developed is an interactional one which is well suited for understanding AA as a voluntary association.

Although Madsen gives an excellent account of some aspects of AA, he does not develop support for his usage of the crisis cult label. Thus he appears to use the term as an attention-getting device rather than as a scholarly assessment.

Nonetheless there are certain outcomes that result from use of the crisis cult model. One is Madsen's focus on the newcomer, the convert in crisis cult terms. Another is his stress upon decidedly spiritual aspects of the AA program. Third is emphasis on the visionary experience of an AA cofounder. These phenomena are significant features of crisis cults and they are worthy of attention. But they are not necessarily the important features of

AA for many of its members. For example, there are AAers who do not know about the "spiritual experience" of the cofounder. For those who do, it is apparently not a topic of concern since it is rarely discussed.

These remarks should not be construed as wholly negative. Madsen's use of the crisis cult term is a clue to a more comprehensive anthropological approach to the problem at hand. A crisis cult is a kind of voluntary association. As a concept, voluntary association has breadth suitable for the study of AA. Voluntary associations may be operationally defined as social units whose members have freely chosen to join the group (Brown 1973). As a concept, voluntary association directs attention not only to newcomers and founders but to the entire scope of interaction among members.

For present purposes interaction among recovering alcoholics has been studied by a traditional anthropological fieldwork procedure, participant observation. Hence the following discussion makes little use of AA literature. Quotations are from AAers' verbal interaction during AA meetings, although many of these quotations originate in AA literature.

Before discussing the AA meeting as an interactional setting I shall consider whether AA membership is actually voluntary and I shall show that the central aim of AA is achieved in a manner that contrasts with the activities of crisis cults.

Voluntarism

The voluntary aspect of recruitment might be questioned since many AAers indicate that they were coerced to attend their first AA meeting. This is especially true of people who attend a few meetings under court orders.

Nonetheless, assertions made by AAers evidence the fundamentally voluntary nature of the association for people who consider themselves members. Most explicit is the saying, "AA is for those who want it, not those who need it." A sentence from the book *Alcoholics Anonymous* is often quoted in conversations: *"If you want what we have . . .* you are ready to take certain steps" (1955:58; italics mine).

The unpressured acceptance of newcomers further underscores the voluntary aspect of AA. Though it is often said, "no one gets here by mistake," the newcomer who is not sure he wants sobriety is told to go out and try some more controlled drinking. This is a simple recognition that an alcoholic must want sobriety before the program will work for him.

Powerlessness

Madsen asserts that AA members, like crisis cult members, believe in the supernatural in order to feel they have "control in a situation that otherwise seems uncontrollable" (1974a:27, also in this volume: 382). Seeking control does characterize crisis cults, especially cargo cults. The motivation for joining AA is to gain control over a seemingly uncontrollable behavior. But AAers do not themselves seek to exert this control over their situations. AAers seek a relationship with the supernatural in order to cease managing their own lives. This is an important contrast with the measures used by crisis cults to remedy uncontrollable situations. Cargo cult members attempt, for example, to control airplane landings. But AAers seek to discontinue all controlling behaviors by delegating the management of their lives to some higher power, usually a supernatural power.

The AA concept of control differs significantly from the concept of control presented to drunkards by the rest of society. The active alcoholic is often advised to control drinking, develop some backbone, or strengthen moral character. Sober members joke about the unsuitability of such advice. Its inappropriateness is that it enables the alcoholic to repeat his self-destructive behavior. As the victim of an overwhelming compulsion to drink, the alcoholic who attempts to control his drinking himself is bound to fail. AA, in contrast, tells the newcomer that his life is unmanageable and that it is ridiculous for him to try to manage it. The genius of AA is that it insists that an alcoholic is powerless and that such powerlessness must be conceded. Admission of powerlessness and discouragement of controlling behaviors have significant practical consequences. Whereas cargo cultists do not effect airplane landings, AAers do maintain sobriety. By deliberately denying the ability to control their lives, AAers' former drunken situations are brought under control.

The positive evaluation of the absence of control was indicated in the description of the newcomer who is never forced to want sobriety. Similarly, sober members do not attempt to control each other. One member may advise another, if asked, but no one is resented for not following advice. During a meeting members may mention their attempts to manage the lives of family and friends. Such managers are reminded that the desire to control others may lead to drinking.

Most importantly, abstinence is not considered a kind of control. The individual who comes to AA in order to control his drinking will be disappointed. AAers insist that abstinence is possible only when powerlessness is conceded. AA offers supportive interaction in which powerlessness comes to be positively valued.

The AA Meeting: An Interactional Context

The principles of voluntarism and powerlessness were discovered in the verbal activity of AA members. Turning now to the context of that verbal interaction, I will describe some pertinent aspects of AA meetings. The type of meeting to be considered is the discussion meeting.[1]

Most discussion meetings have a chairman. There is no authority attached to that role. He simply opens and closes the meetings and calls on assembled members to speak, one by one. The person who plays the role of chairman may change from week to week, or less frequently depending on the desires of the group. Such desires are made known in casual conversation, before or after the hour-long meeting. The chairman is not necessarily the person who has maintained sobriety longest. This role and other responsibilities do not serve to rank members, for they are alternately shared by all.

The chairman directs only the sequential order in which members' contributions are heard. Though he may suggest a discussion topic, no one is obliged to address it.

The chairman opens the meeting and identifies himself as an alcoholic, as do other members when they are called upon. Comments from some members indicate that this self-labeling serves as a leveling device. Whatever differences exist among members, they share a fundamental similarity as alcoholics.

As the chairman calls on one and then another member, each talks about anything he cares to discuss. If he does not want to talk, he simply "passes." Usually each member gives a brief monologue.

Despite the large amount of "experience, strength, and hope" verbalized during AA meetings, the format of meetings is nonconversational. Thus the term "monologue" is used in this discussion. Member's monologues are put "on the table," with or without reference to anything said by the previous speakers. One person may describe a recent traumatic event in his life. The next speaker may discuss something trivial by comparison. This does not mean that the traumatized member is ignored in favor of minor concerns. Members are not talking past each other. The net result of an evening's monologues is to level the highs and lows of all members. Such leveling is of practical significance to members who assert that despair and elation are equally dangerous to sobriety.

The one-at-a-time format is not rigidly followed. For example, one alcoholic couple reveals the brittle nature of their relationship by interrupting and commenting on each other's monologue. This is an extreme example, yet it illustrates the tolerance that members extend to each other. This couple displayed such "deviance" for a year yet no one voiced objection to their departure from the standard format.

It was indicated above that the act of self-labeling as "alcoholic" operates as a leveling device. In keeping with this, length of sobriety is rarely mentioned by an alcoholic in his self-labeling. Contradictory notions exist as to the importance of sheer length of sobriety. Thus, if a member mentions his term of sobriety he is likely to add, "the person who got up earliest today is the one who is sober longest." The saying "one day at a time" is taken seriously. There is similar meaning in the expression, "we are all just one drink away from a drunk."

Most discussion group monologues have the structure, "what I was like, what happened, and what I am like now." Contrary to Madsen's comparison of the AA member to the religious convert, "what I am like now" is rarely in stark contrast to "what I was like." "What I am like now" often consists of a list of character defects that have been carried over from drinking days. In further contrast to religious converts, AAers attest to a long process of personal improvement. Many long-term members indicate that their personal growth and development did not begin with the onset of abstinence. Some say that all they did in the early years of sobriety was "not drink and come to meetings." Older members advise newcomers to "take it easy" and "don't compare your insides with other peoples' outsides." Hence I suggest that, in the minds of sober alcoholics, the interactional sphere of AA is more crucial to sobriety than a philosophical or theological sphere. Attending meetings and observing other sober alcoholics is more important than introspection or reading AA literature. Interaction with sober alcoholics is valued by members. Interaction, not philosophical tenets, is the most appropriate focus of investigation.

Egalitarian Interaction

Much of the foregoing discussion characterizes AA as an egalitarian group. In egalitarian groups members are not ranked. Rights and privileges do not accrue to members differentially. Leadership is flexible and does not constitute authority. The egalitarian nature of AA contrasts with the hierarchically structured society within which it exists. Despite members' remarks that "AA has the largest admission fees of any organization in the world," no one who desires sobriety may be excluded.

The egalitarian nature of AA corroborates some assertions made by Bateson (1971). For Bateson, AA philosophy provides drinkers with relationships of complementarity as opposed to the competitive, risk-taking relations that lead the drinking alcoholic again and again to challenge the power of the bottle. Bateson comments that AA is an excellent illustration of a Durkheimian religious system, i.e., a system in which concepts of how man relates to God are directly reflected in patterned human interaction. According to Bateson, the AA notion of God is a higher power that neither rewards nor punishes. Bateson concludes that this idea of God is paralleled in the "strictly democratic" interactions among members, as these interactions are outlined in AA literature.

Though discussion here has focused on people rather than theology, members often remind each other, "AA is a spiritual program." Interpretation of this statement is up to the individual. An individual may identify his higher power as "God," as the AA group itself, or whatever he chooses. By focusing on interaction of members "on the ground" this discussion stresses the social aspect of spirituality. The social manifestation of spiritual principles seems more important to AAers than theological notions. This is borne out in a member's remark: "AA is here, not to save your soul, but to save your ass." Like sobriety itself, any spiritual growth attained by members must be shared rather than kept to oneself. It is said that "you can't keep it unless you give it away." "It" is best shared in the interactional context of meetings.

It is possible to provide only a sketch of AA meeting interaction here. Other aspects of relationships among recovering alcoholics are significant for understanding the recovery process. Description of interaction before and after meetings as well as more refined analysis of interaction during meetings is needed.

Conclusion

An aim of this paper has been to clarify the importance of group interaction for recovering alcoholics. It is not my intention to give artificial primacy to the study of interaction over study of values.

Ideational and interactional realms are inextricably linked. But it does seem that the understanding of currently proliferating self-help groups will be more reflective of members' perceptions if investigators scrutinize on-the-ground interaction of members rather than the literature of the groups.

Fieldwork methods have been developed by anthropologists for the study of small groups of non-Western peoples. These methods, especially the participant observation technique, are equally fruitful for the study of groups in industrialized societies. But anthropological labels such as "crisis cult" that were devised to categorize specific non-Western phenomena must be used cautiously when extended to urban, Western peoples.

Note

1. "Brands" of AA are varied in different parts of the United States. Consequently, the description of a discussion meeting herein characterizes the type found in a single midwestern community; however, similarities have been observed in discussion meetings elsewhere.

Alcoholism and the Irish
Dermot Walsh

That the Irish and alcohol do not mix, or mix too well, has been known for a very long time. Literary and historical sources give impressive support to this contention. Thus the historian, MacLysaght, from an extensive study of sources declares, "Drunkenness seems to have been a national weakness at most times. Allusion is made to it by almost all authorities I have consulted on morals, manners and customs, native and gaelic as well as Anglo-Irish or English and continental" (1950:72). Many travelers in Ireland, English and continental, and such well known commentators as Dunton (1699), Fynes Moryson (1904), Sir William Petty (1927), and Arthur Young (1892) have all commented on the prevalence of excessive drinking and drunkenness in seventeenth- and eighteenth-century Ireland. An Irishman, Doctor O'Grady (1923), in his biography of Thomas Wentworth, the Earl of Strafford, Lord Deputy for Ireland under Charles I from 1632 until 1640, has assembled a great deal of evidence to show the prevalence of excessive drinking in Ireland in the first half of the seventeenth century.

That this excessive drinking was not the prerogative of any one class is indicated by Richard Head's observations of the Irish gentry in which he says that "if you, on a visit to them, do not drink freely then they think they have not made you welcome; so that a man knows not how to take leave until he is unable to stir a foot." (1647). Professor J. C. Beckett in *The Making of Modern Ireland* (1966) asserts that "the country gentry of eighteenth-century Ireland have passed into popular history as they are portrayed in the pages of Sir Jonah Barrington and Miss Edgeworth; and the picture as generally perceived is at least as true as such pictures commonly are. Hundreds of gentlemen and half-gentlemen, however impecunious themselves, however wretched their tenants, lived lavish and riotous lives. The resident gentry, wrote a critical observer in the 1770s, enjoy their possessions so thoroughly, and in a manner so truly Irish, that they generally become beggars in a few years' time, by dint of hospitality and inadvertence. But even 'Beggary,' did not necessarily bring this gay life to an end; for the cost, in terms of money, was inconsiderable. Servants' wages were a mere trifle; provisions were produced on their own lands or obtained on credit; the universal practice of illicit distillation meant that whiskey was plentiful and cheap; smuggled brandy and claret were easily come by. To entertain their neighbors, and be entertained by them, at drinking and field-sports, was almost the sum total of their activities, and probably formed a fair index of their notions of social responsibility and public duty" (Beckett 1966: 181–82).

Sir Jonah Barrington himself, a most interesting observer of contemporary life, in his "personal sketches" separates the gentry of Ireland into three classes thus:

1. Half-mounted gentlemen
2. Gentlemen, every inch of them
3. Gentlemen to the backbone [1968]

Barrington in a sketch entitled "Irish Dissipation in 1778" describes attending a party where he says numerous toasts of buttered claret were consumed and each guest voluntarily surrendered a portion of his own reason in bumpers to the duty of his neighbor's toast. Claret flowed, bumpers were multiplied, and Barrington goes on, "My reason began gradually to lighten me of its burden and two rattling pipers, a jigging fiddler and twelve voices in twelve different keys all swelling in one continuous unrelenting chime was the last point of recognition which Bacchus permitted me to exercise for my eyes began to perceive a much larger company than the room actually contained, the lights were more than doubled without any virtual increase in their numbers and even the chairs and tables commenced dancing a series of minuets for me." He remembered no more until "at noon, next day, a scene of a different nature was exhibited. I found, on awakening, two associates by my side in as perfect insensibility as that from which I had just aroused" (1968: 43–44).

McCarthy in his book *Irish Land and Irish Liberty*, written in the early twentieth century, says, "Amongst the Irish Catholics, drink is the synonym for hospitality. It stands alone and is not associated with food. Every festive meeting, every social call, every business transaction, must be wet, as they say, with a drink. The man that does not stand a drink is considered a mean man; the man that gives drink freely in his own house and pays for it for others in public-houses is a 'decent fellow.' There is a kind of veneration for the man who has spent a fortune or ruined a career by drink; and people expatiate on the great things he might have done, if it were not for drink." (1911).

Thus the heroic spirit of Ireland insisted that there was no more honorable way in which a man, be he rich or poor, might ruin his career and even his life than by drink.

No doubt some of these pictures of Irish drinking were exaggerated for literary effect by people such as Barrington and heightened by the natural antagonism of English visitors such as Arthur Young.

This heroic spirit, however, was to be countered in the nineteenth century by the abstinence or temperance movements. There were sporadic and usually local attempts to establish such movements, generally by men of religion, in various parts of Ireland and Harrison in his recent book *Drink and the Victorians* (1971) tells us that the first antispirits society was founded in the Quaker meeting house in New Ross in the early 1830s. Both in Ireland and in England Quaker influence in leading temperance movements was very strong. However, earlier attempts at the formation of temperance societies in Ireland are on record and the Ulster Temperance Society was founded in 1829. However, the temperance movement in Ireland really got under way with the arrival on the scene of Father Theobald Mathew (1790 to 1856). Father Mathew was a Capuchin priest from Cork and his own account of his conversion to the temperance movement reveals "it was the Quakers in Cork who were always asking me to do something about the people's temperance societies" (Harrison 1971). Shortly afterwards he embarked on his career as an advocate of temperance in 1838. According to the Dictionary of National Biography, as quoted by Connell (1968), Mathew was credited with administering more than five million pledges to nearly half the adult population of Ireland (although Longmate in *The Water Drinkers* contends that many of these lapsed within a short time) "with such effect that a taste for music replaces a taste for tippling; that the spirit revenue fell from one million, four hundred and thirty-five thousand pounds in 1839 to eight hundred and fifty-two thousand pounds in 1844; that twenty thousand bankrupt publicans left the country; and the police idled for want of crime" (Longmate 1968). Mathew was associated with the liberator Daniel O'Connell during his massive public campaigning for the repeal of the Act of Union of 1800. They often appeared on the same platform and commanded audiences of hundreds of thousands of people. Of course O'Connell's gift of oratory and appeal are legendary and together they must have provided many a stimulating evening. Thousands and thousands were reported as joining O'Connell and Mathew on their knees in taking the abstinence pledge at these meetings.

Father Mathews's English campaigns were equally successful and Harrison tells us that Father Mathew was feted by London society, defended by London police, championed by Irish peers, and that Lord Stanhope, the earl of Arundel, publically took the pledge from him before London crowds in 1843, and Lord John Russell addressed a meeting designed to raise money for him. However, the widespread parliamentary support for Mathew may have been not entirely without self-interest for the English at this time had the mistaken notion that a sober Ireland might be less troublesome than a drunken one, and the cynical might note that Mathew was in 1847 awarded a government pension. Father Mathew died in 1856. Eight years later a statue to him was unveiled in Cork, but within a few years, on three of the four corners of the same square, stood public houses. It was said that at least Father Mathew had his back to them.

The next notable development in the nineteenth-century Irish abstinence story was the formation by a Jesuit priest, Father Cullen, of the Pioneer Total Abstinence Association in the year 1889.

With the establishment of a national system of mental hospitals throughout Ireland during the nineteenth century from 1830 to the 1880s, to provide specifically for the lunatic poor who were previously housed either in poorhouses or prisons, increasing numbers of individuals were admitted for alcoholism. A survey of the hospital registers at the time shows that "intemperance and whiskey" were frequently given as supposed causes of patients' insanity. However, it wasn't until the next century that the Mental Treatment Act of 1945 gave formal recognition to alcoholism as a specific disorder requiring treatment and acknowledged that it was sometimes a characteristic of this disorder that the patient did not realize that he was ill and needed treatment by providing for the compulsory admission and detention of alcoholics in mental hospitals as addicts.

During the 1950s and in the 1960s there were significant improvements in the therapeutic facilities available for alcoholics, particularly in private psychiatric hospitals and later in local authority hospitals, and the impact of these improved facilities is already apparent from the results of some studies that will be mentioned.

The first European branch of Alcoholics Anonymous was established in Dublin in November 1946, and since then the organization has continued to grow and there are now meetings of Alcoholics Anoymous held in 150 centers in Ireland.

In 1961 the minister for health, Mr. Sean MacEntee, established a Commission of Enquiry on Mental Illness and this commission reported in 1966. Concerning alcoholism, the commission declared itself satisfied "on the basis of the experience of psychiatrists practising in Ireland and daily dealing with its effects, that the problem of people who cannot control their consumption of beverages containing alcohol is a very serious one which requires immediate attention."

The commission report did not neglect the need of research—"the commission recommends that sample surveys both of Irish drinking patterns and of the probable prevalence of alcoholism would be of great value in assessing the extent of the problem created by the abuse of alcohol."

National concern at the problem of alcoholism in this country bore practical fruit when, following a visit by Marty Mann, the Irish National Council on Alcoholism was established following informal meetings of psychiatrists and laymen in early 1966. Mr. Richard Perceval, whose work for the council since its inception has been of such magnitude and success, was appointed executive director in July 1966, and the council was registered as a company in December 1966. The council received a grant through the minister of health, the late Mr. Donagh O'Malley, of 2,000 pounds and since then it has been able to continue its work through the munificence of the nineteen health authorities and private donors. Early in 1967 registered offices were opened in Dublin and Mrs. Mary O'Hagan was appointed as social worker in charge of the advisory services of the council.

From the research point of view it is true to say that until recent years there had been little research into the problem of alcoholism in Ireland. However, in 1965 the Medico-Social Research Board was established to enquire into the influence of social factors on medical problems in Ireland. One of the activities of the Medico-Social Research Board has been to take over from the Department of Health the National Psychiatric In-Patient Reporting System which was established in 1963. Thus the board has been able to monitor the numbers and the characteristics of patients entering psychiatric hospitals for the treatment of alcoholism over the years. This activity has given us the basis for some assumptions with regard to the incidence of alcoholism in this country. However, these figures relate only to hospitalized illnesses and hence indicate only the lower limit of incidence of the conditions. We have not had in this country an adequate community survey of these conditions and so the upper limit of their incidence must remain hypothetical. However, in regard to the lower limit, as measured by first admissions to psychiatric hospitals, the following data may be of interest. In 1965 there were 699 first admissions to Irish psychiatric hospitals with a diagnosis of alcoholism or alcoholic psychosis. Numbers of first admissions then continued to rise steadily up to 1969 when there were 1,181 first admissions for alcoholism and alcoholic psychosis to Irish hospitals. This represents an increase of 69 percent from 1965 to 1969, and a rise in rates per 100,000 of population from 24 in 1965 to 41 per 100,000 of population in 1969. In 1969 admissions for alcoholism comprised almost 16 percent of all first admissions to psychiatric hospitals. First admissions for alcoholism among males alone accounted for over 28 percent of all male first admissions. The disease expectancy based on the 1970 first admission rates and the 1966 population, gives a risk of 3.8 percent for all people surviving to age 65—that is to say that almost 4 out of every 100 people in Ireland will be admitted to a psychiatric hospital for alcoholism at least once in his or her lifetime. When the risk is calculated for males alone the figure is practically doubled. These are striking figures indeed and compare with corresponding figures for England and Wales for 1969 for "alcoholism and all other addictions combined," of 0.7 percent for males and 0.2 percent for females (Great Britain, Dept. of Health and Soc. Sec. 1969). The shortcomings of first admissions to hospitals as indicators of incidence and prevalence of alcohol are well known. As an example, a limited community survey of alcoholism in a Dublin working-class housing estate of 40,000 persons in 1966 and 1967, by Kearney, Lawlor and Walsh (1969), indicated that a very substantial degree of alcoholic drinking was not being treated at all indicating that there was a large gap between the upper and lower limits of the extent of the condition. Accordingly, the 70 percent increase between 1965 and 1969 must be interpreted with caution. At the polarities or extremes of interpretation it may be that the increase in first admissions to hospital exactly mirrors a similar increase in the extent of the problem in the community. At the other extreme it may be interpreted as meaning that there has been no increase in the extent of the problem in the community but that substantially more people are entering hospital for treatment for the condition. Some measure of support for this latter interpretation is given by examination of the changes in first admission rates for other diagnoses in the same time period of 1965 to 1969. Thus the percentage increase in first admissions for all psychiatric conditions from 1965 to 1969 was of the order of 22.4 percent. The increase in first admissions for schizophrenia has been low, only 2.3 percent; for manic depressive psychosis 11 percent; for organic psychosis 12 percent. The overall increase for all psychotic conditions, whether functional or organic has been 8.5 percent. On the other hand, there has been an increase of 38 percent for psychoneuroses and 63 percent for personality disorder. Accordingly, a tentative hypothesis suggests that the changes in first admission rates to Irish psychiatric hospitals over this five-year period may indicate an increase in willingness of persons to seek hospital treatment for milder psychiatric disorders. The study of alcoholism in a working-class housing estate by Kearney, Lawlor, and Walsh already mentioned, had indicated that a good deal of working-class alcoholism went untreated because working-class alcoholics refused treatment. In local authority hospitals the first admission increase from 1965 to 1969 was from 258 first admissions to 560 first admissions, an increase of 117 percent; whereas for private hospitals the increase was from 441 first admissions to 621, an increase of 41 percent. This confirms that a greater number of working-class people are accepting treatment in local authority hospitals and that it is this increase in working-class admissions which accounts for the greater part of the 69 percent increase observed from 1965 to 1969. If this hypothesis is true it represents a very rapid and heartening change for the good in the changed community attitude towards alcoholism and the willingness of persons to seek treatment for the condition. Whether treatment will prove effective is something which we cannot evaluate at the moment, but it is worth noting in passing that since April 1972 the National Psychiatric In-Patient Reporting System has introduced record linkage and so it will be possible to follow cohorts of hospitalized alcoholic patients over time and therefore to give some indication as to prognosis and change in prognosis for the condition.

Evidence of the Irish susceptibility to alcoholism has also come from countries outside Ireland. The data from the United States and from the United Kingdom seem fairly consistent on this point, that is that of all ethnic groups the Irish are most susceptible to alcoholism, whether measured by first admissions to hospital, or, as in the case of the study of Hyde and Chisholm, rejectees for army enlistment in the United States (1944). In 1970 admissions to psychiatric hospitals in England and Wales were classified by place of birth and so it is possible to examine the first admission rates to the hospitals of England and Wales of those who on admission gave Ireland as their birthplace. I am indebted to Dr. Brothwood of the Department of Health and Social Security for data for 1970 which show the first admission rate for "all other nonpsychotic disorders" (a group which consists of I.C.D. No. 302 sexual deviation, 303 alcoholism, 304 drug dependence, 305 physical disorders of psychogenic origin, 306 special symptoms, 307 transient situational disturbances, 308 behavior disorders of childhood, and 309 mental disorders not specified as psychotic associated with physical conditions) to be 49 per 100,000 of population (of a total first admission rate of 126 per 100,000 of population for all diagnoses) for Irish-born patients first admitted to psychiatric hospitals and units in England and Wales in 1970. Of this group of disorders—which excludes alcoholic psychosis—alcoholism almost certainly accounts for the majority and so it is fair to assume that the first admission rate for the Irish in England is probably as high as it is among the Irish in Ireland and compares with a first admission rate of 10 per 100,000 of population for "alcoholism and other addictions" among the native-born in England and Wales in 1970.

Duffy and Dean (1971) have investigated the frequency of cirrhosis of the liver from a large Irish autopsy series of almost eight thousand and found that fifty-eight of these deaths were from cirrhosis. They had done so because the official incidence of cirrhosis of the liver from certified deaths in Ireland is low. Their study found that although the rate of death from cirrhosis among the autopsies was higher than the certified death rate from cirrhosis, it was still low by international standards.

Professor Wilson, head of the Department of Pharmacology in Trinity College, has for some time been investigating the mechanisms involved in the taste for alcohol. As he says, "One of the principal factors which characterizes the consumption of alcohol among individuals and races is the taste for drink." He has been concerned with investigating the relationships between alcohol consumption and food intake and the relationships of human taste threshold to alcohol and its implications. Professor Wilson sees the relationship of individual human variation to alcohol taste threshold as a link in the chain between the external environment and the physiological mechanisms which ultimately lead to alcoholic addiction. Professor Wilson and his colleagues have also been studying the effect of group size and composition on the differential preference of ratios for water and alcoholic solutions.

The per capita consumption of alcohol in Ireland has by international standards been low. Thus in 1966 the Irish per capita consumption of alcohol per head of population aged fifteen and over was 5.8 litres of pure alcohol compared with 5.9 for the United Kingdom, 7.6 for the United States, 11.3 for West Germany, and 20.8 for France, all for the same year. On the other hand, the Irish per capita consumption is rising steadily. Thus the annual consumption in gallons of pure alcohol per head of total population rose from 0.67 in 1953 to 1.05 in 1970, an increase over this time period of 58 percent.

In 1953, 77 percent of total intake (excluding wine) came from beer and 23 percent from spirits; in 1970, 68 percent of intake was from beer and 32 percent from spirits.

Walsh and Walsh (1970) concluded from a study of alcohol consumption time trends in Ireland that with rising level of income, the quantity of alcohol consumed per head of population would grow rapidly and that spirit consumption would increase more rapidly than beer consumption, and that with increasing income most of the growth will be due to a very rapid growth of spirit consumption. One of the most serious problems created by dependence on alcohol, and one frequently prominent in the etiology of serious depressive psychiatric illness in families of poorer socioeconomic groups, is shortage of money and consequent heavy indebtedness. If expenditure on alcohol is a sizable proportion of total income the amount available for food, rent, clothing, and other necessities may be insufficient to meet minimal requirements. Walsh and Walsh examined the economic aspects of alcohol consumption in Ireland with international comparisons. The result of these investigations, based on household budget enquiry data and national income data from the United Nations national accounts yearbook, were that in the Irish Republic in 1970 expenditure on alcoholic beverages as a percentage of total personal expenditure on goods and services was over 11 percent and the next highest country for which data are available was Austria in 1967 with 7.68 and France, which in 1965 had a figure of 6.45 (Walsh and Walsh 1970).

These financial income data support the view that an unusually high percentage of Irish personal expenditure is devoted to alcohol. While this is largely due to the high price of alcohol in Ireland relative to income per person, it does indicate that the Irish attach great importance to alcohol consumption. If the price of alcohol continues to increase more rapidly than the general price level, it appears likely that the proportion of total expenditure devoted to alcohol will also continue to rise.

In recent times there has been a growing consensus that the science of sociology can complement the study of the historical development of attitudes and the study of individual and national psychologies by attempting to study the cultural and social determinants of drinking. Thus the study of normal drinking habits is added to the older study of problem drinking—though these are clearly complementary. Attitudes, then, in various cultural and social settings, are the product of a racial or national history, and understanding of these attitudes may lead to preventive, educational, and public health measures.

The first approach of this type undertaken in Ireland was initiated when the minister for health, Mr. Sean Flannagan, made a grant of 1,500 pounds to the Department of Psychiatry, U.C.D., supplementing 500 pounds that had already been donated by the Irish National Council on Alcoholism, towards funding a research fellowship for two years. The research fellow was Miss Joyce Fitzpatrick and her work was carried out in conjunction with a joint research committee of the Irish National Council on Alcoholism, the Department of Psychiatry, University College Dublin, and the Medico-Social Research Board. Her work entitled "Drinking among Young People" concerned a study of the attitudes and practices of two hundred young Dubliners, and on the conclusion of this two-year project the Irish National Council on Alcoholism, the Department of Psychiatry, University College Dublin, the Medico-Social Research Board, and later the Department of Social Science, University College Dublin, joined with the Medical Council on Alcoholism of Great Britain in undertaking a joint Anglo-Irish project.

I have, in a very superficial way, tried to review the Irish addiction scene in its historical context, in the development of the heroic tradition of Irish drinking followed by the abstinence movements of the nineteenth century, the provision of treatment facilities, the setting up of suitable mental health legislation to deal with the problem, and more recently the awareness of professional workers and of central and local authorities, of the need for research into the extent and the origins of the alcoholic problem. I have briefly described some of the research activity that has been undertaken and that is proceeding in this country. I think it is clear that these activities, whether thereapeutic, research, or preventive, undertaken in the last two decades in Ireland, indicate the concern with what is a characteristically Irish problem, the moving away of public attitudes from accepting a stereotype of Irish role-fulfillment towards a standpoint of responsible public attitudes to the problems of alcoholism.

The Great Jewish Drink Mystery

Mark Keller

It is particularly appropriate for me to speak on the great Jewish drink mystery, for I happen to have created it—as a modern topic, that is. Let me tell you how it happened.

In the early 1940s, what was to become the famous Yale (and now is the Rutgers) Center of Alcohol Studies was just beginning to take shape. It had no name yet, but Dr. Howard W. Haggard, the director of the Yale Laboratory of Applied Physiology, had begun to collect a staff of nonphysiologists who were interested in alcohol and in the study of its problems. One day as I sat by his desk, he quite suddenly fired a surprise question at me: Suppose there was a chance to do some research on the causes of drunkenness or alcoholism. Did I have any ideas for any kind of fresh research direction? And at the moment, stimulated to make a good impression on the big boss, I succeeded in touching the right button on my unconscious computer, and out came an idea. I said: "Dr. Haggard, everybody naturally thinks the secrets of alcoholism can be learned from alcoholics, that if one studies them the right way, the mystery of why they become alcoholics will be uncovered. Maybe. But wouldn't it be a good idea to study those who don't become alcoholics? I mean such a group as the Jews. It happens that practically all Jews do drink, and yet all the world knows that Jews hardly ever become alcoholics. Why? What protects them? If we could discover that, wouldn't it be a masterly clue?"

Dr. Haggard, a lightning-fast thinker, replied immediately: "All right, Mr. Keller—and suppose we discover why the Jews don't become alcoholics. How are we going to convert 150 million Americans to Judaism?"

But after we finished laughing over his witticism—which was to prove astoundingly insightful—Dr. Haggard did not neglect this idea, and he raised the first substantial research money to study Jewish drinking. Out of this came a number of studies at the Yale Center, including Ruth Landman's study (1952) of drinking by children attending religious schools, and especially Charles Snyder's dissertation, *Culture and Sobriety* (1954)—renamed, when published, *Alcohol and the Jews* (1958).

In the meantime, at Harvard, another bright graduate student in sociology, Robert Freed Bales, had gotten interested in this subject, and long before Snyder—whose excellence is not manifested in speed—was ready to publish, Bales got his Ph.D. with a dissertation (1944) based on the hypothesis of a "fixation factor" in alcohol addiction, derived from a comparative study of Irish and Jewish social norms and drinking behaviors.

And on the west coast, Donald Davison Glad tackled this problem from still another but closely allied angle, and produced a dissertation (1947a) and a publication (1947b) describing the attitudes toward drinking, and the practices, of Irish and Jewish boys in the United States, as compared with differences in rates of inebriety among adults in these population groups.

Undoubtedly my suggestion that Jewish drinking should be studied was founded on the repeated encounter of references to the sobriety or temperance of the Jews, the absence of drunkenness or alcoholism among them. Immanuel Kant (Jellinek 1941) had written about it in Germany, and had even bothered to formulate an explanatory hypothesis about it—philosophically profound but psychologically naive. In England the great Dr. Norman Kerr (1888) had remarked upon the absence of inebriety among the Jews, and in the United States, Robert Hunter (1904) and Morris Fishberg (1911). Cheinisse (1908) and Durkheim (1897) wrote about it in France. In Russia it is alluded to in a fascinating tale by the great folklorist, N.S. Leskov (1957) in a story about "Immortal Golovan," a folk hero beloved among the peasantry. Mystical powers were attributed to Golovan. He was supposed to have acquired the bezoar stone, which warded off the plague. Because he used his powers only for good, his irreligiosity was tolerated. Even such "un-Christian behavior" as giving milk to the Jew Yushka for his children was overlooked, since the peasants assumed his motive was to extract from the Jews their two valuable secrets: that of the Judas lips, which enable one to speak falsehood in court; and that of the hairy vegetable, which enabled the Jews to drink without getting drunk!

I will not repeat the extensive documentation (Snyder 1954) of the observations of Jewish sobriety in country after country after country.

Since the Jews, after all, are more likely to eat a piece of herring with their drink than a slice of mandrake—I imagine that's what the hairy vegetable was supposed to be—some other protective factor must be at work.

I hope you do not expect me to reveal that magnificent secret on this occasion—though if I knew it, I would. I shall try to review briefly what has been studied and proposed and supposed. My main contribution will be to point out the area or the time on which I think research is most needed, where I think the secret is wrapped up. And along the way I hope to call attention to some materials which have not been attended to by the academic researchers thus far.

Bales (1944) compared Irish with Jewish drinking ways, on the basis of documentary evidence. He found it possible broadly to characterize the drinking of the Irish as convivial; that is, the mainly sought effect was achieved through the pharmacological action of alcohol. The Jews, by virtue of cultural practices effective from infancy, acquired a ritual attitude toward drinking, and learned to use it chiefly for communion. The pharmacological effect of alcohol was secondary and could not be allowed to become dominant, as that would frustrate the fundamental motive. Thus the Jews could not permit themselves drunkenness. They were fixated on sobriety in drinking. Obviously, people who don't get drunk can hardly acquire the condition of alcoholism. The protective culture phenomenon is inherent in the religion, in the practice of sanctifying important rites, especially the rites of passage, by drinking wine and blessing it—at circumcision, when the infant boy is given his first taste of the ceremonial wine; at the transitions from weekdays to Sabbaths and festivals, in the kiddush, and back again to the weekdays in the habdalah; at the wedding ceremony, when the man and his bride drink wine from the same cup; and on other valued occasions. The inculcated ritual attitude toward drink is carried over into everyday life, so that the abuse of drink would be unthinkable. That, very briefly, is the essence of Bales' hypothesis.

Snyder (1958) went out into the community to study. He surveyed a randomly formed sample of the Jews of a New England city. He also analyzed the responses of a sizable sample of Jewish students in the Straus and Bacon (1953) college drinking survey, dividing them into four categories of religious attitude or affiliation: Orthodox, Conservative, Reform, and Secular. Among the population and among the students alike, the experience of intoxication was on a continuum, with those most adhering to orthodox or religious practices experiencing the least intoxication. This in spite of the fact that the Orthodox tended to drink most frequently. After considering some alternative hypotheses, Snyder concluded that Bales in essence was right. The culture of the Jews, as influenced by the religion, acted as an inhibitor of drunkenness. A drunkard was defined by Jews as alien. Snyder believed he saw some indications that as acculturation proceeded, as orthodoxy waned and secularism waxed, signs of an increased rate of alcoholism among Jews were emerging.

D. D. Glad (1947b) studied attitudes of Jewish and Irish boys and discovered quite distinctive differences undoubtedly related to their background. The Irish boys thought of drinking as promoting fun, pleasure, conviviality; the Jewish boys thought of it as socially practical and religiously symbolic and communicative.

Always it seems to come to the same thing: the Jewish culture, dominantly influenced by the religion, evokes attitudes which inhibit drinking to drunkenness, even while it encourages frequent but controlled drinking.

In fairness I should warn that, while a variety of alternate psychological, sociological, and anthropological hypotheses have been considered and sometimes tested by these and other theorists—Glad, for example, tested the parental-permissiveness hypothesis but found no support for it—one important biological hypothesis has been brushed aside rather cavalierly by the social scientists: that the Jews may have some sort of genetic immunity to alcoholism. As an observer not committed to either side I must say that the reasoning against the purely biological hypothesis is less than conclusive. Insofar as this reasoning is based on the fact that no biological necessary cause of alcoholism in anybody has yet been discovered, the position is negatively sound enough, but a door to doubt must be kept open, for biology has by no means yet spoken its last word on this subject. Insofar as the antibiological reasoning is based on the notion that Jews are not a genetic unity, it is practically on a level with superstition. Of course the Jews are not a pure "race," like laboratory stocks of mice. But they constitute a sufficiently inbred strain or group of strains to have a substantial number of genetic traits in relative frequency; and a genetic trait which could influence the chances of alcoholism—if such a thing existed at all—could well prevail among Jews. But in the present state of knowledge, it would be hardly anything but superstition to adopt a genetic hypothesis, while ignoring the powerful indications of psychology and sociology.

Now I have reviewed the state of knowledge briefly and at this point it seems appropriate to ask: What is the great mystery? After all, it seems only a question of genetic versus cultural immunity, and in due time the researchers will presumably resolve the issue.

The great Jewish drink mystery which I have in mind is not just why don't the Jews get drunk today, but how did they get this way. I refer to the historical fact that the ancestors of the Jews were a bunch of renowned topers. Somehow, at some time, they reformed, or they gave it up—I mean gave up drunkenness, for they never gave up drinking. When did this happen? And how was it accomplished? If we could know that, might it not be the masterly clue we are looking for? Anyhow, my curiosity would be gratified.

Again, not to raise false hopes, I must warn that I am not about to deliver the answer. I don't know it. I am going to try to elucidate the problem and to pinpoint the time and place where I think the answer should be sought.

That the ancestors of the modern Jews were copious drinkers, rather like the French of recent times, is well documented in the Bible. I assume that—after the archaeological discoveries of recent years—and the discrediting of much of the pseudoscholarship of the "Higher" Bible Criticism, I need not take time to demonstrate the reliability of the Biblical record. In a very old part of it, the earthly blessing of the main tribe of the Hebrews, the Judah clan, whose totem, the lion-image, survives to this day at the holiest place in every Orthodox synagogue, reads in part as follows: "Binding his foal unto the vine, and his ass's colt unto the choice vine, he washes his garments in wine, and his clothes in the blood of grapes. His eyes shall be red with wine . . ." (Gen. 49:11–12). In other words, wine should flow more freely than water. It did, too, in the fruitful hills of Israel and Judaea. The much later Proverbist, too, included, among the rewards of virtue, "So shall thy barns be filled with plenty, and thy presses shall burst out with new wine" (3:10). And the inhabitants did not use the wine just for washing their garments or as a primitive Murine for their eyes. In very early days we find the high priest Eli readily mistaking Hannah, as she was whispering her prayers at the holy shrine, for a common drunkard (1 Sam.1:13–15). And all throughout, the Prophets inveigh against drunkenness as against a rampant evil, typified by Isaiah: "Woe unto them that rise up early in the morning that they may follow strong drink, that tarry late into the night, till wine inflame them!" (5:11). And again, "Woe unto them that are mighty to drink wine, and men of strength to mingle strong drink" (5:22). That sounds like long and hard drinking—and the Prophets were no temperance preachers in the modern sense, they never protested against drinking.

Right down to the destruction of the two kingdoms, to the exile of the Judaeans into the near lands, such as Egypt, and the farther lands, such as Babylonia, near the end of the sixth century B.C., the rich grape harvests were converted into wine, and copious drinking was the practice of many. There is a tendency to distinguish the Hebrews from the Canaanites. But this is like distinguishing the Normans from the French, or the Bulgars from the Slavs. The Hebrews were Canaanites, and multitudes of them repeatedly, as was the common practice in the ancient world, chose to honor the worship of other Canaanite gods than the One who was in the beginning the particular God of the Hebrew clan. Those other Canaanite gods, even Baal and Asherah, Dagan and Anat, and others, had interesting and attractive forms of worship— orgiastic festivals frowned upon by the peculiar Deity of the Hebrews, orgies intended to ensure the fertility of man and land, and in which drunkenness was blessed rather than rebuked.

What followed upon the first great national catastrophe, when an important segment of the population was taken captive into exile over twenty-five hundred years ago, is an essential part of the mystery which is my topic. The interesting fact is that from that time on we almost hear no more of drunkenness among the Jews. But it is not as simple as all that.

The Biblical account stops with the return from exile after only a few generations, and the resumption of a national form of life. We need to try to examine what happened to drinking during the first exile period and, after the restoration, during the time of the Second Temple.

How did the Jews behave with respect to drinking during that first exile? I cannot give an exact answer. I emphatically call attention to that period and this question because it is possible that it was then that drunkenness vanished or began to decline among the Jews. Perhaps it was connected with the disappearance of the Canaanite gods. If so, it is obviously of the utmost importance to understand what happened and how it happened.

Actually, there is some indication that the Jews in the Babylonian exile had not lost their interest in wine. The Midrash Rabbah on the Book of Esther attributes the catastrophe of Haman's plot to the fact that eighteen thousand five hundred Jews attended the great feast of Emperor Ahasuerus, "and they ate and drank, and became drunk, and were corrupted" (Chap. 7).

A Midrashic statement is not necessarily historical. It could have been invented by a rabbi several hundred years later, in approved exegetic style, for homiletic purposes. But the Midrash is full of historical as well as fanciful stories, and there is no reason to assume that a record or oral tradition did not survive which described the participation of the Perso-Median Jews in the grand empire festival, and which included an account of their excess in drinking. Wine was apparently plentiful, and as yet we have no evidence that copious drinking and drunkenness had been given up by the exiled Jewish population. Even if the Midrash is not based on a known fact but on an assumption that the preexilic behavior was continued, it is a reasonable assumption. Evidently the earliest authors of the idea that the Jews got drunk at the feast of Ahasuerus did not think that the preexilic drunkenness was abolished by the mere fact of exile.

We have no right to think so either—not until we acquire some evidence about it. But this may be the last reference to widespread drunkenness among the Jews.

We come then to the return, beginning in 537 B.C. We know from the Biblical record that only a minority returned to the land of Israel, and under the leadership of Ezra and Nehemiah, after much hardship and delay, they succeeded in building the Temple anew and established a distinctive national-cultural life. The high point of this restoration was the formal adoption of the Bible itself, the Torah, as the national constitution. The significant consequence was the rise of a new nonpolitical national leadership, of unsurpassed influence: the Scribes, the Bookmen, the Men of the Great Assembly, later the Pharisees and the Talmudic rabbis.

The remarkable thing about the ensuing period is the paucity of historical record. There are so few contemporary records of the next several hundred years that a historian must weep. It seems especially grievous when one reflects that the national leadership was assumed by a class known by the name of *soferim:* scribes!

In my opinion, from all that I can make out—and I have not researched in depth but have only skimmed what materials came to hand—it is during this period that drunkenness really was banished from Jewish life. It is in this time span, not more than two hundred years, between the establishment of the Second Temple and the reappearance of the Jews on the scene of world history, which happened with the advent of Alexander of Macedonia and the start of the Hellenistic epoch, that the basis of Jewish sobriety was firmly laid. For when the historical record becomes ample again, we no longer find any evidence of drunkenness, in a people who still cultivated the vine, still poured out libations of wine to God, drank at many ceremonies, and drank with pleasure.

In this period the scribes, whose leaders constituted the famed Men of the Great Assembly, as successors to Ezra the Scribe, firmly established the institution of the synagogue, the "little sanctuary" in every community, which became a center of local worship and learning so mingled that worship and study could hardly be told apart. They established popular education, education for the common people. They democratized their own class: anybody, not just a hereditary priest or Levite, could become a scribe and a member of the Great Assembly—later a pharisee or a rabbi. They preserved the traditions and compiled and edited the sacred texts, and fixed the ritual practices and composed liturgic formulas and benedictions. One of their embellishments was to fix the rule that the pronouncement of the advent of the Sabbath, on Friday eve—the Sanctification of the Sabbath— the kiddush—should be recited over a blessed cup of wine. The regular and popular ceremonial drinking of wine, apart from its continued use in sacrificial libations in the Holy Temple, was their initiative. Was it in association with and in consequence of these developments—the remolding of the whole culture, and the embedding in that religious culture of a particular sort of use of wine and a particular attitude toward drinking—that drunkenness declined remarkably? I think we must at least suspect this.

Not, however, that drunkenness was forgotten. Indeed, it continued to be a matter of concern, and continued to be feared— as I shall attempt to show. And if remembered, and if still feared, then we must assume that it was still sometimes manifested, as we should expect. There were still winebibbers, as the phrase in Matthew suggests (11:19). But no longer was inebriety common, no longer a national trait and problem. Drinking was under control. In due time, the control was to become so well established that even the fear and all but the formal remembrance of drunkenness was to vanish, as I hope to show, and the behavior was to become an attribute of the others, the non-we's, the non-Jews—as Snyder has shown.

It is in the Midrashim and the Talmud that we find the post-Biblical indications of the disappearance of drunkenness but the survival of the fear of it.

I believe it is subtly illustrated in the rhymed toast which Rabbi Akiba (first century) recited over each cup of wine at the grand feast he gave when his son was ordained: "Wine and life in the mouth of scholars, life and wine in the mouth of students." It sounds cautionary. It says, as we drink, we must remember that for finished scholars, adults, wine may take precedence over that which is our life (the Torah, the substance of scholarship), but for younger men, life—learning—must take precedence, drinking must be secondary. Even as he offered wine he had to offer this caution.

But the survival of the fear of drunkenness seems exquisitely illustrated in the ancient formula, doubtless going back to the days of the Great Assembly, for initiating a ceremonial benediction over a cup of wine, as at kiddush, or habdalah, or for the grace after meals. We read: " . . . he [the precentor, exhibiting the cup of wine in his hand] is required to say, *sabre maranan, hayayin mishtaker*" (that is, "By your leave," or "Attention, my masters, wine causes drunkenness!"); the text continues: "and he says this out of fear; but they respond, *le-haiim*" (that is, "It's for life," or "for health" (Beth Joseph, sec. 167). It seems to me enormously significant that the introductory formula to the use of the cup of blessing should have been a warning of the danger of intoxication in the use of wine, and that he who was to drink it should have required the permissive toast of the company, assuring him that this use was approved, safe, for life and health.

Equally interesting is that, in due course, this cautionary formula vanished! Among western Jews, the kiddush begins with the *sabre*, "attention, please," and proceeds to the benediction of the wine without waiting for any response. The danger of intoxication is not mentioned. Among the Sephardic Jews, when the precentor opens with *sabre*, the company still respond, as of yore, *le-haiim,* "to life" or "to your health"—but the warning of intoxication which necessitated this response has disappeared everywhere. I take this banishment of the warning to be the sign that not only widespread inebriety, but practically any drunkenness, and even the fear of it, had vanished.

There are other signs, in the rich rabbinic literature of the middle ages, that drunkenness was no longer feared. Best of all these I like the discussion, in a sixteenth-century work, of the problem of dilution of wine. The ancient custom, well established in the times of the Men of the Great Assembly, and repeatedly confirmed in the Talmud, required strictly that wine be drunk, diluted; surely a precaution related to the surviving fear of drunkenness. Even kiddush wine, which was required to be "fit for libation"—and libation wine was absolutely undiluted—had to be diluted for drinking. Indeed, anyone who drank undiluted wine was assumed to be a drunkard. Thus we find the Talmud ruling that the accused "rebellious son," among other wrongful acts, must have drunk a given large quantity of wine in one draft before he could be found guilty; however, it had to be diluted wine. For, if he had drunk so much undiluted wine, then he must be a drunkard—and a drunkard could not be held responsible. But great medieval authorities ruled that the European wine (i.e., of France or Germany) need not be diluted: "Our wines are much better undiluted since they are not so strong" [as the wines of the ancients], one wrote (Aruk ha-Shulhan, sec. 272) and another: "Our wines are not strong and are better when not diluted" (Lebush ha-Hur:91).

These rulings verge on the fantastic. These wise rabbinic authorities were so firmly convinced that the European wines were weaker, less intoxicating, than the wines of their ancestors, that they went so far as to reform the law fixed by the highest ancient authorities and hallowed by more than two millenia of custom. Why should they think the modern wines comparatively so weak? I can only guess it was because, on the one hand, they knew their ancestors used to get drunk on wine, and on the other hand, any Jew getting drunk on the local wines was unheard of. Perhaps it was naive that they should have failed to realize that the difference was not in the strength of the beverage but in the motivation of the drinking. Their ancestors drank for the purpose of getting drunk, and managed with diluted wine; their contemporaries did not wish to get drunk, and hence they could safely drink wine undiluted.

Along the same line, sixteenth-century authorities discussing the use of the newly available distilled spirits for the lesser kiddush on the Sabbath morning (called the Great Kiddush), note the difficulty of fulfilling the requirement to quaff the quantity of a *reviit* (the displacement of 1.5 eggs) of distilled spirits. "In the case of brandy," Rabbi Jacob ben Samuel wrote, "it is not customary to drink so much at once" (Responsa, Beth Jacob, no. 57).

Indeed, it is abundantly evident that it was no longer customary to drink enough of anything that would cause intoxication, and the Jewish authorities simply no longer seriously feared that anyone might.

I believe I have shown three significant developments relevant to the disappearance of inebriety among the Jews. One is the banishment of the pagan gods of Canaan, to whose worship orgiastic drinking had been attached. The second is the development of the religious culture, with the Bible, the Torah, as constitution, along with the institution of the local synagogue as a place of popular education as much as worship. Third is the positive integration of drinking in religiously oriented ceremonials in the home and synagogue, including meals and rites of passage. The integration of moderate drinking with most religious actions, and most important activities with religion, may have gone hand in hand with the displacement of the pagan gods and their ways, including the interest in orgiastic drinking. When the alien paganism of the Greeks came upon the scene in the Hellenistic era, the bulk of the people rejected its allurements. They had no doubt their own ways were better. Sobriety was indeed fixed in Jewish culture. If we can elucidate the means by which this was effected more explicitly than I have been able to do, we might have the "answer."

Dynamics of Drinking in an Austrian Village
John J. Honigmann

Comparative anthropological and sociological research on drinking has enhanced our understanding of the part drinking plays in social life (Pittman and Snyder 1962). The best of these studies trace in detail the functional concomitants of drinking and in so doing demonstrate drinking to be intricately connected with other parts of a cultural texture. Snyder (1958) adopts a forthrightly configurational point of view. He shows how moderation in drinking is maintained by the warp and woof of a culture, by the paramount values of Jewish Orthodoxy.

I have two purposes in this paper: first, to demonstrate how drinking (the apparently simple custom of downing alcoholic beverages) integrates with other parts of a cultural configuration and, second, in doing so to describe drinking in a German-speaking, central European village in Austria. My approach will not adhere fully to the configurational method of Ruth Benedict and Margaret Mead, who see a culture as possessing an overall pattern, or a highly inclusive value premise, that bestows characteristic form to the parts and molds personality. (Snyder's study of alcohol and the Jews illustrates in only slightly modified form Benedict's concept of pattern, though he does not acknowledge this.) Mostly I will employ another concept of configuration, regarding a way of life as an interrelated system, an organization of interdependent parts.

One implication of a configurational view of drinking is clear. It will be hard to eradicate drinking from a culture in which it is strongly interwoven with several areas of living without undertaking simultaneously a revolutionary readjustment of values, such as might follow from a religious conversion. Protestantism has been revolutionary in this sense in some Latin-American communities (Willems 1955). Resistance to change would arise not only from the functional contributions drinking makes economically, psychologically in the form of anxiety reduction, and socially by intensifying social solidarity; it would also come from all the meanings that have come to be associated with the act by virtue of its satisfactory occurrence in a variety of contexts, from the degree to which it has come to be viewed as necessary or appropriate in the performance of other behaviors, and from the way it is accepted from an early age.

Availability and Consumption of Alcohol

To a visitor from the United States, where alcohol is treated with nearly the same caution as guns, drugs, and germs, western Europeans are amazingly casual about drinking. The American realizes by comparison how his land is unable to accept drinking easily but instead surrounds it with restrictions, curtails it by difficulties, and conceals it from public view. Europeans' far more accepting attitudes are indicated by sidewalk cafés, by beer hawked through trains, by the beer and other alcoholic beverages sold from stands at railroad stations, and by the ease with which strong drinks can be obtained even in places that readily admit children. These traits do not suggest much conflict or ambivalence over the use of alcohol.

A person living in the Enns valley community of Altirdning, Steiermark, needs no official permit to buy domestic and French brandies, rum, or schnapps. He can obtain them in the general stores located in the community and in the market town two miles distant. In the *Markt* he can select a bottle from the open shelves of the self-service stores. These establishments also sell liter bottles of beer and wine; the former are as cheap as or cheaper than Coca Cola and fruit sodas. He can bring his own bottle to the wine-dealer's shop in the *Markt* and have the young lady measure into it wine, brandy, schnapps, pure alcohol, or liqueur. A small table in the place invites him to sample before he buys. In the bakery café's garden or inside near the espresso machine and ice cream counter he can order bottled beer, choose from a display of Austrian wines and imported aperitifs, or select from a wider variety of Austrian liqueurs, some of them tasting as exotic as their names. At another *Markt* café, undistracted by Sunday morning church bells, townsmen play chess seated with goblets of wine at a window overlooking the square and the Catholic church.

Altirdning, with its eight hundred permanent residents (exclusive of college students), lacks a café but provides enough business for four *Gasthäuser* or taverns. Two operate in the community's nucleus—the village of Altirdning proper. Another tavern keeper has enterprisingly built his establishment in a hamlet half a mile from the center, almost next door to a new federal agricultural college. During the academic term the all-male enrollment brings him considerable business. The fourth *Gasthaus* is in a farmhouse that lies high on a hill. Its vista attracts a few paying guests in the summer and draws local folk who are free on a Sunday afternoon. My generalizations will be confined mainly to the two village taverns. Here clients drop in briefly while a horse is being shod or an agricultural machine repaired at the blacksmith's, on their way home from work, or for more leisurely drinking in the evenings after supper. Customers are mostly male and eighteen years old and over. *Gasthäuser* are small, and with the exception of Saturday night they are also never crowded. This means that most of the time they are actually patronized by only a small proportion of the resident youths and men. A few women, with or without escorts, visit them on Saturday and Sunday evenings, but otherwise women attend only as members of a wedding or funeral party.

A *Gasthaus* has three kinds of rooms, each appropriate to a somewhat different facet of the role played by tavern drinking in the culture. The *Saal* is large enough for a whole wedding party—perhaps fifty guests—to receive an elaborate meal; space also allows dancing to a live orchestra. At funerals, upon returning on foot from the cemetery, members of the bereaved family invite kinsmen and close friends to share a goulash in the *Saal*. Otherwise the room is closed. There is also a guest room, but in Altirdning taverns this, too, is rarely opened except for strangers or to accommodate a society meeting, at which the members drink beer or wine as they complete their agenda. Its intended purpose, that of receiving customers or "guests," is preempted by the family kitchen, which is more convenient, cozier, and warmer in winter. Here, amidst her laundry and cooking, with her children watching or helping depending on their age, the *Wirtin* serves guests at one or two large tables that also provide the family board. She will cook a scrambled egg or fill an order for bread and sausage, but she does not provide full meals. Both taverns are family enterprises. Since their owners also operate dairy farms, there are times when neither husband nor wife can be spared to serve. At such times the street door remains locked, or a daughter may take over her mother's role at milking time. In the evenings, however, from seven to ten o'clock or later—much later on Saturdays, for in the unpoliced village nobody takes closing rules seriously—*Wirt* and *Wirtin* both sit with their guests, though the latter still does most of the serving.

People recognize the vested interest of the *Wirtin* in seeing that her guests drink—even to excess. She is doubtless able to predict some of the consequences of intoxication, for, like others in the community, she knows her customers' family lives quite well, including the strains dividing wives and husbands who show alcoholic tendencies. (Only four or five cases of heavy or compulsive drinking came to my attention, and not all problem drinkers regularly drink in *Gasthäuser*.) The *Wirt* and *Wirtin* remain tolerant of drunkenness, whatever they may think of the actual behavior sometimes shown. Rarely do they themselves drink; and wisely so, for it takes a clear head to keep track of how much they serve and to collect the right sum when a guest is ready to pay.

As in every house, once the electric lights go on, the curtains of the *Gasthaus* are drawn, shutting off the kitchen from the street. Inside, a table draws the guests together. They even sit tightly bunched together if company is heavy, for everybody hates to be first at an as yet empty table. Even in the *Saal* and guest

room, a group concentrates around one table, or else several tables
are pushed together to make a single group. This is a major distinction between a *Gasthaus* and a *Markt* cafe, where small tables
keep people apart like strangers. In a tavern group, over their beer
bottles and glasses, eighth-liter glasses of wine, small schnapps, or
soft drinks, everyone joins freely in the general conversation if he
wishes. Under a haze of cigarette smoke, speaking in the Styrian
dialect, the company circulates local news and retails with comments items read in a newspaper or heard on the radio. Farmers
discuss weather, hay, and their cows' illnesses. They appraise the
conduct of absent community members and sometimes criticize it.
They recall past incidents and thus keep some of them memor-
able—not alone for the benefit of overseas strangers.

Frequently the evening ends with someone becoming the
butt of sharp, persistent teasing and an object of wit. In his ri-
postes he tries to find an opening with his own wit, searching for a
vulnerable spot in those who have joined the game. If, for example, he is a woodcutter, and allegations are made about how
little work is done by those who spend the week isolated in the
mountains supposedly cutting trees, he ridicules the occupations
of his accusers. But they refuse to become defensive, pressing
their own attack by leveling more and more absurd charges
against the butt. Or a man may be accused of having fathered an
excessive number of children out of wedlock and of failing to
contribute anything to their support. Another may be derided for
his ineptness at mountain climbing, especially if he has dared to
suggest that he has exceptional skill. Others will tell him where
his skills actually lie. Always the object is to provoke a defensive
response, to stir the victim to defend himself, and to make him
angry. Mostly the butt of such humor—never is he a person highly
respected in the community—takes the jibing in fairly good grace,
and once he or others are ready to leave everybody exchanges
farewells with the greatest friendliness. If drinking continues long
enough, group singing breaks out: Styrian and German folksongs
or rhythmic marching songs recalled from the First or the Second
World War. Risque stories are told, despite the presence of the
Wirtin's children. Village humor is unsubtle, and the appreciative
laughter that follows a good story rings hearty and loud. An evening filled with wit and laughter is *lustig*, gay. *Lustigkeit* or gaiety
is what people want from a *Gasthaus* and from alcohol.

Partially different clienteles favor the two village taverns.
The owner of one of them, a man seventy years of age, reveals
considerable contentment with what he has accomplished in life.

A former burgomeister, he has held the respect of his contemporaries despite having served under the occupying Nazis, for whose policies the local people had little affection. He does not oppose progress, although for him the most significant time dimension is the past. His ambitions are modest, and his dairy farm remains one of the least modernized. He is one of a very few men who stop producing milk for the dairy during the summer and instead drive most of their cows to a mountain meadow (*Alm*) for a milkmaid to tend in the old-time manner. The butter and cheese she makes he uses at home or sells to friends. His tavern attracts a steady clientele of older men, farmers, and community leaders, though on occasion some of these also patronize his neighbor's tavern. Around his table nobody is reminded of his empty glass; *Wirt* and *Wirtin* become so involved in conversation that they even forget to serve.

The other tavern belongs to a mature but younger man who, like his wife, is eager for progress and impatient with the community's arrested economic growth. He would like to see the council take steps to beautify the streets to attract a profitable tourist trade. The *Wirtin* plies her trade diligently, promptly pointing to an empty glass with the suggestion that the customer might want it refilled. The regular guests are younger, unmarried, and more inclined to consist of "workers," i.e., men who hold nonagricultural jobs. Economic development, they say, would increase such jobs locally. Now they must travel considerable distances to work. The *Wirt* has an attractive daughter who is approaching marriageable age, and this helps to augment his clientele, whereas the brusque manner of the other tavern keeper when he counters what he regards to be the brash assertions of youth may have the opposite effect. In any event, congenial company is sought for drinking, and the good *Gasthaus* company reciprocally invites men to drink.

Undoubtedly men can drink more cheaply at home, and they do; but the *Gasthaus* provides additional gratification, notably sociability and gaiety. Alcohol and *Gasthaus* form part of a single pattern. Though men are free to order soft drinks, they usually do not, owing in part to their preference for the taste and effects of alcoholic beverages and in part to the meaning they attach to them, a subject to be considered later. *Gasthaus* drinking has more functions than those I have suggested, but I need not examine them since my aim is to note the cultural factors that help to sustain drinking in Altirdning.

Opportunities for sociable drinking and gaiety also exist outside the *Gasthaus*. Summer excursions to an *Alm* or mountain meadow, where nowadays mostly calves and a few low-yielding cows are economically pastured, inevitably call for purchasing schnapps or beer from a milkmaid. She augments her income by keeping on hand a small stock of beverages, especially for Saint Anna's and Assumption days, the traditional holidays for mountain excursions (Honigmann 1964b). Pre-Lenten balls and summer garden festivals, designed to raise money for enterprises like the *Markt* band, the kindergarten, and the community's volunteer fire fighters, involve considerable drinking and varying degrees of intoxication. Drinking is associated with them almost by definition; the sales of alcohol swell the profits of the sponsoring organizations. At garden festivals women sell schnapps and liqueurs in rough replicas of the mountain huts used by milkmaids for summer dairying. To boost trade, pretty girls in the hut offer a kiss in exchange for a glass of liqueur; then, hardly surreptitiously, they pour out most of their drink, merely touching their lips to the rim. Balls and festivals attract a large proportion of young people from neighboring communities. Hence these events constitute major occasions for courtship. Young men do much of the drinking. They not only grow increasingly gay as the afternoon or evening wears on, but they also grow bolder and sometimes become involved in fights. Girls drink alcoholic beverages cautiously or stay wholly with soft drinks.

Home, too, presents a chance to drink. At mealtimes the family drinks bottled beer, bought in a tavern or general store; beady, dry sugared must, made in autumn by fermenting apples or pears; or simply tea spiked with rum or schnapps. Some families buy their must from a farmer with an extra supply of good quality, from the nearby Capuchin monastery, or from dealers at a cost of about sixteen cents for two liters. Must, drawn from cool cellar barrels, is a casual drink, excellent for quenching thirst or washing down a meal. Even so, it is not consumed on the hay meadows because its alcoholic content produces too much relaxation for heavy work. Farm wives each year prepare a supply of refreshing, unfermented raspberry juice for use by haymakers.

Visitors to a home are honored with a glass or two of alcohol: a mug of cool must; or, somewhat more formally, schnapps to be sipped from small glasses; or, if it is the Christmas season, a glass of liqueur. Formal visiting, however, does not often occur; not even kinsmen exchange dinner invitations.

Some women prepare their own schnapps, often from cherries, making it in licensed tax-free quantities. An excise officer calls to unseal and reseal the still, but rumor has it that ways exist for circumventing alert official eyes. Homemade schnapps is contributed to the pre-Lenten balls, where bottles of it are raffled off; a winner and his friends consume their prize on the premises. Women also make liqueurs, purchasing pure alcohol along with extracts (coffee, cherry, and others) to flavor it. Some farmers make wine from homegrown cherries or from the wild elderberries that grow profusely in the vicinity. Beer, however, has not been homemade as long as informants can recall. Formerly, when farmers could afford to drink relatively little beer beyond a small barrel bought for the Christmas holidays, it was produced locally by numerous small breweries. In today's more affluent times beer has become the most popular drink, and nearly all of it bears the labels of two large national plants.

Ceremonies and Drinking

We shall see that attitudes toward alcohol are complex. To drink intoxicants is relished for the release and the *Lustigkeit* it brings. But one should drink only in moderation. Most persons in Altirdning manage to confine the intoxicating properties of alcohol within acceptable limits. Having learned to drink in approved fashion, they are able to participate successfully in the many ceremonial situations to which alcohol properly belongs. Such ceremonies include calendrical religious holidays, Sundays, and rites of passage like funerals and weddings. As already noted, the pattern of some religious feast days calls for a visit to an *Alm* or mountain meadow, where drinking is very much in order. At Easter the emphasis is placed on festive eating, an activity to which drinking is readily assimilated. Procession days, notably Corpus Christi, understandably generate exceptional thirst; so after the march the men drop in at a *Gasthaus* before going home to dinner. The *Markt* band, to which several inhabitants of Altirdning belong, always plays in processions and then continues in formation to a favorite tavern where its members can refresh themselves. Sundays bring a thriving business to *Gasthäuser* in the *Markt* as well as in Altirdning. From mid-morning on the men drop in, first on their way home from Mass and later to help fill the leisurely afternoon.

Many special observances bound up with certain holidays demand alcohol. For example, St. Nicholas Eve brings a call from the horribly masked Grampus armed with a whip and from the bishop dressed in white who distributes candy and presents to awed children. These personages must be offered a drink. Successive draughts of schnapps make the evening gay for both the players and those who accompany them. At Epiphany, women armed with brooms impersonate the legendary old woman to whom go children who die before they can be baptized. Their symbolic service of brushing the table and floor wins them a glass of schnapps in every house they visit. Christmas and Easter provide special reasons for visiting a *Gasthaus*. At Christmas, the members of the savings association assemble in the guest room of a tavern to eat and drink the festive dinner toward which they have contributed throughout the year. At Easter, tavern keepers give their clients colored eggs decorated with decals. Young men use these in a game. One flings a shilling piece to see if it will stick in an egg which another holds; if it does, he not only retrieves his money but wins an egg.

The custom whereby a funeral party after the burial adjourns to a *Gasthaus* for a small meal and liquid refreshment has already been mentioned. Since practically the whole community respectfully follows one of its mature members to the cemetery, it would be difficult for the bereaved family to entertain everyone, and consequently only selected guests are invited. At the wake, however, a household offers coffee, beer, or wine to each person who visits the bier to offer his condolence. The tavern is felt to be a particularly suitable setting for commemorating a man renowned for his *Lustigkeit* and his frequenting of *Gasthaus* kitchens. We heard of two men who had ordered gay funerals for themselves. The mourners duly honored the request of one of them, staying late at the tavern and leaving exhilarated. The other man, however, still lives.

Alcohol impinges at many points of a wedding, especially that of a farmer, starting with the bells rung to wake the bride and send her off—by which services the noisemakers earn a snack and drinks—and ending with the evening wedding feast celebrated in a tavern's *Saal*. Wine constitutes a sacramental element in the church service and is delivered to the altar by the wine dealer in liter flagons along with glasses. As the marriage service concludes, the priest blesses the wine at the altar and then, still in his vestments, clinks glasses and drinks with the couple. Meanwhile the sacristan fills additional glasses that are lined up on the communion rail. As the priest departs, the invited guests move forward from their pews to toast and drink with the bride and groom. Each person takes only a small sip before passing his glass on to the next. Now, in an atmosphere choked with tearful emotion, the first congratulations are spoken. After the service the wedding party drives off to visit some scenic spot, such as a mountain meadow,

and calls in at taverns en route there as well as on the way back to
the village, where the wedding feast is yet to be celebrated.
Villagers awaiting the party's return may bar the street and act out
more or less embarrassing scenes of the groom's and bride's lives.
To get past them, the wedding party pays the actors a two-liter
bottle of wine or a case of beer. The interval before the couple
actually sit down to eat is a dangerous one, for either or both may
be kidnapped and taken off to another *Gasthaus* to be held for
ransom. Once again the ransom consists of drinks.

These examples by no means exhaust the role of alcohol in
holiday and other ceremonies; they merely illustrate it. The annual round and ceremonial points in the individual life cycle call
for drinking as war calls for weapons. Alcohol is an intimate part of
a configuration.

Children and Alcohol

Parents do not shield their children from alcohol, although they do
reveal definite ambivalence about youngsters' drinking. Actually,
it is impossible completely to insulate a child from alcohol in a
community where drinking occurs on so many occasions, both
public and private. A youngster gains his earliest awareness of
alcoholic beverages from his elders at home. As he does so, he
also learns that caution and moderation should govern their use.
He discovers that alcohol stands in a special class of objects. For
example, when he is eating with his parents, he reaches, as children of two or three will, confidently toward his father's glass of
beer or sweetened must or the cup of sugared tea into which his
mother has just poured rum or schnapps. He learns that, in contrast to other occasions when he demands something from the
table, his wish is not directly gratified. Adults dissuade him from
his request or perhaps try to distract him with a substitute. Con-
fusingly, however, a grandfather may indulgently permit him to
sip his cup or glass, despite the mother's clear annoyance. Formerly she, too, might have been more tolerant; we heard that a
generation or two ago mothers sometimes sent babies to sleep
with a pacifier steeped in schnapps. Nowadays, however, the
young farm mother has learned "advanced ways" (as the people
themselves put it) from the year she spent away from home as a
girl at a domestic-science school or from the year or two spent as a
maid in a well-to-do urban family. She objects to serving alcohol
to a two-year-old because she has learned that it causes harm in
the early years and because she shares the popular belief that

young children are quick to relish alcohol, especially in the form of beer and wine, and are therefore prone to drink injurious amounts.

I have not yet had time to trace the gradual change in parental attitudes toward drinking as the children grow older, but it is clear that by the age of seven or eight their objections have grown considerably milder and their ambivalence is less pronounced. Drinking becomes a bit more permissive, though adults still ration it by sips from their own glasses or, as at a picnic or fair, directly from the mouth of a bottle. From such rationing, casual as it may be, children are reminded that alcohol stands in a special category of things. Jokes about drinking to excess and becoming drunk reiterate a similar warning message. By the age of eight a girl or boy is considered old enough to be sent to fetch beer from the *Gasthaus* kitchen and thus comes to learn about that orbit of drinking. By the age of fifteen a child has graduated from sips and receives his own modest glass of must, beer, or wine, particularly on ceremonial occasions. Two or three years later, normal adult quantities go to him by right. A girl, after cycling to her aunt's house on a hot day, drinks a full liter of dark beer, which women prefer to light beer because it is sweeter. A boy, for reasons connected less with appetite than with the socially approved image of masculinity, begins calling at a *Gasthaus*. Young men whom we happened to observe when they were beginning their drinking careers often chose soft drinks, but after few months or a year graduated to beer, particularly on Fridays and Saturdays when their friends congregated in the *Gasthaus*. Weekend drinking at this age may lack something in moderation, with the result that women's tongues cluck and they ask rhetorically what such a youth will make of himself. We have not yet had an opportunity to follow up the two or three youths whose drinking careers we observed over two summers. Barring any drastic change in culture patterns, however, and allowing for idiosyncrasies, they will settle down to moderation, judging from the prevailing pattern of moderation observed by most of their seniors.

The child of a tavern keeper, growing up as he does where his mother daily serves her guests, is exposed to considerably more drinking and drunkenness than other children. He also begins to handle alcohol earlier; serving bottles of beer and pouring glasses of wine at the age of ten to twelve is for him the equivalent of the chores into which other children are inducted. Summer festivals offer all children an opportunity to observe, with conspicuous demonstrations, the intoxicating properties of alcohol.

Nor are they shielded from such learning, which is a vital part of growing up. The *Alm* hut with its stock of schnapps and liqueurs may even be the only place at the festival that sells fritters spread with Styrian cheese; a child who wants this popular snack must push his way into the noisy hut and up to the crowded counter, where a serving woman takes the warm coin from his clenched fist. The drunken clanging of the cowbell in the *Alm* hut at a festival also helps arouse childish curiosity. At one of these Sunday afternoon summer affairs I spied two ten-year-old boys sampling a foaming glass of beer—dubiously, it must be added, rather than with any pronounced sign of pleasure. The dance band at a lively festival plays indefatigably, with only brief respites for the musicians to refresh themselves from the beer bottles at their feet. Unmarried girls beyond puberty and young married women circulate in constant demand as dance partners. Festivals and balls bring out new skills in girls, not only in dancing but in unoffensively warding off the unwelcome attentions too intensely lavished on them by emboldened partners. They teach girls about another side of alcohol and suggest a partial reason for the moderate drinking characteristic of women.

The Ideology of Drinking

Attitudes, beliefs, and sentiments about alcohol act as an ideological charter that controls and rationalizes drinking. The ideology itself is shaped and reinforced by the very situations that employ alcohol and conjoin its use with physical and social concomitants. In other words, drinking and associated behavior condition ideas about alcohol; ideas concerning alcohol in turn condition drinking. Over time, of course, the circle is not unchangingly regenerated, for people learn new ideas and also encounter new experiences while drinking. Fed into the system, these alter either drinking behavior or, in the case of new drinking experiences, the attitudes, beliefs, and sentiments pertaining to alcohol and its use. It is not my purpose, however, to account for change but rather to describe how a given pattern of drinking persists in a culture.

Probably the most important attitude motivating drinking in Altirdning is the explicit recognition, already referred to, that alcohol touches off gaiety and promotes exuberance. An informant revealed this attitude when he explained that a group will have a few drinks together *so dass sie lustig werden,* so that they will become gay. A similar explanation was given for a funeral party visiting a *Gasthaus.* As one informant expressed it, the somber part of the ceremony is now over, and a bit of drinking relieves the mourners' depression, bringing them a sense of relief. Drinking is thus valued for its ability to stimulate pleasant feelings—gaiety—rather than solely for its intrinsic meaning, although intrinsic significance also attaches to alcohol in certain ceremonies and on the *Alm.* Established contexts of drinking, like the *Gasthaus,* are therefore supposed to be gay. Men are likely to be disappointed if they find the tavern company quiet and may attempt to provoke greater stimulation, e.g., by trying to rouse a song.

Folksongs themselves reiterate the release and gaiety that drinking is expected to unloose, as well as the congeniality ideally found in a drinking group. The ideology of drinking distinctly implies that it is a social activity: alcohol is drunk at meals, with guests, at festivals and balls, at weddings, after burials, on picnics, and in taverns. These are occasions that people define as pleasant. Good times and alcohol, the charter predicts, go together. This predominant sentiment connected with drinking was voiced in one way or another more often than negative attitudes concerning immoderate drinking.

Popular thought associates drinking with the male sex. In fact, it forms an essential component of the masculine role as culturally defined. Hence it is an entirely proper activity for young men to adopt as they pass into manhood. As background, it is worth noting that in Altirdning sex roles are frequently interchangeable; women often work alongside men in jobs too big or time-consuming for men to perform alone. Thus dairying, the major economic activity of the community, is a family enterprise in which husband and wife cooperate very closely. In the use of alcohol, nevertheless, sex roles diverge sharply. We knew no man who abstained from alcohol. Such a man would be dubiously regarded, for he would not be fulfilling all the expectations of his status. "A man who drinks only milk," one woman said picturesquely, "and never goes to the *Gasthaus* isn't really a man." She could not explain why, though she added that an occasional visit to a tavern allows a man to mix with masculine company. No similar evaluation is attached to whether a woman drinks or not.

The charter associates alcohol with health, and this is a culture where health is a matter of concern. Without being hypochondriacal, everybody can cite certain hygienic folk beliefs: rules of eating, dangerous and beneficial foods, and things to do or take—like herbal teas—to relieve indisposition. Alcohol fits into this body of folklore. There are folk medicines made at home with an alcohol base. Generally speaking, used in moderation, alcohol is considered healthful. Schnapps gives strength (Reiterer 1915). It relieves fatigue, for example, when one has been working strenuously or mountain climbing. Unlike cold drinks, it prevents chilling of an overheated body and hence avoids the danger of contracting a cold from too quick cooling. Wine, too, is healthful— red wine more than white, we learned. A woman on a visit from Vienna explained that after the Second World War the abundant use of wine held epidemics in the city in check, the alcohol combating disease germs. Alcohol is harmful only for young children, and this, it appears, is a recently acquired idea to which not everyone subscribes. The hygienic properties ascribed to alcohol by the ideology contribute further to the positive feeling tone enveloping its use. Even excessive drinking is viewed not so much as dangerous to health as destructive to social relationships. Danger lies more in the behavior attending alcohol's immoderate use than in its inherent nature. This enables us to understand why so little ambivalence is associated with alcohol itself, why it is employed by adults so freely and openly, and why it is so readily accessible.

Alcohol nevertheless arouses alarm when it is used immoderately or compulsively so that drinking begins to conflict with other responsibilities. Though they are too relaxed to be compulsive, the inhabitants of Altirdning are a duty-conscious people who regard it as important to fulfill social expectations and to play their roles as well as possible. Excessive drinking obtrudes on this value. Furthermore, it wrecks family and social relationships with consequent great distress. Paula Grogger (1947: 21), the modern Styrian poetess, notes this:

Mannslust ist Weiberweh.
Sein Rausch ist dein Straf. . . .

Folk theory views the excessive craving for alcohol in two ways. Sometimes alcoholism is attributed to intense emotional stress, occasioned, for example, by an incurable illness that leaves no hope. At other times it is ascribed to heredity, to the transmission from father to son of a tendency to drink compulsively. Emotional problems are blamed for one man's heavy drinking, and inheritance is held to cause another's, particularly if the latter seems to have nothing to be distressed about. Drunkenness itself earns men no disapproval; in fact moderate intoxication is the very basis for gaiety. Even a confirmed alcoholic's intoxicated behavior evokes good-humored amusement up to a point, though the charter hardly condones his plight. Regardless of its source, a man's drunkenness is accepted so long as he retains control over his acts and stays in good humor. A woman, however, cannot without disgrace risk any evidence of being drunk. Attitudes circumscribe feminine *Lustigkeit* much more narrowly than men's. Hence a woman must manage to be gay with the aid of much smaller quantities of alcohol than a man consumes, lest she reach what in her husband would be merely an acceptable degree of tipsiness. Immoderate drunkenness—intoxication that can no longer be called tipsy, in which a man loses his ability to evaluate and control his acts, and wherein he becomes aggressive—arouses annoyance and even repugnance. Drinking to this extreme occurs uncommonly, though I saw it two or three times, once in a young woman.

The community recalls witnessing the epitome of disapproved drunkenness in the personnel of the Soviet Red Army who occupied the area for a short time as the last war ended and before United States troops took over. Apparently the Russian soldiers, in their drunken behavior, went far beyond anything that the people had ever experienced. Fear of the consequences made their drinking the most traumatic aspect of the Soviet occupation. For safety, the Austrians hid their stocks of alcohol and swore to search parties that they did not possess a drop. Some villagers, on the other hand, used schnapps as a precious medium to buy favors from the occupying army. Recollections of Russian drunkenness have become part of the charter, reinforcing by contrast the meaning of moderation and the expectation that the use of alcohol will lead to gaiety rather than uncontrolled behavior.

Conclusion

Drinking in Altirdning is maintained by the ready availability of alcohol, by the rewards that accrue from joining a congenial *Gasthaus* company, by the expectation of drinking at meals and on ceremonial occasions, and by the acceptance of these and other uses of alcohol from childhood on. It is also guided and controlled by the attitudes, beliefs, and sentiments attached to alcohol's use. Basic to an understanding of the community's style of drinking is the expectation that alcohol will be used moderately. For men to drink moderately means not to avoid intoxication but to watch carefully the degree of intoxication reached. Drinking, an element of culture, is sustained by other parts of the cultural configuration. Better said, the dynamics of drinking resides in the total web of drinking itself.

How French Children Learn to Drink

Barbara Gallatin Anderson

Visitors to France—even those with some knowledge of life in Mediterranean cultures—are often startled by the great amount of wine drinking they find. Frenchmen everywhere drink with unflagging dedication and a quiet passion. For two years, my husband and I lived in the Seine-et-Oise village of Wissous, an area ten miles from Paris. As anthropologists, we were struck by the tenacity with which villagers clung to their old drinking habits, specifically wine drinking, despite considerable pressure from the government to abandon or at least cut down on their alcohol consumption. In particular, we were interested in finding out just how these drinking practices were transmitted to the village children.

Our two daughters, Andrea and Robin, then seven and two, were with us, and our son, Scott, was born there. We participated in the village life and, where possible, penetrated behind the scenes, gathering information about village customs. Of course, the questions we asked about children's drinking habits presented problems. The questions had to be very specific, yet apparently off the cuff. Eventually we incorporated them into a rather elaborate questionnaire on child care in general.

On the questionnaire, we asked people what every member of the household had eaten or drunk in the past twenty-four hours—at home or away from home. When feasible, we called at the villagers' homes during meal hours. Our interest was in what they had drunk, but we tried to give our questions no particular emphasis. We were as scrupulous in our attention to the kinds and quantities of foods they ate as we were in cataloging the beverages they drank. We administered these questionnaires and conducted follow-up interviews beginning in late February and ending in late April—a period of increasing warmth, which lowered the amount of drinking slightly. (To the villagers, cold weather is often a rationale for wine drinking.)

Now, our interest lay specifically in the village's socially accepted drinking practices. For the French, this amounts to a study of wine drinking. Our findings: adult male villagers consumed approximately 1.58 quarts of wine per day. Women drank more than half a quart. The averages for children, however, could not be estimated—for reasons that will become clear later.

Our village was representative of France, where the total consumption of *pure* alcohol for the year 1955 (our study was done in 1957–59) averaged 23.78 quarts per person, or 32.1 for adults over twenty. This average for adults was 16.9 quarts more than was consumed that same year by the world's second-largest wine-consuming country—Italy. The Danes drink only 3.17 quarts of pure alcohol per year. Americans drink 9.29 quarts.

According to the French government's figures, 15 percent of France's men are alcoholics, and 30 percent consume alcohol in amounts dangerous to their health. The government's National Institute of Hygiene has said that very active manual workers should not drink over one liter (1.057 quarts) of wine per day. Yet many sedentary workers, who are advised not to drink more than half a liter per day, drink a whole liter—as much as the most active workers. Alcoholism, to the average Frenchman, is identified only with reeling drunkenness.

Children Encouraged to Drink

Now, how does this receptivity to wine drinking take shape in the children of the village? In other words, how is wine drinking enculturated?

First of all, in Wissous, a positive value is attached to wine. People view wine drinking as an act of virility. Men and families cannot socialize without wine. For a host not to offer wine is at best impolite.

In addition, wine is thought to have nutritive value. One reason: Throughout the schools, the very active wine lobby distributes blotters that carry highly dubious statements. One such blotter states that a liter of wine (12 percent alcohol) has nutritive value equivalent to 850 grams of milk, 370 grams of bread, 585 grams of meat, or 5 eggs. The blotter has a drawing of a scale with a wine bottle balancing these foods.

Wine is also believed to be necessary for working. While at work, a manual or farm worker must have wine at fairly regular intervals. The body can best endure prolonged muscular exertion, it is alleged, with the sustained, revitalizing support of wine. Strong men have a propensity for drink. It is nature's way—"C'est comme ça."

Finally, wine may not be purer than any other drink, but Frenchmen think it is. In fact, the alcohol in wine is widely believed to compensate for the unsanitary conditions under which it, and many other food products, are prepared.

These beliefs about wine are strongest among the peasants. The few upper-middle-class families of Wissous also link wine drinking to vigor. But they are more likely to stress moderation, and they drink less wine than the peasants. The moderation of the upper-middle-class, however, does not appear to extend to *apéritifs* and *digestifs*. They drink considerably more of these than the other villagers do, at home and in cafés.

In contrast with the positive value placed on wine, the French place a negative value on western Europe's two major *non*alcoholic drinks: water and milk. The Wissous village spring water, which flows from two central fountains, is potable, but little is drunk (except in coffee), especially by the men. The local attitude is that, although a certain amount of water drinking is inevitable, water takes second place to almost any other beverage. As one of the subway signs posted by France's powerful wine lobby puts it, "Water is for frogs."

In its campaign against the wine lobby, the French government has recently turned to building the image of fruit juice. Government ads show popular sportsmen drinking fruit juice with apparent gusto. But the wine lobby is still far more successful than any other lobby in France at carrying its message to the people.

As for milk, a precept firmly adhered to by all classes is summed up in a popular 1947 book on child care: "Milk should never constitute the mealtime drink." This book also states that "the quantity of milk drunk in a day should not exceed half a liter, under risk of digestive troubles such as diarrhea." In this regard, the villagers run no risks. When children stop taking the breast or the bottle, and stop eating the *bouillies* (thin milk mushes) of babyhood, they rarely drink milk at all, except in café au lait, chocolate, or the milk-thinned mashed vegetables called purées.

Of course, the fact that milk is unrefrigerated, especially in the villages, does nothing to increase its appeal. And though it is pasteurized, it is *not* homogenized. When poured, it goes clunk-clunk in uneven globs. And in warm weather, it has a strong, almost curdled flavor.

During the time we lived in Wissous, milk was delivered to the village in huge tin urns, and poured into bottles by the grocer. Unknown to him, I once followed him to the back of his shop and saw him slosh a dirty bottle around in a tub of cold water before filling it with milk.

A book on practical child-raising, known in the village since the early twenties, differs little in its warnings about milk, but acknowledges that children cannot be "bad off" if they drink milk almost exclusively for the first two years. I quote: "One can also give at mealtime a half-glass of water lightly reddened with wine, or some beer or cider very diluted with water." In general, the recent literature is more cautious. It suggests, as a more suitable time for introducing children to alcoholic beverages, four years of age rather than two.

Wine Introduced as "Reddened Water"

Here, then, is our major point: wine drinking begins while the child is still in near-infancy. And government efforts to show that wine hurts children run into a semantic trap. A child does not drink *wine:* he drinks "reddened water."

To the French, the consumption of wine in quantities of less than a fourth of a quart is equivalent to abstinence. The mother of a boy of twelve will tell you, though the boy may be sitting across from you with a glass of the diluted wine in his hand, that her son does not drink at all. By this, she means that his "reddened water" contains only a couple of soupspoons of wine.

One day I bought refreshments for my daughter and her eleven-year-old playmate at a café. The playmate ordered and drank a bottle of beer. It surprised me a little, because her mother had told me that the girl did not drink. But I am sure that, to the mother, her child's minimal and irregular intake did not constitute drinking.

If parents are drinking wine, beer, or cider, they give some—diluted with water—to their children. The younger ones sip beer or cider from a parent's glass. As they get older and more demanding, they are given small glasses of their own.

Children of lower-class homes drink more wine than children of middle-class homes, and they start drinking when they are younger. One mother even reported putting a drop or two of wine in a baby's bottle to "fortify" the milk. Generally, though, wine is first offered when the child is two or more, can hold his own glass quite safely in his hand, and can join the family at table.

In short, wine drinking is already a habit before French children are old enough to reflect about it. If they do begin to assess their drinking practices, it is against a cultural backdrop where all the answers are value-loaded. Under the circumstances, it is hardly surprising that the campaigns in France against wine drinking—led by teachers, social workers, and specialists in child welfare—have met with little success, and that in the past quarter-century the drinking patterns of French villagers, despite much social change and many social pressures, have hardly changed at all.

Alcohol and Soviet Society

Walter D. Connor

If, in a nation where comprehensive statistics on social problems are rarely if ever published, legislative action and press attention to such problems may be taken as an indication of the seriousness with which they are regarded, then the Soviet Union's alcohol problem is serious indeed. On April 8, 1967, the supreme soviet of the RSFSR approved a decree, On Compulsory Treatment and Labor Reeducation of Habitual Drunkards (Alcoholics).[1] This decree, which went into effect on September 1 of the same year, provides for one- to two-year terms in special "treatment-labor" medical institutions for excessive drinkers who violate "labor discipline, public order, and the rules of the socialist community." The new institutions were subordinated not to the Ministry of Health but to the RSFSR Ministry for the Preservation of Public Order (MOOP, now renamed MVD). While it contained a number of significant departures from earlier legislation, the decree's most important point was its "preventive" emphasis. Previously an offending drunkard had to be on trial for a crime in a people's court before proceedings for compulsory treatment could be instituted. But the need to reach the drunkard before he committed a serious offense had been argued over recent years in the press and in Soviet legal periodicals.

In 1969 two signed articles by Soviet scholars long concerned with crime and alcoholism were published. On March 29 *Pravda* published a contribution by Professor Iu. M. Tkachevsky of the criminal law department at Moscow State University, a large part of which was devoted to a proposal for the establishment of a "public" organization to continue the efforts of the All-Union Council of Antialcohol Societies, which ceased to function in 1930. Two months later, on May 27, *Izvestiia* included an article by Professor A. A. Gertsenzon, a veteran criminologist and section head at the All-Union Institute for the Study of the Causes and Elaboration of Preventive Measures of Crime, referring to Tkachevsky's article and strongly favoring the establishment of a new antidrunkenness society. Gertsenzon complained that the "liquidation" of the earlier antialcohol organization had been "without sufficient reasons." In 1966 the collective volume *Alcoholism: The Path to Crime*, published under the auspices of the institute with Gertsenzon as responsible editor, had strongly recommended the establishment of such an organization. However, no action has yet been taken (as of July 1971) to implement these recommendations.

The legislative changes and the more recent calls for organizational innovation indicate a growing concern with the problems of alcoholism and drunkenness and a dissatisfaction with the measures hitherto employed to deal with them. State and party bodies have generally shared responsibility for conducting "antialcohol propaganda" with medical personnel on the local level. Low priority has apparently been assigned to the task, and the propaganda itself has been of low quality. The proposed antialcohol society would evidently assume these functions. In addition, there is evidence that the decision to broaden the application of compulsory treatment in institutions under police management accords with a feeling that psychiatric hospitals do little for drunkards who are also "hooligans" and that a system which requires inmates to work (and in which deductions are made from their earnings to cover costs of treatment and maintenance—such "care" is not free) is more suited to the treatment of persons who are held to be basically to blame for their afflictions.

Quantitative data on alcohol consumption per capita in the USSR are sketchy and dated, but of interest nonetheless. In 1956 the *Bol'shaia meditsinskaia entsiklopediia* reported an annual consumption rate of 1.85 liters of absolute alcohol per capita for 1948–50. This placed the USSR last among thirteen listed nations, well below France's figure of 21.5 liters per capita, and the 5.1 for the United States. While much is made of the fact that this represents a decline from a consumption rate of 3.41 liters per capita during the years 1906–10 in European Russia, reduction in consumption has been a *general* trend. The USSR dropped from twelfth to thirteenth place in per capita consumption between 1906–10 and 1948–50. (All of the countries reporting in both the 1906–10 and 1948–50 periods underwent a decline: in Italy an even greater proportional reduction took place, from 18.29 liters to 9.2.) Referring to the "high" consumption in the 1906–10 period, Soviet sources also note that in consumption of strong liquor (vodka), Russia was fifth among countries reporting (*Alkogolizm* 1966).

For more recent years, indirect evidence indicates an increase in consumption. The 1965 production figures for ethyl alcohol (assuming that about 40 percent of such production is used in the manufacture of 40 percent alcohol beverages and the rest devoted to industrial use) indicate that in that year there were approximately ten liters of such strong liquor available per capita for a population of 231 million (Mironenko 1967). This represents a significant increase over 1950 when slightly more than four liters were available per capita (see Eason 1968). Although the estimates do not take account of probable increases in export and industrial use, they are impressive. It should be noted that these figures do not include wine and beer, and also that given the high concentration of drinking among adolescent and adult males the average annual intake of the *drinker* is bound to be higher. This hypothesized growth finds some reflection in a 1966 observation that over the course of ten years in Moscow Oblast, sales of alcoholic beverages had grown 2.2 times, and vodka sales had exceeded the growth rate of other alcoholic beverages by 15–20 percent (*Alkogolizm* 1966).

The persistence of illegal distilling (*samogonovarenie*) increases the need to qualify available consumption figures. A study of rural areas in the RSFSR in 1927 found that the rural population consumed an average of 7.5 liters of *samogon* per capita each year, and that 80 percent of their alcohol consumption was in this form. A more recent study in the late 1950s, though it gave no data on how widespread the offense was, found it enduring. Small-scale production (up to two liters) accounted for 37.7 percent of the offenders, while 5.3 percent were apprehended after producing over ten liters. Of all offenders, 78.5 percent had used "special apparatus" for the distilling (*Alkogolizm* 1966).

This article addresses itself first to the drinking practices and attitudes widespread in the USSR—what may be called a Russian "drinking culture." The adjective "Russian" is advisable in this context. The republics of the Caucasus and the Muslim areas of Central Asia differ in historical background, attitudes toward alcohol, and types of alcoholic beverages most frequently consumed. There is a lack of Soviet data on contemporary ethnic differences in this regard, and therefore what is said of the European areas cannot be extended without modification to Central Asia, the Caucasus, and areas where non-Slavic populations are concentrated. Subsequent sections deal with the perceived social costs of alcoholism, the gap between "official" and popular attitudes, and the present state and future prospects of the Soviet "struggle" with problems of excessive drinking.

The Drinking Culture

One of the most striking elements in Russian drinking behavior is the multiplicity of occasions with which drinking is associated. In the sphere of popular, "unofficial" values alcohol is a virtually indispensable adjunct to many events, and is a direct refuge from tension or pain-creating situations. Persistent complaints in the press about the practice of payday drinking bouts by factory workers, which often end in brawls with co-workers and family "scandals" when the intoxicated worker returns home minus some of his wages, indicate one of the most frequent occasions for "convivial" drinking. V. E. Rozhnov, in a book addressed to members of the armed forces, enumerates some other occasions:

> One bought a pair of shoes—he has to "wash it off," he won on a lottery ticket—he also must "wash it off," he got an apartment or a bonus—how can he not "wash it off"? Is a child born, did someone die, did there occur some sort of misfortune, or, on the other hand, some happiness, is someone going away on vacation, or returning from a health resort—many begin to drink because of these "occasions." [1969: 35–36]

Important events in family life provide another stimulus for the sort of excesses deplored by those who write about the problem of drunkenness. *Pravda* recently noted on two separate occasions the large amount of money spent, and workdays lost, because of large wedding celebrations on collective farms, which include "drinking bouts lasting many days and involving large numbers of people and in which . . . an unhealthy competition in plying the guests with liquor has been conducted" (6 April 1969). Thus it is no surprise that the Soviet nondrinker often finds himself at odds with the rest of the company in social situations. The teetotaler, or the person who is unshakable in his resolve to drink only moderately, does so at the risk of offending his companions, of being considered something less than a "real man." Obstinate refusal to drink under these circumstances is often regarded as a real insult, as well as "peculiar" behavior (Rozhnov 1969; see also Tkachevsky 1966, Levin 1963). Strenuous also is the route of the reformed drinker, whose "friends and relatives" often provide the push to send him "off the wagon" (Levin 1963). One of the leading Soviet medical specialists in alcoholic problems notes that in one survey of alcoholic "backsliders" 42.2 percent of the cases were attributable to the influence of companions or relatives who persuaded the patient to have a drink (Segal 1967).

Drinking remains largely a male activity (cases of alcoholism are "still encountered" among women, but "very seldom" [Bogdanovich 1967; Rozhnov 1969]), and "socialization" in drinking practices often begins early. A father who, over his wife's objections, gives his five-year-old son a glass of wine argues, "let him get used to it . . . he's got to be a real man" (Bogdanovich 1967:49). Teenage factory workers soon become accustomed to payday drinking with "veterans" in their shops. A refusal to participate is often viewed as "bad form." The intoxication which often follows the "workers' baptism" accompanying the first payday occasionally lands the youth in the arms of the militia.

Soviet journalists and pamphleteers are content to denounce these phenomena as "survivals of the past," but they in fact point to the existence of a Russian "drinking culture"—an historically deep-rooted complex of attitudes and practices involving the use of alcohol, which also has its roots in the conditions of contemporary Soviet life. Studies of the drinking patterns of other ethnic groups have shown the intricate relations of norms and values concerning alcohol use, and the incidence of drunkenness and alcoholism (e.g., Bales 1962; Snyder 1962). Drinking, when closely linked with religious ritual, as among Jews, or when viewed as an integral part of meals, as the consumption of wine is among Italians, rarely takes on pathological dimensions, even when the population shows a high annual per capita consumption rate. The relatively high rate of alcohol pathology among the Irish, on the other hand, has been explained, at least in part, on the basis of the *absence* of social contexts for drinking that integrate it into religious or family life, along with the presence of the idea of drinking as a masculine activity, something which affirms one's manhood and solidarity with one's fellows, and as an approved means of increasing one's gaiety or deadening one's sorrow. Such may be true as well of the Russian case.

Research in the West has pointed to "dependency conflicts" in the male life cycle as important elements in the etiology of alcoholism (e.g., McCord and McCord 1960). For a variety of reasons "dependency needs" (for maternal warmth, response, nourishment, protection) acutely felt by male children may be inconsistently and sporadically fulfilled in the family setting. Although "legitimate" for young children, such needs conflict with the "model" image of the adult male—in the USSR as well as in the West—as a mature, productive, and independent adult, whose duties consist largely of satisfying the needs of wife and children. For those whose childhood dependency needs are satisfied, the transition to the adult male role is relatively easy. For the unsatisfied the transition is fraught with difficulties. Consciously or subconsciously, dependency needs, now regarded as "illegitimate" and "feminine," are suppressed, and are disavowed through adoption of decisively "masculine" behavior patterns—sometimes extremely aggressive behavior, and sometimes, where the culture makes it available, heavy drinking, a "man's prerogative." The warmth and solace that many find in drinking may provide a means, if a dangerous one, of satisfying the dependency needs still felt.

Although Soviet researches are not conducted in this perspective, it merits attention. Problems of divorce, desertion, parental conflict, and the like are widespread in Soviet as in American society, and presumably have an important impact on parental abilities to satisfy dependency needs. Given the existence of some segment of the male population whose childhood needs remain unfulfilled, and the demands on them, as on other Soviet men, to provide support for dependents in much the same manner as in the West—to be, within the scope of their jobs, "achievers"—it is not difficult to imagine some seeking the refuge that a manhood-affirming drinking culture offers.

In addition, heavy drinking can be viewed as an "escape" mechanism. Crowded housing, low wages, high-priced consumer goods, and other problems result in a certain level of dissatisfaction, especially among the working classes who feel the burden most directly. Frustrations over limited opportunities for upward mobility as social class boundaries become harder to cross and the feeling of being "stuck" in uninteresting jobs add to the stress. But escape mechanisms are not in abundance in Soviet society for those who would seek them. Emigration to lands where perceived opportunities are greater is rarely an alternative. Nor do involvement in organized religion and the adoption of a perspective minimizing the significance of worldly problems seem to be viable solutions for many adult males, even leaving aside the issue of governmental atheism. Alcohol, however, is available. Its use to cope with stress is culturally permissible. It can provide the solitary drinker with the oblivion which is the most radical temporary form of escape. Heavy drinking in convivial groups can provide a sense of camaraderie, of effortless interaction with others, which many find lacking in modern urban society, whether Soviet or not.

These are some suggestions concerning the causes of Soviet alcoholism. To determine the relative significance of a drinking culture, dependency conflicts, and the demand for escape mechanisms is a knotty methodological problem, as well as one for which we lack the requisite data. It can only be said that each of the factors discussed is bound to be important, and that none can be ignored.

The Social Costs of Alcohol

Soviet calculations of the social costs of drinking fall into three broad categories: public order (delinquency and crime), the economy (industrial accidents, waste, etc.), and what might be loosely termed the "quality of life"—the effects of alcohol abuse on family life and leisure.

Scattered statistics report a high rate of violent crimes committed "in an unsober state." For the nation as a whole, statements are made that "70 percent of all crimes" and "more than 80 percent of all hooligan acts" are commited by intoxicated persons (*Izvestiia* 2 March 1958:4; Banshchikov 1958:32). Nonviolent property crimes are often traced to alcohol, notably embezzlement and theft by employees who need money for liquor (Gurvich 1958). In another vein, the illegal distilling of alcohol is itself a major category of crime in some areas. Data from a study of crime for the years 1953–63 in a district in Belorussia show that one out of three offenders "brought to criminal responsibility" was engaged in illegal distilling (Kondrashkov 1966).

The relatively unregulated sale of alcohol to minors, and the social pressures on (especially) the less-educated young workers to "be a man" and drink, have given rise to concern over the connection between alcohol and delinquency. The authors of an article on the subject report that "in the course of talks with 356 youths, held in a labor colony for juveniles, it was found that almost half of them had committed [their] crimes in a state of intoxication, 78 percent admitted that they had continually used alcoholic beverages up to the time of arrest, [and] 33 percent had violated the criminal law with the purpose of getting money for them" (Vaisberg and Taibakova 1968:101).

The concern over drunkenness as a cause of crime is not usually directed at the person whose intoxication is casual, who "under the influence" does things he would otherwise abhor. Some writers even doubt that such a person exists: "Even in a state of intoxication, a person does not do anything that is utterly foreign to his nature; possessed of high and strong moral principles he will not, even under the influence of alcohol, commit an immoral act" (Sakharov 1961:232). The major worry is rather that the long-term "degradation" of the personality that results from habitual heavy drinking leaves the drinker susceptible to immorality and crime (Sakharov 1961:235). Some support for this view is found in a research study which showed that only 17 percent of the persons studied who had committed crimes while intoxicated did *not* have a long alcoholic period before their offense. The other 83 percent were "chronic alcoholics" (*Alkogolizm* 1966).

Although comprehensive figures on the number of man-hours lost and injuries sustained on the job because of drunkenness are not available, the indications are that alcohol plays an important role in these areas. *Nedelia* reports that a "study" in Gorky showed violations of labor discipline to be connected with drunkenness "in sixty-six instances out of a hundred" (24–30 July 1966:2). In March 1964 the party secretary of a lathe-building plant complained that workers' and technicians' drinking sprees had caused the loss of over a thousand man-hours—"enough for six new lathes" (*Sovetskaia Rossiia* 1964:4). Workers who are tempted to drink at lunchtime are continually warned that anything but complete sobriety in operating large machines can lead to serious injury (Rozhnov 1969), and antialcohol writers also strive to convince the many who feel they "work better" after a drink that their sense of increased capability is not matched by any increase in productivity, but leads often to a higher rate of spoilage (Banshchikov 1958).

The economic impact of rural illegal distilling is also seriously felt. The use of sugar, grain, beets, and potatoes in the production of *samogon* exacerbates agricultural problems, as does the loss of workdays on collective farms because of overindulgence.

A host of family problems is attributed to excessive drinking by husbands and fathers. Tkachevsky claims that 40 percent of all divorces are caused by the drunkenness of one of the spouses. Mistreatment of children is another major offense. Five years ago, a letter from a twelve-year-old whose father's habitual drunkenness had made home life unbearable was the starting point of a "readers' discussion" in *Izvestiia* which continued for many issues.

As Soviet writers become less reticent to discuss sexual matters, they find that alcohol is connected with many problems in this area. Prolonged impotence from habitual heavy drinking is cited as a source of marital tensions (e.g., Bogdanovich 1967; Rozhnov 1969), and a noted Soviet clinician cites his own researches to show that husbands who drink heavily become "gross" in their approach to intercourse and decrease the pleasure of both partners (Segal 1967). The evils of "casual" sex under the influence of alcohol are stressed for youth; and Rozhnov (1969), in his book intended mainly for members of the armed forces, ominously cites the words of a Soviet venereologist, 90 percent of whose syphilis and 95 percent of whose gonorrhea patients contracted the diseases while drunk.

The increase in leisure time available to many in the Soviet Union is accompanied by concern in some quarters that the time will be used "unprofitably." Among unprofitable uses, drinking is considered a major one. After the establishment of the five-day workweek, weekend liquor sales were reported to have increased as much as 25 percent in Moscow (*Literaturnaia gazeta* 13 Dec. 1967). Even those who engage in "healthy" athletic activity, such as swimming, may endanger their lives by combining it with drinking—Tkachevsky notes that 63 percent of all individuals in Moscow Oblast who drowned in 1968 (which should include a large number of swimmers) were intoxicated. The peril to sports careers from drinking is detailed in a number of Soviet books and pamphlets, with stories of the moral and physical downfall of athletes who develop a liking for the "green serpent" (e.g., Rozhnov 1969; Bogdanovich 1967).

Official Values and Popular Opinion

The gap between official attitudes toward drinking and "private" or popular opinion seems to be a wide one. The regime's values form the basis for a scale of evaluation in which a citizen is found "good" insofar as he embodies the qualities of the "new Soviet man"—sober, methodical, industrious, and committed to productive work and participation in the "public life" of Soviet society. A statement such as the following one can only be understood as an exhortation in the "indicative-imperative" style of Soviet writing: "Soviet man, the builder of the new Communist society, the sovereign ruler of his own native land, has firm confidence in tomorrow, and does not need drunkenness" (Gurvich 1958:11). The attitudes which cause so many Soviet citizens to deviate from this ideal are worth attention. Beyond the fact that most men drink, it is clear that drunkenness is viewed by many without any particular feelings of censure or disgust. A pamphlet writer complains that the struggle with alcoholism would enjoy greater success "if there were not connivance and an indifferent attitude toward it on the part of the public" (Tkachevsky 1966:n.9). The belief that alcohol is an indispensable element in the celebration of family events and holidays is seen as a major cause of alcoholism. One Soviet treatise cites studies indicating that in a large majority of cases the family backgrounds of alcoholics and drunkards revealed tolerance or acceptance of drunkenness (Segal 1967).

Certain "widespread beliefs" are another target of the writers and propagandists—among them, that alcohol is useful and beneficial as a medicine, and that although vodka may indeed be dangerous when drunk continually in large quantities, weaker drinks such as wine and beer may be consumed without fear (Rozhnov 1969; Levin 1963). Party and state officials are also faced with economic objections to their efforts to discourage drunkenness. Appeals to plant and office management to "do something" about the drunkenness of workers off the job brings the response that skilled workers are at a premium, and that even "measures" short of firing that could be taken against an offender may cause him to quit. An official complained that of "several thousand" notifications about employees' public drunkenness in Khabarovsk, only 634 were answered with a reply to the militia that "measures" had been taken.

In attempting to convince the public at large of the evils of drinking, the regime encounters at least three major problems. First, the web of popular attitudes that define drinking as "manly" and a necessary adjunct to conviviality is hard to penetrate. Such attitudes, as one doctor notes, "are extremely hard to overcome in an adult, especially when the majority of those around him also use alcoholic beverages" (Segal 1967:546). Nor has antialcohol persuasion linked itself effectively to other positive values in the drinker's consciousness. Rhetorical appeals on the basis of "patriotism" and civic dignity have scant effect. Warnings about the dangers of illness to the drinker and genetic harm to his offspring are closer to his personal concerns, but are often met with disbelief that such could happen to him (these "scare" tactics have generally not been successful [Lemert 1962]). Appeals to the drinker not to jeopardize the happiness of his family conflict with his conviction that at home, at least, he should be allowed the mode of relaxation he wishes.

The second major difficulty encountered in attempts to convince the public of the dangers of drinking is the inconsistent treatment of the subject in various media and in lectures. Most antialcohol tracts are completely against the use of alcohol, but articles in the press often make a distinction between beer and wine on the one hand and stronger drink on the other—thereby, in the minds of critics, encouraging the use of the former. In view of the counterproductive experience of both the Russian Empire and the Soviet state with "dry laws," prohibition is rejected as a solution. Yet such a refusal may be somewhat hard for Soviet citizens, accustomed to government intervention in many aspects of "private" life, to comprehend. "If," asked an occasional drinker's wife in a letter to a Soviet editor, "alcohol is so bad, why isn't it prohibited?" Proalcohol messages in the entertainment media also cause concern. Cinema heroes are frequently criticized for heavy drinking on the screen and the impression of enjoyment they convey. Even *Komsomol'skaia pravda,* in a discussion of proposed regulations to curtail holiday drinking, turned them down on the grounds that it would be "inconceivable" to thus "emasculate" celebrations (9 Oct. 1965).

The third obstacle antialcohol forces face lies in the characteristics of the "target" audience. Persons with drinking problems are frequently said to be those who have "little culture," little formal education, and relatively unskilled jobs. Many give "boredom" as a reason for their drinking. To the degree that this is true, these "escapist" drinkers are unlikely to pay much attention to antialcohol messages, or, for that matter, any other exhortations from official sources.

Weapons in "The Struggle"

In pressing the fight against drunkenness and alcoholism, the state has "armaments" roughly divisible into four categories: (1) antialcohol propaganda, (2) the mobilization of "public" pressures, (3) compulsory treatment, and (4) measures that are primarily medical. (The last category will not be discussed in detail here.)

Perhaps the most interesting thing about the antialcohol propaganda presented in the Soviet media and lectures is the dissatisfaction with it, which can be expressed in two not wholly consistent complaints: it is largely ineffective and unconvincing, and there is not enough of it. The announced objectives of this propaganda are, first, to form public opinion to view drunkenness as an "alien" and harmful phenomenon, and, second, to involve the "public" in the struggle against it (Orlovsky 1963). In concrete form, antialcohol propaganda fluctuates between generalized appeals to the Soviet citizen's personal and social dignity and relatively crude "scare tactics," such as the description, with illustrations, of pathological changes in the stomach and liver from long-term drinking (e.g., Rozhnov 1969). "Case histories," replete with stories of broken families, lost jobs, and ruined lives, are another feature of the propaganda in pamphlets and newspapers.

Some of the standard claims made by propagandists are problematic. Often it is said that moderate drinking leads almost inevitably to heavy drinking (e.g., Lerman 1958; Banshchikov 1958; *Sovetskaia torgovlia* 12 May 1959). Many audiences find this hard to believe, and even those specializing in propaganda find themselves complaining about it: " 'Rivers begin from a stream'—they repeat, in every way, this favorite proverb. The numerous exceptions to this rule compel one to have doubts about its infallibility. . . . The majority of those who have gotten used to contenting themselves with small doses, despite the 'prognosis,' do not change for the rest of their lives" (*Meditsinskaia gazeta* 16 July 1963).

Even more debatable is the frequent assertion that heavy drinking has a direct, physical influence on offspring—accounting for the birth of many weak-witted and physically handicapped children (see Rozhnov 1969). Only rarely explored is the possibility that the academic and emotional problems of the children of alcoholics are attributable not to direct physical consequences but to early home environments reflecting parental pathologies (Segal 1967).

Much of the face-to-face propagandizing in factories, apartment complexes, and the like is done by persons who have no medical knowledge, or by lower-echelon medical workers who may themselves find the content of their message difficult to believe. B. M. Segal, author of the most comprehensive recent Soviet work on alcoholism, notes that the low effectiveness of propaganda in combatting the deep-rooted proalcohol traditions of the population may be partly due to the propagandists' own lack of "internal convictions of the correctness of their appeal" (1967:546).

Mobilization of the public as a force for the correction and rehabilitation of drunkards presents real problems, and complaints about public apathy are more frequent than praise for their civic-spiritedness in intervening with drunkards. Thus the account which follows of a worker reformed by the censure of his fellow workers probably represents more the ideal than the typical situation:

> One day when he appeared in the shop drunk he was put into the "workers' circle." At first Vladimir was cocky.
> "I got drunk; so what? I did it with my own money, not yours. What business is it of yours?"
> But the workers began to speak, one after another. The "circle" came to life and got excited, and it was as if a refreshing wind were blowing around Vladimir. He began to sober up right before their eyes. His arrogance vanished as if by magic. He began to defend himself, then to make excuses, then to repeat, and finally he broke down and burst into tears. He swore on his honor that he would never do it again, and he has kept his word. He is now on a par with the leading production workers. [*Izvestiia* 29 Aug. 1965:4]

On the other side of the coin, management, workers, the Komsomol, and even the militia are criticized for the lack of concern they frequently show in a hands-off attitude toward drunkards.

"Compulsory treatment" and the network of institutions that provide it represent a "tough" approach to alcoholics. As noted earlier, it is aimed at those whose alcohol problems have already made them violators of public order—though not necessarily criminals. Nonetheless, it seems likely that under the new legislation persons committed who have not been brought to "criminal responsibility" will be living alongside those who are convicted felons. It is instructive that (1) the "treatment-labor *profilaktorii*" which existed before the new legislation, and the "treatment-labor institutions" to be set up under it, are administered by the MVD, (2) the period of confinement in the RSFSR statute is one to two years, and at least half of the "sentence" must be served before a patient can be released, and (3) attempted escape from these institutions is a criminal offense, for those committed who are *not* felons as well as those who are. With the exception of the added element of "special medical treatment," the characteristics of these institutions—a "regime" of confinement, "labor reeducation," and "political-upbringing work"—sound the same as those of the corrective-labor colonies for criminal offenders. Since construction of facilities for the new institutions seems to be lagging, it may be assumed that much, if not most, of "compulsory treatment" is still carried out in the "treatment-labor" divisions of corrective-labor colonies.

Little can be said about the success of compulsory treatment, for not much information has been made public. Segal discusses the relatively positive results of compulsory treatment in the "closed narcological division" of the North Kazakhstan Oblast psychiatric hospital, but has little to say about the newer institutions just getting into operation (1967). From all indications, the compulsory treatment institutions reflect a punitive attitude toward the alcoholic, which many doctors share with the public-order authorities. But as well as answering the call for a "crackdown," these institutions may also reflect economic considerations. Complaints are still frequently voiced about habitual drunkards who commit themselves voluntarily to psychiatric hospitals for treatment, sometimes as often as once a year, and resume their old habits when released. They receive their medical care free, do no work in the hospitals, and receive sick-leave pay in addition. A psychoneurologist describes one person in this category:

> After drinking up his last kopeks, a drunkard is placed in the comfortable conditions of a psychiatric clinic. . . . After a few days of treatment with modern medicines the alcoholic's symptoms of psychic derangement disappear, as a rule, and he is transferred to the

category of the so-called "conscious ill." And then a perfectly
healthy lug begins literally making fun of people who are really
sick. As soon as he is discharged, the drunkard "washes off" his
sick leave payments, and everything starts all over again. [*Izvestiia*
1 Oct. 1968:5]

It seems probable that many such "lugs" are classifiable as "violators" under the language of the compulsory treatment decree. If
so, the state may well regard treatment-labor institutions, where
inmates are made to work and deductions are made from their
earnings for the cost of their care and maintenance, as a more
suitable environment for them than a psychiatric hospital.

One other "front" in the war against drunkenness involves
the structure of retail trade in alcohol and the attempts to control
drinking by price manipulation and setting limits on times and
places for the sale of liquor. By the mid-1950s gradual price de-
creases and increasing income had made vodka cheaper, and the
increase in numbers of establishments selling it added to the
problem of growing consumption. Administrative regulations in
many large cities attempted to limit sales, and by 1961 it was
claimed that alcoholic beverages could no longer be purchased in
communal dining rooms and snack bars—two major sources (Sokolov 1961). Violations of these regulations were, however, frequent,
and remain so. Since the sales plans of eating establishments
where liquor can be served concentrate on the high-profit items,
alcohol is often "pushed" in these places to a degree that draws
complaints from those who see the economic forces here as working counterproductively (*Komsomol'skaia pravda* 10 Sept. 1961).

It is, in fact, easier to detail the problems encountered in
enforcing such regulations than to specify their provisions, since
most of these regulations are promulgated on a local (city) level
and are "administrative" in nature. Writing in *Izvestiia* in 1958, a
doctor praised the Moscow city soviet for an ordinance prohibiting
the sale of vodka in market stalls, but complained about its weak
enforcement (*Izvestiia* 2 Mar. 1958). In 1961 the Rostov city soviet's Trade Administration limited restaurants to serving no more
than one hundred grams of vodka to a customer and prohibited its
sale in dining rooms and cafés, but left the sale of wine and
brandy completely unregulated (*Komsomol'skaia pravda* 10 Sept.
1961). As samples of apparently widespread provisions, one
source cites the prohibition of the sale of vodka in fish, meat, fruit,
vegetable, dairy, and dietetic stores, in all eating places (excluding restaurants), in railroad stations and airports, as well as before
10:00 A.M. and to minors (*Alkogolizm* 1966). The volume of com-

plaints indicates that many of these regulations are honored mainly in the breach.

The considerable income the state receives from alcohol, however, may limit how far it is willing to go to restrict trade. The collective volume *Alcoholism: Path to Crime* (1966) contains among its concluding proposals certain ones for the "furthest development" of sale restriction measures on "strong drink" and for a gradual substitution of some other source for the income the state now derives from alcohol. There is little evidence that much action has been taken on either proposal.

The Future

The foregoing survey of popular values, official attitudes, and the measures employed to combat drunkenness and alcoholism in the USSR leads us to the question, What of the future? Is there any evidence that measures now in effect or recently proposed will affect the problem significantly? As economic conditions continue to improve over the nadir reached in the years immediately after World War II, one might expect a decline in purely "escapist" drinking. But the whole pattern of complaints about the drinking behavior of factory workers and kolkhozniks seems to reflect a stable "drinking culture," many elements of which are traceable, in both the urban and rural populations, to peasant life in the nineteenth century. That so much of this culture survived the revolution and the migration of the population to the cities is not surprising. Studies of the drinking behavior of Irish, Jews, and Italians show that generally their respective high and low potentials for alcohol pathologies also survived large-scale immigration to the United States.

Thus many of the measures discussed seem destined for little success. "Antialcohol propaganda" reiterates the same appeals in each year's crop of books, pamphlets, and films, and seems as far as ever from gaining mass attention in an effective way. Segal is certainly correct that the identification of drinking with manliness and conviviality in so many minds is one of the major factors in the low effectiveness of the propaganda directed against alcohol, but the "scare tactics" the propagandists use in referring to the physical consequences of alcoholism are exactly the sort he warns against (1967). The inertia evident in most of this pamphleteering suggests that the "formula" used now, ineffective as it may be, will endure.

What is true of antialcohol propaganda seems all the more

true of attempts to enlist the "public" (with the possible exception of some women) in the struggle on any mass scale. Such "popular" social control mechanisms as the comrades' courts and people's volunteers (*druzhiny*), although they may enjoy public support in some of their dealings with petty "hooligans" and the like, have yet to make a large dent, apparently, in the problems within their provinces. Any All-Union Society for the Struggle with Alcoholism which depends on unpaid volunteers for its "mass" work will be likely to encounter the same problems as the comrades' courts and, more so, the *druzhiny*—"assignment" of personnel to duties under party or trade-union pressures rather than "volunteering," and a consequent lack of interest in and, wherever possible, avoidance of the work involved. Since the average citizen is less concerned about drunkenness than crime and directly "antisocial" behavior, there is little to be expected from such organizations, if established.

Compulsory treatment in the institutions referred to earlier is aimed at the isolation and "cure" of those with serious drinking problems and antisocial behavior. It appears that the lines between the treatment for this category and for "garden variety" criminals (short of repeated offenders) are loosely drawn (with the exception of the medical treatment the former are to receive). Experiences with compulsory treatment in the past were not the kind that would inspire confidence. Whether longer sentences under the new legislation will prove more effective remains to be seen. "Punitive" approaches to problem drinkers are rarely successful, and it seems a vain hope that this one will be more effective than medical measures of a chemical or psychiatric variety. (With regard to the more strictly "medical" approaches, Segal notes that the average "cure" is "not long," and that in one-third of all cases "recidivism" occurs early [1967:533].)

One cannot say definitely that the Soviet alcohol problem is increasing. Perhaps it has "stabilized." However, the tone of government pronouncements and the language of antialcohol propaganda make it clear that it is not decreasing. As is true of crime and delinquency, the problem of alcoholism is not one that menaces the stability of Soviet society on the whole. But it does reflect the limited ability of a government never notably reluctant to intervene in the everyday lives of its citizens to modify widespread behavior patterns when these patterns are supported or tolerated by the mass of the people.

Notes

1. The two categories—"habitual drunkard" and alcoholic—in the statute's title are not clearly distinguished in Soviet writings. A rough distinction between "drunkenness" as a behavioral concept relevant to public-order concerns and "alcoholism" as a medical concept can be made, but it obscures the reluctance of Soviet writers to call alcoholism simply a "disease." For our purposes, the terms can be taken as roughly interchangeable and as signifying a person whose involvement with alcohol has seriously impaired his social, economic, or civic functioning.

Conclusions
Mac Marshall

The preceding articles show some of the myriad ways persons in various cultures consume and symbolize the consumption of alcoholic beverages. The authors offer details on who drinks, the settings in which drinking occurs, attitudes toward drunks, expectations about drunken comportment, and the kinds of alcoholic beverages imbibed. Commentary also is given by many of these authors on the presence or absence of drinking pathologies and social disruption caused by drunken persons. In all this cross-cultural detail it is not always easy to discern the more general rules and relationships that recur from society to society. My purpose, therefore, in this conclusion is to present some of the more important generalizations about alcohol and humanity that derive from the preceding articles. I shall phrase these generalizations as hypotheses that hopefully will stimulate further and more specific research. Wherever possible I will point out those articles in this book that support or refute the general rule.

1. *Solitary, addictive, pathological drinking behavior does not occur to any significant extent in small-scale, traditional, pre-industrial societies; such behavior appears to be a concomitant of complex, modern, industrialized societies.* A number of authors specifically note the absence of solitary and addictive drinking in small-scale social systems (e.g., Madsen and Madsen [regarding Tecospan], Lemert, Nason, and Westermeyer in Section V, Hutchinson [regarding traditional Bantu society], and Netting). Other writers document the presence of this form of drinking pathology in more complex, industrialized societies (e.g., Sargent, Madsen, Sadler, Walsh, Anderson, and Connor). Finally, several authors provide evidence of the onset of limited amounts of addictive drinking by individuals outside of group settings in "modernizing" situations where social systems have become transitional between small-scale traditional and large-scale modern societies

451

(e.g., Madsen and Madsen [regarding Tepepan], Doughty, and Yawney [regarding East Indians in particular]). The only case in this volume that appears to contradict this generalization is that of the Hopi (Kunitz et al.). The Hopi live in a small-scale, traditional, preindustrial setting, and yet solitary, addictive drinking appears to be the rule among them. Apparently this results from a very high degree of ambivalence about alcoholic beverages.

2. *Beverage alcohol usually is not a problem in society unless and until it is defined as such.* Nonmoralistic attitudes toward alcoholic beverages generally seem to accompany non-pathological uses of such beverages, and vice versa. Yawney, for instance, observes that East Indians in Trinidad, who are ambivalent about alcohol and practice religions opposed to alcohol use, suffer a much higher incidence of alcoholism than blacks in the same country, who accept drinking and drunkenness and adhere to religions that do not moralize about alcohol. One of Lurie's main points is that the moralistic stances on American Indian drinking adopted by whites have contributed to the perception of a problem where one does not always exist. Westermeyer in section III reinforces this point, and Lemert reaches a similar conclusion when commenting on the French view of Society Islanders' drinking and the islanders' own views on the matter. Several writers also show that when alcoholic beverages are viewed as a "nonproblem" they usually are not a problem (e.g., Carstairs, Singer, Netting, and Keller).

3. *When members of a society have had sufficient time to develop a widely shared set of beliefs and values pertaining to drinking and drunkenness, the consequences of alcohol consumption are not usually disruptive for most persons in that society. On the other hand, where beverage alcohol has been introduced within the past century and such a set of beliefs and values has not developed completely, social—and sometimes physiological—problems with ethanol commonly result.* There are numerous examples in this volume of peoples who have known alcoholic beverages for centuries and who have integrated these beverages into the fabric of their lives in nondisruptive and positive ways (e.g., Madsen and Madsen, Doughty, Yawney [regarding blacks], Westermeyer in Section V, Carstairs, Singer, Netting, M. C. Robbins [regarding banana beer], Keller, Honigmann in Section VII, and Anderson). On the other hand, some peoples who have possessed alcoholic beverages for a long time have begun to develop alcohol problems under the press of rapid social change (see, for example, Sargent and Hutchinson). Walsh demonstrates that the

Irish present an unusual case where a widely shared set of beliefs and values exists that fosters and reinforces individual and social problems with alcoholic beverages. Many North American Indian tribes (e.g., Lurie) and the Samoans (Lemert) illustrate instances where social and physiological problems with alcohol are consequent on insufficient time to develop a widely shared set of assumptions about the place of alcohol in society.

4. *The amount of pure ethanol in the beverage consumed bears little or no direct relationship to the kind of drunken comportment that results; i.e., one cannot assert that the stronger the beverage the more disruptive the comportment.* Singer discusses the lack of boisterous and violent behavior among Chinese drinkers even though they consume beverages quite high in ethanol content. By contrast, Irish beer drinkers, whose beverage is relatively low in ethanol, are well known for rowdy and aggressive drunkenness (Walsh). Other instances where ethanol content of the dominant beverage consumed varies independently of the kind of drunken comportment described are presented by Madsen and Madsen, Lurie, Nason, Schwartz and Romanucci-Ross, Westermeyer in Section V, Netting, and Anderson.

5. *All societies recognize permissible alterations in behavior from normal, sober comportment when alcoholic beverages are consumed, but these alterations are always "within limits." The limits for drunken comportment usually are more lax than those prescribed for sober persons in the same situations.* The articles in this volume confirm the generalization summarized above which derives from MacAndrew and Edgerton's (1969) cross-cultural study of drunken comportment. Particularly good discussions of the limits on drunken behavior are provided by Lurie, R. H. Robbins, Lemert, Nason, Schwartz and Romanucci-Ross, Yamamuro, Sargent, Hutchinson, Netting, M. C. Robbins, and Honigmann in Section VII.

6. *Beverage alcohol usually is defined as a social facilitator (i.e., as a substance that promotes friendship, camaraderie, social solidarity, etc.), and this belief may persist despite considerable evidence to the contrary.* The contrast pointed to in this general statement is illustrated in Madsen and Madsen's comparison of Tecospan and Tepepan. In both communities alcohol is defined as a social facilitator. In Tepepan alcohol contributes to social divisiveness, violence, and addiction, whereas in Tecospan it promotes social solidarity and is never accompanied by in-group aggression or addiction. Other instances where alcohol is viewed as a social facilitator are given by Doughty, Lemert, Nason, Yama-

muro, Sargent, Westermeyer in Section V, Carstairs, Hutchinson, Netting, Honigmann in Section VII, and Connor.

7. *Socially disruptive drinking occurs only in secular settings. When alcoholic beverages are used in sacred or religious contexts they seldom produce socially disruptive drunken comportment, unless such comportment is considered an appropriate part of the religious worship.* The most dramatic example in support of this generalization is provided by Keller. However, this general rule also is underscored by Madsen and Madsen for Tecospan, by Leacock for the Afro-Brazilian cult, by Yamamuro for traditional Japanese drinking, and by Netting and M. C. Robbins for two unrelated African societies. Moreover, Carstairs's data give the impression that the same hypothesis might hold for drug substances other than ethanol, such as cannabis.

8. *Beverage alcohol is used for festive, ceremonial, or ritual celebrations the world over.* Mention of this fact appears frequently in the literature. It is important to note that these occasions are explicitly nonsacred or nonreligious in nature, and that they provide a special atmosphere within which drinking takes place. Documentation of this hypothesis is found in the articles by Doughty, Yawney, Lemert, Nason, Yamamuro, Westermeyer in Section V, Carstairs, Singer, Hutchinson, Netting, Keller, Honigmann in Section VII, and Connor.

9. *Where opportunities for group or community recreation are few and alcoholic beverages are available, alcohol consumption will become a major form of recreational activity in a community ("the boredom rule").* While persons consume alcoholic beverages for a host of reasons, this generalization makes the point that "recreational drinking" often occurs when other forms of recreation are either absent or relatively inaccessible. This can be seen in Madsen and Madsen concerning Tepepan, in Yawney concerning the rumshops of Trinidad, in Nason's descriptions of yeast parties on Etal, and in Walsh's discussion of the Irish "heroic tradition."

10. *Typically, alcoholic beverages are used more by males than by females and more by young adults than by preadolescents or older persons. Hence in any society the major consumers of beverage alcohol are most likely to be young men between their mid-teens and their mid-thirties.* Confirmation of this generalization comes from many different articles as well as from cross-cultural research conducted by Child, Barry, and Bacon (1965). Specifically, the following studies reprinted in this volume support these differences: Madsen and Madsen, Doughty, Kunitz

et al., Lemert, Nason, Schwartz and Romanucci-Ross, Sargent, Westermeyer in Section V, Carstairs, Midgley, Netting, Walsh, Honigmann in Section VII, Anderson, and Connor.

11. *Not only do males usually drink more and more frequently than females, but males' drunken comportment usually is more exaggerated and potentially more explosive than that of females, regardless of relative ethanol consumption.* Obviously, this generalization has as much to do with cultural expectations about the differing behavior of the sexes as it does with drunkenness. Examples of this come from Madsen and Madsen's description of "macho" mestizo males in Mexico, Lemert's discussion of Samoan drinking, Nason's observations of drinking on Etal Atoll in Micronesia (cf. also Marshall 1979), and Connor's comments on alcohol use in the Soviet Union.

12. *The drinking of alcoholic beverages occurs usually with friends or relatives and not among strangers. Where drinking among strangers does take place, violence is much more likely to erupt.* Madsen and Madsen describe how drinkers from Tecospan, who never aggress against each other when inebriated, frequently become violent drunks when away from their home village. Further support for this generalization is found in the articles by Doughty, Nason, Westermeyer in Section V, Hutchinson, Netting, and M. C. Robbins.

13. *Peoples who lacked alcoholic beverages aboriginally borrowed styles of drunken comportment along with the beverages from those who introduced them to "demon rum."* This generalization derives from MacAndrew and Edgerton's (1969) study and is supported by material on North American Indians and Pacific Islanders reported in this volume (see especially Dailey, Lurie, Lemert, Marshall and Marshall, and Schwartz and Romanucci-Ross).

14. *When alcoholic beverages are defined culturally as a food and/or a medicine, drunkenness seldom is disruptive or antisocial.* This generalization is supported by data from Mexico with regard to pulque (Madsen and Madsen); Peru with regard to *chicha* (Doughty); China with regard to Chinese wine (Singer); Nigeria with regard to local beer (Netting); Uganda with regard to banana beer (M. C. Robbins); Austria with regard to schnapps and wine (Honigmann in Section VII); and France with regard to wine (Anderson). Interestingly, among the societies described in this volume distilled beverages are nowhere thought of as a food and in only one case are distilled beverages mentioned as having medicinal value (schnapps in Austria; Honigmann, Section VII).

15. *Alcoholic beverages are the drug of choice for a majority of persons in any society, even if alternative drug substances are available.*   Several examples in support of this finding may be found in the preceding articles. Alcohol has supplanted kava as the drug of choice in much of Polynesia and in parts of Micronesia (Lemert and Marshall and Marshall), and it has begun to replace betel in the Admiralty Islands (Schwartz and Romanucci-Ross). Westermeyer in Section V and Singer comment on the preferential use of alcohol over opium for most persons in two different Asian societies. Carstairs's material on cannabis use by Brahmans only partially contradicts the above generalization. Regrettably, reliable data on the concurrence of tobacco and alcohol use in other cultures are lacking at this time, although the smoking of tobacco is known to frequently accompany the drinking of alcohol in many societies.

16. *Once alcoholic beverages have become available in a society, attempts to establish legal prohibition have never proven completely successful.*   In spite of this fact, efforts to force legal prohibition continue to be made; for example, recent laws to this effect have been enacted in India and in Truk District of Micronesia. Illustrations of the failure of prohibition appear in Madsen and Madsen (Spanish efforts in Mexico), Westermeyer in Section III (American Indians in the United States), Lurie (French efforts in "New France"), Lemert (colonial efforts in Polynesian societies), Marshall and Marshall (missionary attempts in Micronesia), Nason (Etal Atoll, Micronesia), Schwartz and Romanucci-Ross (Papua-New Guinea), Yamamuro (Japan), and Connor (the Soviet Union). The only "prohibition" against alcohol consumption that seems to work in human society is that taken on *voluntarily* by the drinker himself—often for religious reasons (e.g., Midgley; cf. Madsen and Sadler).

In the introduction I noted that a full understanding of the complex relationships between human beings and alcoholic beverages will never be realized until biological, psychological, and sociocultural data are all taken into account. The articles in this volume, and concluding generalizations, make it plain that what people believe alcohol to be (e.g., a disinhibitor, a food, a medicine, a social facilitator, a sacred or a secular substance) greatly influences the ways they behave once they ingest it. It is clear that sociocultural understandings of alcohol use and abuse by themselves will not solve the mysteries or the problems of alcohol abuse and alcoholism. It is equally certain, however, that efforts to comprehend why some persons in some societies drink addictively and destructively will never succeed until serious account is taken of the beliefs surrounding the behaviors that result following alcohol consumption. The contributors to this volume have made many such beliefs clear for societies other than our own, and in many cases they have also provided insights that—suitably modified—may assist in the development of more effective alcohol treatment programs in those societies where alcoholism exists. It remains for us to take the lessons learned from cross-cultural studies of alcohol use and apply them to problems in our own society. It is my hope that this volume will contribute in some small measure toward this worthy goal.

Bibliography

Abegglen, J. G.
  1958   *The Japanese factory: aspects of its social organization.* New York: The Free Press.
Aberle, David R.
  1967   The psychosocial analysis of a Hopi life-history. In *Personalities and culture,* edited by R. Hunt. Garden City, N.Y.: Natural History Press.
Abu-Laban, B., and D. Larsen
  1968   The qualities and sources of norms and definitions of alcohol. *Sociology and Social Research* 53: 34–43.
Adler, A.
  1931   *The pattern of life.* New York: Cosmopolitan Book Co.
Alcoholics Anonymous
  1955   *Alcoholics Anonymous.* New York: Alcoholics Anonymous, World Services, Inc.
  1957   *Alcoholics Anonymous comes of age: a brief history of A.A.* New York: Alcoholics Anonymous Publishing, Inc.
Alexander, F.
  1963   Alcohol and behavioral disorder, alcoholism. In *Alcohol and civilization,* edited by S. P. Incia. New York: McGraw-Hill.
Alexander, James M.
  1895   *The islands of the Pacific. From the old to the new.* New York: American Tract Society.
Alkogolizm: put' k prestupleniiu.
  1966   Moscow.
Allardt, E.
  1957   Drinking norms and drinking habits. In *Drinking and drinkers,* by E. Allardt, T. Markkanen, and M. Takala. Helsinki: Finnish Foundation for Alcohol Studies.
Allen, G.
  1965   Random and nonrandom inbreeding. *Eugenics Quarterly* 12: 181–98.
Ames, C. G.
  1934   *Gazeteer of Plateau Province.* Jos: Jos Native Authority.
Asahi consumer's survey
  1965   Tokyo: Asahi News.
Assagioli, R.
  1971   *Psychosynthesis: a manual of principles and techniques.* New York: The Viking Press.

459

Australia
1964   From rum-running and wool-gathering to a billion dollar business. *Australia* 2:12–15.
Babcock, C. G.
1963   Reflections on dependency phenomena as seen in *nisei* in the U.S. In *Japanese culture: its development and characteristics*, edited by R. J. Smith and R. K. Beardsley. Chicago: Aldine.
Bacon, Margaret; Herbert Barry III; and Irving L. Child
1965   A cross-cultural study of drinking practices. Pt. 2. Relations to other features of culture. *Quarterly Journal of Studies on Alcohol*, supp. no. 3, pp. 29–47.
Bacon, Selden
1944   *Sociology and the problems of alcohol.* New Haven: Yale University Press.
1945   Alcohol and complex society. In *Alcohol, science and society.* New Haven: Yale University Press. Reprinted 1962. In *Society, culture, and drinking patterns*, edited by David J. Pittman and Charles R. Snyder. New York: John Wiley & Sons.
1958   Alcoholics do not drink. *Annals of the American Academy of Political and Social Science* 315: 55–64.
Bailey, W.
1967   Primary drug addiction. *Medical Opinion and Review* 3: 82–91.
Bales, Robert F.
1944   The "fixation factor" in alcohol addiction: an hypothesis derived from a comparative study of Irish and Jewish social norms. Ph.D. dissertation, Harvard University.
1946   Cultural differences in rates of alcoholism. *Quarterly Journal of Studies on Alcohol* 6: 480–99.
1962   Attitudes toward drinking in the Irish culture. In *Society, culture and drinking patterns*, edited by D. J. Pittman and C. R. Snyder. New York: John Wiley & Sons.
Banfield, Edward C.
1958   *The moral basis of a backward society.* Glencoe, Ill.: The Free Press.
Banshchikov, V. M.
1958   *Alkogolizm i ego vred dlia zdorov'ia cheloveka.* Moscow.
Barber, B.
1941   Acculturation and messianic movements. *American Sociological Review* 6: 663–69.
Barnett, M. L.
1955   Alcoholism in the Cantonese of New York City, an anthropological study. In *Etiology of chronic alcoholism*, edited by O. Diethelm. Springfield, Ill.: Charles C. Thomas.
Barrington, Jonah
1968   *The Ireland of Sir Jonah Barrington*, edited by H. B. Staples. London: P. Owen.
Barry, Herbert, III
1968   Sociocultural aspects of addiction. *Addiction States* 46: 455–71.
Barth, Fredrik
1969   Pathan identity and its maintenance. In *Ethnic groups and boundaries*, edited by Fredrik Barth. Boston: Little, Brown & Co.

Bascom, Willard R.
1950 Ponape: the cycle of empire. *Scientific Monthly* 70: 141–50.
Basham, A. L.
1954 *The wonder that was India.* New York: Grove Press.
Bastide, Roger
1958 *Le Candomblé de Bahia.* Paris: Mouton & Co.
1960 *Les religions Africaines au Brésil.* Paris: Presses Universitaires de France.
Bateson, Gregory
1971 The cybernetics of "self": a theory of alcoholism. *Psychiatry* 34: 1–18. Reprinted 1972. In *Steps to an ecology of mind.* New York: Ballantine.
Baudelaire, C. P.
1860 *Les paradis artificiels, opium et haschisch.* Paris.
Beardsley, R. K.; J. W. Hall; and R. E. Ward
1959 *Village Japan.* Chicago: The University of Chicago Press.
Beattie, J.
1958 The blood pact in Bunyoro. *African Studies* 17: 198–203.
Beckett, J. C.
1966 *The making of modern Ireland 1603–1923.* London: Faber.
Bellah, Robert N.
1957 *Tokugawa religion: the values of pre-industrial Japan.* New York: The Free Press.
Belshaw, Cyril S.
1950 The significance of modern cults in Melanesian development. *Australian Outlook* 4: 116–25.
Benedict, Ruth
1934 Anthropology and the abnormal. *Journal of General Psychology* 10: 59–82.
1947 *The chrysanthemum and the sword.* London: Secker & Warburg.
1959a Anthropology and the abnormal. In *An anthropologist at work,* edited by Margaret Mead. Boston: Houghton Mifflin Co.
1959b Psychological types in the cultures of the Southwest. In *An anthropologist at work,* edited by Margaret Mead. Boston: Houghton Mifflin Co. (First published in 1930 in *Proceedings of the Twenty-Third International Congress of Americanists.*)
Berreman, Gerald D.
1956 Drinking patterns of the Aleuts. *Quarterly Journal of Studies on Alcohol* 17: 503–14.
Berreman, J. V.
1950 The escape motive in alcoholic addiction. *Research Studies of the State College of Washington* 18: 139–43.
Blakeslee, George H.
1921 Japan's new island possessions in the Pacific: history and present status. *The Journal of International Relations* 12: 173–91.
Blum, R., and E. Blum
1964 Drinking practices and controls in rural Greece. *British Journal of Addiction* 60: 93–108.
Bogdanovich, L. A.
1967 *Zhizn' nachinaetsia segodnia.* Moscow.

Bollig, P. Laurentius
    1927   Die Bewohner der Truk-Inseln. Religion, leben und kurze
            grammatik eines Mikronesiervolkes. *Anthropos Ethnologische
            Bibliothek* 3: 1–320. Munster: Aschendorff.
Borden, Charles A.
    1961   *South sea islands.* Philadelphia: Macrae Smith Co.
Bourguignon, Erika
    1965   The theory of spirit possession. In *Context and meaning in cul-
            tural anthropology,* edited by Melford E. Spiro. New York: The
            Free Press.
Bradfield, Stillman
    1963   *Migration from Huaylas: a study of brothers.* Ph.D. disserta-
            tion, Cornell University.
Brand, C. M.
    1968   The Indians of the Cape Peninsula. *Journal of Social Research*
            17: 83–94.
Bridge, Cyprian
    1886   Cruises in Melanesia, Micronesia, and Western Polynesia in
            1882, 1883, and 1884, with visits to New Guinea and the Loui-
            sades in 1884 and 1885. *Proceedings of the Royal Geographical
            Society and Monthly Record of Geography,* n.s. 8: 545–67.
Brody, H.
    1970   *Indians on Skid Row.* Ottawa: Northern Science Research
            Group, Department of Indian Affairs and Northern Develop-
            ment, Publication 70–2
Bromage, W. H.
    1892   Blackbirds of the Pacific. *The Weekly Examiner* (San Francisco).
            20 October 1892.
Bromberg, W., and T. C. Rodgers
    1946   Marihuana and aggressive crime (in naval service). *American
            Journal of Psychiatry* 102: 825–27.
Brown, D. E.
    1973   Voluntary associations: a further comment. *American Anthro-
            pologist* 76: 309–12.
Bruun, Kettil
    1959   Significance of role and norms in the small drinking group for
            individual behavioral changes while drinking. *Quarterly Jour-
            nal of Studies on Alcohol* 20: 53–64.
Bunzel, Ruth
    1940   The role of alcoholism in two Central American cultures. *Psy-
            chiatry* 3: 361–87.
Burridge, Kenelm
    1969   *New heaven, new earth: a study of millenarian activities.* New
            York: Schocken Books.
Burton, Roger V., and John W. M. Whiting
    1965   The absent father and cross-sex identity. In *A reader in compa-
            rative religion,* edited by William A. Lessa and Evon Z. Vogt.
            New York: Harper & Row.
Canadian Alcohol and Drug Addiction Research Foundation
    1966   *Culture and alcohol use: a bibliography of anthropological
            studies.* Ottawa.

Cancian, Frank
  1965   *Economics and prestige in a Maya community.* Stanford: The
         Stanford University Press.
Cape of Good Hope
  1874   *Blue book on native affairs*, G. 27–1874.
  1875   *Blue book on native affairs*, G. 21–1875.
  1880   *Blue book on native affairs*, G. 13–1880.
  1884   *Blue book on native affairs*, G. 3–1884.
  1898   *Blue book on native affairs*, G. 42–1898.
  1903   *Blue book on native affairs*, G. 29–1903.
  1904   *Blue book on native affairs*, G. 12–1904.
Cape of Good Hope, House of Assembly Papers
  1883   *Report and minutes of evidence of the Commission on Native
         Laws and Customs* (G. 4–1883), pars. 2381–84, 5096, 4322–24.
  1894   *Further minutes of evidence and report of the Labour Commis-
         sion* (G. 3–1894), pars. 14708, 20, 800–20, 805.
Cape of Good Hope, Labour Commission
  1893   *Minutes of evidence of the Labour Commission* (G. 39–1893),
         pars. 5092–94, 1150–51.
Cape of Good Hope, Report on Natives
  1908   Report on the occupation of land by natives in areas not set
         apart for them (G. 46–1908).
Cape of Good Hope, Select Committee
  1883   *Report of the Select Committee on the Port Elizabeth Native
         Strangers Location Bill* (A. 10–1883), par. 144.
Carstairs, G.
  1926   *The Hindu.* Edinburgh.
Carstairs, G. M.
  1953   The case of Thakur Khuman Singh: a culture-conditioned crime.
         British Journal of Delinquency 4: 14–25.
  1954   Daru and bhang: cultural factors in the choice of intoxicant.
         Quarterly Journal of Studies on Alcohol 15: 220–37.
  1957   *The twice-born.* London: Hogarth Press.
Catanzaro, D. G.
  1967   Psychiatric aspects of alcoholism. In *Alcoholism*, edited by
         David J. Pittman. New York: Harper & Row.
Caudill, William
  1959   Observations on the cultural context of Japanese psychiatry. In
         Culture and mental health, edited by Marvin K. Opler. New
         York: Macmillan.
Chafetz, Morris E.
  1964   Consumption of alcohol in the Far and Middle East. *New En-
         gland Journal of Medicine* 271: 297–301.
Chafetz, Morris E., and H. W. Demone, Jr.
  1962   *Alcoholism and society.* New York: The Oxford University
         Press.
Cheinisse, L.
  1908   Médicine sociale. *La Semaine Médicale* 28: 613–15.
Cherrington, E. H., ed.
  1924   *Standard encyclopedia of the alcohol problem.* Westerville,
         Ohio: American Issue Publishing Co.

Cheyne, Andrew
1852   *A description of islands in the western Pacific Ocean* . . . London: J. D. Potter.
Child, Irvin L.; Herbert Barry III; and Margaret K. Bacon
1965   A cross-cultural study of drinking. Pt 3. Sex differences. *Quarterly Journal of Studies on Alcohol,* supp. no. 3., pp. 49–61.
Chiñas, Beverly L.
1973   *The Isthmus Zapotecs: women's roles in cultural context.* Case Studies in Cultural Anthropology. New York: Holt, Rinehart & Winston.
Churchward, W. B.
1888   *"Blackbirding" in the South Pacific; or, the first white man on the beach.* London: Swan Sonnenschein & Co.
Clinard, Marshall B., ed.
1964   *Anomie and deviant behavior: a discussion and critique.* New York: The Free Press.
Coale, George L.
1951   A study of chieftainship, missionary contact and culture change on Ponape 1852–1900. M.A. thesis, University of Southern California.
Codere, Helen
1950   *Fighting with property.* Monographs of the American Ethnological Society, no. 18. Seattle: The University of Washington Press.
Cohen, Yehudi A.
1964   The establishment of identity in a social nexus: the special case of initiation ceremonies and their relation to value and legal systems. *American Anthropologist* 66: 529–52.
Comess, L. J.; P. H. Bennett; and T. A. Burch
1967   Clinical gallbladder disease in Pima Indians; its high prevalence in contrast to Framingham, Massachusetts. *New England Journal of Medicine* 277: 894–98.
Connell, K. H.
1968   *Irish peasant society.* Oxford: Clarendon Press.
Cooper, H. Stonehewer
1880   *Coral Lands.* Vol. 2. London: Richard Bentley & Son.
Cooper, John M.
1948   Alcoholic beverages. In *Handbook of South American Indians,* edited by Julian H. Steward. Vol. 5, pp. 539–46. Bureau of American Ethnology Bulletin 143. Washington, D.C.: Government Printing Office.
Cornell, J. B., and R. J. Smith
1956   *Two Japanese villages.* Center for Japanese Studies, Occasional Papers, no. 5. Ann Arbor: The University of Michigan Press.
Crawford, David, and Leona Crawford
1967   *Missionary adventures in the South Pacific.* Rutland, Vt.: Charles E. Tuttle Co.
Crosby, E. Theodora
1899   The Caroline Islands and their people. Unpublished manuscript.

Curley, R.
  1967   Drinking patterns of the Mescalero Apache. *Quarterly Journal of Studies on Alcohol* 28: 116–31.
Dakin, William J.
  1934   *Whalemen adventurers.* Sydney: Angus & Robertson.
Dana, Julian
  1935   *Gods who die. The story of Samoa's greatest adventurer* [George Westbrook], *as told to Julian Dana.* New York: Macmillan.
Deekin, Richard
  1912   *Die Karolinen.* Berlin: Wilhelm Süsserott.
de la Mare, W. J.
  1924   *Desert islands.* London.
Deloria, Vine, Jr.
  1970   *Custer died for your sins.* New York: Macmillan.
Demory, Barbara
  1974   The commercialization of sakau (Ponapean kava). Paper read at the Third Annual Meeting of the Association for Social Anthropology in Oceania, 13–17 March 1974, Asilomar, Pacific Grove, California.
De Vos, George
  1963   Deviancy and social change: a psycho-cultural evaluation of trends in Japanese delinquency and suicide. In *Japanese culture: its development and characteristics,* edited by R. J. Smith and R. K. Beardsley. Chicago: Aldine.
Dewar, J. Cumming
  1892   *Voyage of the Nyanza.* Edinburgh and London: William Blackwood & Sons.
Dhunjibhoy, J. E.
  1930   A brief résumé of the types of insanity commonly met with in India, with a full description of "Indian hemp insanity" peculiar to the country. *Journal of Mental Science* 76: 254–64.
Doane, E. T.
  1874   The Caroline Islands. *The Geographical Magazine* 1: 203–5.
Dodds, E. R.
  1956   *The Greeks and the irrational.* Berkeley and Los Angeles: The University of California Press.
Dore, R. P.
  1958   *City life in Japan.* Berkeley and Los Angeles: The University of California Press.
Doty, Richard G.
  1972   Guam's role in the whaling industry. *Guam Recorder,* n.s. 2: 20–27.
Doughty, Paul L.
  1963   Huaylas: un distrito en la perspectiva nacional. In *Migración e integración en el Perú,* edited by Henry F. Dobyns and Mario C. Vásquez. Lima: Editorial Estudios Andinos.
Dozier, Edward P.
  1966   Problem drinking among American Indians: the role of sociocultural deprivation. *Quarterly Journal of Studies on Alcohol* 27: 72–87.

Drucker, Phillip
    1966   Rank, wealth, and kinship in the Northwest Coast Society. In *Indians of the North Pacific Coast,* edited by Tom McFeat. Seattle: The University of Washington Press.
Duffy, G. J., and G. Dean
    1971   The reliability of death certification of cirrhosis. *Journal of the Irish Medical Association* 64(417): 393–97.
Dunton, J.
    1699   *Dublin scuffle (including conversation in Ireland).* London.
Du Plessis, I. D.
    1944   *The Cape Malays.* Cape Town: Maskew-Miller.
Durkheim, Emile
    1897   *Le suicide.* Paris: Alcan.
Du Toit, Brian M.
    1964   Substitution: a process in culture change. *Human Organization* 23: 16–23.
Eason, Warren
    1968   Population changes. In *Prospects for Soviet Society,* edited by Allen Kassof. New York: Praeger.
Eduardo, Octavio da Costa
    1948   *The Negro in northern Brazil.* Monographs of the American Ethnological Society, no. 15. New York: J. J. Augustin.
Efron, Vera, and Mark Keller
    1964   Selected statistical tables on the consumption of alcohol, 1850–1963, and on alcoholism, 1930–1960, with a bibliography of sources. New Brunswick, N. J.: Publications Division, Rutgers Center of Alcohol Studies.
Erasmus, Charles J.
    1961   *Man takes control.* Minneapolis: The University of Minnesota Press.
Evans-Pritchard, E. E.
    1940   *The Nuer.* London: Oxford University Press.
Everett, Michael W.; Jack O. Waddell; and Dwight B. Heath, eds.
    1976   *Cross-cultural approaches to the study of alcohol: an interdisciplinary perspective.* World Anthropology Series. The Hague: Mouton.
Fallding, H.
    1964   The source and burden of civilization illustrated in the use of alcohol. *Quarterly Journal of Studies on Alcohol* 25: 714–24.
Farkas, Gary, and Raymond Rosen
    1976   Effect of alcohol on elicited male sexual response. *Journal of Studies on Alcohol* 37: 265–72.
Farrell, Andrew, transcriber
    1928   *John Cameron's Odyssey.* New York: Macmillan.
Fawcett, J.
    1836   *An account of an 18 months' residence at the Cape of Good Hope in 1835–6.* Cape Town.
Ferguson, Frances Northend
    1968   Navaho drinking: some tentative hypotheses. *Human Organization* 27: 159–67.

Ferreira de Camargo, Candido Procopio
1961 *Kardecismo e Umbanda.* São Paulo: Livraria Pioneira Editora.
Field, Peter B.
1962 A new cross-cultural study of drunkenness. In *Society, Culture and Drinking Patterns,* edited by D. J. Pittman and C. R. Snyder. New York: John Wiley & Sons.
Finsch, O.
1886 Die Marshall-Inseln. *Die Gartenlaube* 34:37–38.
1893 *Ethnologische Erfahrungen und Belegstücke aus der Südsee.* Vienna.
Firth, Stewart
1973 German firms in the western Pacific Islands, 1857–1914. *Journal of Pacific History* 8: 10–28.
Fischer, John L., and Marc J. Swartz
1960 Socio-psychological aspects of some Trukese and Ponapean love songs. *Journal of American Folklore* 73: 218–25.
Fishberg, Morris
1911 *The Jews: a study of race and environment.* New York: Scott.
Fletcher, C. Brundson
1970 *Stevenson's Germany. The case against Germany in the Pacific.* New York: Arno Press and the *New York Times.*
Forbes, R. J.
1954 Chemical, culinary, and cosmetic arts. In *A history of technology,* edited by Charles Singer et al. Vol. 1. New York and London: Oxford University Press.
Foster, George M.
1967a The dyadic contract: a model for the social structure of a Mexican peasant village. In *Peasant society: a reader,* edited by Jack M. Potter, May Diaz, and George M. Foster. Boston: Little, Brown & Co.
1967b *Tzintzuntzan: Mexican peasants in a changing world.* Boston: Little, Brown & Co.
Fox, Ruth
1967 Conclusions and outlook. In *Alcoholism, behavioral, research, therapeutic approaches,* edited by R. Fox. New York: Springer Publishing Co.
Freund, Paul, and Mac Marshall
1977 Research bibliography of alcohol and kava studies in Oceania: update and additional items. *Micronesica* 13: 313–17.
Friedl, Ernestine
1956 Persistence in Chippewa culture and personality. *American Anthropologist* 58: 814–25.
Friend, The
1850 *The Friend, a journal devoted to temperance, seamen, marine and general intelligence* (Honolulu). 1 September 1850, p. 68.
Gallagher, C.
1968 Islam. In *Encyclopedia of the social sciences.* New York: Macmillan.
Galvão, Eduardo
1955 *Santos e visagens.* São Paulo: Companhia Editora Nacional.

Gautier, Theóphile
   1846   *Le club des hachischins.* Paris.
Gibson, C.
   1964   *The Aztecs under Spanish rule.* Stanford: Stanford University Press.
Gibson, J. E.
   1970   Personal communication.
Gillis, L. S.
   1968   Psychiatric disorder among the Cape Coloured people of the Cape Peninsula. *British Journal of Psychiatry* 114: 1575–87.
Gillis, L. S.; J. B. Lewis; and H. Slabbert
   1965   *Psychiatric disturbance and alcoholism in the coloured people of the Cape Peninsula: report of a psychiatric and socio-economic survey.* Cape Town: Groote Schuur Hospital, Department of Psychiatry.
Glad, Donald D.
   1947a Attitudes and experiences of American-Jewish and American-Irish male youths as related to differences in inebriety rates. Ph.D. dissertation, Stanford University.
   1947b Attitudes and experiences of American-Jewish and American-Irish male youths as related to differences in adult rates of inebriety. *Quarterly Journal of Studies on Alcohol* 8: 406–72.
Glassman, Sidney F.
   1950   Ponape's national beverage. *Research Reviews* (United States Navy Department). July, pp. 16–18.
Gluckman, Max
   1963   Rituals of rebellion in south-east Africa. In *Order and rebellion in tribal Africa.* London: Cohen and West. Originally published by Manchester University Press, 1954.
Goffman, Erving
   1956   The nature of deference and demeanor. *American Anthropologist* 58: 473–502.
   1959   *The presentation of self in everyday life.* Garden City, N.Y.: Doubleday.
   1963   *Behavior in public places: notes on the social organization of gatherings.* New York: The Free Press.
Goldsmith, Robert H.
   1963   *Wise fools in Shakespeare.* East Lansing: Michigan State University Press. First published 1955.
Goodenough, Ward H.
   1963   *Cooperation in change.* New York: Russell Sage Foundation.
Gottheil, E.; B. F. Murphy; T. E. Skoloda; and O. Corbett
   1972   Fixed interval drinking decisions. II. Drinking and discomfort in 25 alcoholics. *Quarterly Journal of Studies on Alcohol* 33: 325–40.
Graves, Theodore
   1967   Acculturation, access, and alcohol in a tri-ethnic community. *American Anthropologist* 69: 306–21.
Great Britain, Department of Health and Social Security
   1969   *Psychiatric hospitals and units in England and Wales. In-*

patient statistics from the mental health enquiry for the years 1964, 1965, 1966.
Great Britain, Parliamentary Papers
1851 *Report from the Select Committee on Kafir Tribes,* xiv (635), pars. 669–70 and 718–19.
1876 Report of the government surveyor, lii (C. 1401), p. 60.
1904 Minutes of evidence of the Transvaal Labour Commission (Cd. 1897), par. 10, 522.
Grogger, Paula
1947 *Bauernjahr.* Graz.
Guilly, P.
1950 Le club des hachischins. *Encéphale* 39: 175–85.
Gulick, Addison
1932 *Evolutionist and missionary, John Thomas Gulick.* Chicago: The University of Chicago Press.
Gunn, Harold D.
1953 *Peoples of the plateau area of northern Nigeria.* Ethnographic Survey of Africa. London: International African Institute.
Gunson, Niel
1966 On the incidence of alcoholism and intemperance in early Pacific missions. *Journal of Pacific History* 1: 43–62.
Gurvich, I. E.
1958 *P'ianstvo gubit cheloveka, nanosit vred obshchestvu.* Moscow.
Gusfield, Joseph R.
1963 *Symbolic crusade, status politics and the American temperance movement.* Urbana: The University of Illinois Press.
Guthrie, W. K. C.
1950 *The Greeks and their gods.* London: Methuen and Co.
Hallowell, A. Irving
1955 *Culture and experience, selected papers.* Philadelphia: The University of Pennsylvania Press.
Halpern, J.
1964 *Economy and society of Laos.* New York: Inblinger.
Hamer, John H.
1965 Acculturation stress and the functions of alcohol among the Forest Potawatomi. *Quarterly Journal of Studies on Alcohol* 26: 285–302.
1969 Guardian spirits, alcohol, and cultural defense mechanisms. *Anthropologica* 11: 215–41.
Hammet, L. U.
1854 Narrative of the voyage of H.M.S. Serpent. *The Nautical Magazine and Naval Chronicle* 23: 57–67.
Hanna, Joel M.
1976 Ethnic groups, human variation, and alcohol use. In *Cross-cultural approaches to the study of alcohol: an interdisciplinary perspective,* edited by Michael W. Everett, Jack O. Waddell, and Dwight B. Heath. The Hague: Mouton.
1977 Cardiovascular responses of Chinese, Japanese and Caucasians to alcohol. Paper read at the NATO International Conference on Behavioral Approaches to Alcoholism, August 1977, Bergen, Norway.

Harrison, Brian
1971   *Drink and the Victorians.* London: Faber & Faber; Pittsburgh: The University of Pittsburgh Press.
Head, Richard
1647   *The Western wonder.* London.
Heath, Dwight B.
1958   Drinking patterns of the Bolivian Camba. *Quarterly Journal of Studies on Alcohol* 19: 491–508. Reprinted 1962. In *Society, culture and drinking patterns,* edited by David J. Pittman and Charles R. Snyder. New York: John Wiley & Sons.
1974a   Anthropological approaches to alcohol: a review. *Journal on Alcoholism and Related Addictions* 10: 24–42.
1974b   A critical review of ethnographic studies of alcohol use. In *Research Advances in Alcohol and Drug Problems,* edited by Robert J. Gibbins, Yedy Israel, Harold Kalant, Robert E. Popham, Wolfgang Schmidt, and Reginald G. Smart. Vol. 2. New York: John Wiley & Sons.
1976   Anthropological perspectives on alcohol: an historical review. In *Cross-cultural approaches to the study of alcohol: an interdisciplinary perspective,* edited by Michael W. Everett, Jack O. Waddell, and Dwight B. Heath. The Hague: Mouton.
1977   A critical review of "the sociocultural model" of alcohol use. Paper read at the Conference on Normative Approaches to Alcohol Abuse and Alcoholism, 26–28 April 1977, San Diego, California; available from the National Clearinghouse on Alcohol Information.
Hellmann, Ellen
1934   The importance of beer-brewing in an urban native yard. *Bantu Studies* 8: 39–60.
1940   *Problems of Bantu urban youth.* Johannesburg.
Hesnard, A.
1912   Note sur les fumeurs de chanvre en Orient. *Encéphale* 2: 40–46.
Hezel, Francis X.
1973   The beginnings of foreign contact with Truk. *Journal of Pacific History* 8: 51–73.
Hickerson, Harold
1971   The Chippewa of the Upper Great Lakes: A study in sociopolitical change. In *North American Indians in historical perspective,* edited by Eleanor Burke Leacock and Nancy Oestreich Lurie. New York: Random House.
Hillery, G. A., Jr., and F. J. Essene
1963   Navajo population: An analysis of the 1960 census. *Southwestern Journal of Anthropology* 19: 297–313.
Holmberg, Allan R.; Mario C. Vázquez; Paul L. Doughty; J. Oscar Alers; Henry F. Dobyns; and Harold D. Lasswell
1965   The Vicos case: peasant society in transition. *The American Behavioral Scientist,* Special Issue, 8(7):3–33.
Hong Kong Annual Report
1969   Hong Kong: Government Press.
Honigmann, John J.
1963   Dynamics of drinking in an Austrian village. *Ethnology* 2: 157–69.

1964*a*   Indians of Nouveau Quebec. In *Le Nouveau Quebec: contribution à l'étude de l'occupation humaine*, edited by Jean Malaurie and Jacques Rousseau. Bibliothèque Arctique et Antarctique. Paris: Mouton & Co.

1964*b*   Survival of a cultural focus. In *Explorations in cultural anthropology; essays in honor of George Peter Murdock*, edited by Ward H. Goodenough. New York: McGraw-Hill.

Honigmann, John J., and Irma Honigmann

1945   Drinking in an Indian-White community. *Quarterly Journal of Studies on Alcohol* 5: 575–619.

1968   Alcohol in a Canadian northern town. Working paper no. 1, Urbanization in the Arctic and Subarctic (mimeographed). Chapel Hill: University of North Carolina, Institute for Research in Social Science.

1970   *Arctic townsmen*. Ottawa: Saint Paul University, Canadian Research Centre for Anthropology.

Horton, Donald

1943   The functions of alcohol in primitive societies: a cross-cultural study. *Quarterly Journal of Studies on Alcohol* 4: 199–320.

1967   The functions of alcohol in primitive societies: a cross-cultural study. Partial reprint. In *Personality in native society and culture*, edited by Clyde Kluckhohn, Henry Murry, and David Schneider. New York: Alfred Knopf.

Hotchkiss, John C.

1967   Children and conduct in a Ladino community of Chiapas, Mexico. *American Anthropologist* 69: 711–18.

Hsu, Francis L. K.

1955   *Americans and Chinese*. London: Cresset Press.

Humphrey, Omar T.

1887   *Wreck of the Rainier, a sailor's narrative*. Portland, Me.: W. H. Stevens & Co.

Hunter, Monica

1936   *Reaction to conquest*. London: Oxford University Press.

Hunter, Robert

1904   *Poverty*. New York: Macmillan.

Hurt, Wesley

1965   Social drinking patterns among the Yankton Sioux. *Human Organization* 24: 222–30.

Hutchinson, Bertram

1956   Early European trade among the South African Bantu. *Revista de Antropologia* 4: 25–39.

1957   Some social consequences of nineteenth century missionary activity among the South African Bantu. *Africa* 27: 160–77.

Huxley, Aldous

1954   *The doors of perception*. New York: Harper & Row.

Hyde, R. W., and R. M. Chisholm

1944   The relation of mental disorders to race and nationality. *New England Journal of Medicine* 231(18): 612–18.

The illicit liquor problem in the Witwatersrand.

1935   Johannesburg.

Izvestiia

1958   2 March, p. 4.

1965   29 August, p. 4.
1968   1 October, p. 5.
James, Bernard J.
1961   Social-psychological dimensions of Ojibwa acculturation. *American Anthropologist* 63: 721–46.
Jansen, M., ed.
1965   *Changing Japanese attitudes toward modernization.* Princeton, N.J.: Princeton University Press.
Japan Handbook, 1965
1965   Tokyo: Rengo Press.
Japan, Ministry of Justice
1962   *Hanzai hakusho* [White paper on crime]. *Tokyo.*
Japan, National Tax Office
1965   *88-kai Kokuzeichō Tōkei Nenkan* [National tax office statistical yearbook, no. 88]. Tokyo.
Japan, Tax Administration Agency
1958   *Sake no shiori* [Guide to alcoholic liquor]. Tokyo.
1960   *Sake no shiori* [Guide to alcoholic liquor]. Tokyo.
1964   *Sake no shiori* [Guide to alcoholic liquor]. Tokyo.
Jastrow, Morris, Jr.
1913   Wine in the Pentateuchal codes. *Journal of the American Oriental Society* 33: 180–92.
Jellinek, E. M.
1941   Immanuel Kant on drinking. *Quarterly Journal of Studies on Alcohol* 1: 777–78.
1960   *The disease concept of alcoholism.* New Haven: The College and University Press.
Jessor, Richard; R. Carman; and P. Grossman
1968   Expectations of need satisfaction and drinking patterns of college students. *Quarterly Journal of Studies on Alcohol* 29: 101–16.
Jessor, Richard; Theodore Graves; R. Hanson; S. Jessor
1968   *Society, personality and deviant behavior.* New York: Holt, Rinehart & Winston.
Jessor, Richard; H. Young; E. Young; and G. Tesi
1970   Perceived opportunity, alienation and drinking behavior among Italian and American youth. *Journal of Personality and Social Psychology* 15: 215–22.
Jhā, Ganganatha
1926   Manu-smṛti. Calcutta: University of Calcutta.
Jones, John D.
1861   *Life and adventure in the South Pacific, by a roving printer.* New York: Harper & Bros.
Joseph, Alice; R. B. Spicer; and J. Chesky
1949   *The desert people.* Chicago: The University of Chicago Press.
Kardiner, Abram
1945   *The psychological frontiers of society.* New York: Columbia University Press.
Kearney, Michael
1972   *The winds of Ixtepeji: world view and society in a Zapotec town.* Case Studies in Cultural Anthropology. New York: Holt, Rinehart & Winston.

Kearney, N.; M. J. Lawlor; and D. Walsh
    1969   Alcoholic drinking in a Dublin corporation housing estate. *Journal of the Irish Medical Association* 62: 140–42.
Kerr, Norman
    1888   *Inebriety, its etiology, pathology, treatment and jurisprudence.* London: Lewis.
Kiwanuka, S.
    1972   *A history of Buganda: from the foundation of the kingdom to 1900.* New York: Africana Publishing Corp.
Klatskin, G.
    1961   Alcohol and its relation to liver damage. *Gastroenterology* 41: 443–51.
Komsomol'skaia pravda
    1961   10 September, p. 4.
    1965   9 October, pp. 2, 4.
Kondrashkov, N. N.
    1966   Analiz raionnoi statistiki prestupnosti. *Voprosy Preduprezhdeniia Prestupnosti,* no. 4.
Koskinen, Aarne
    1953   *Missionary influence as a political factor in the Pacific Islands.* Helsinki: Suomalaisen Tiedeakatemian Toimituksia Annales Academiae Scientiarum Fennicae, 78(1).
Kroeber, Alfred L.
    1948   *Anthropology.* Rev. ed. New York: Harcourt, Brace & Co.
Kunitz, Stephen J.
    1970   Navajo drinking patterns. Ph.D. dissertation, Yale University.
Kunitz, Stephen J.; Jerrold E. Levy; C. L. Odoroff; and J. Bollinger
    1971   The epidemiology of alcoholic cirrhosis in two southwestern Indian tribes. *Quarterly Journal of Studies on Alcohol* 32: 706–20.
Kunitz, Stephen J.; Jerrold E. Levy; and Michael Everett
    1969   Alcoholic cirrhosis among the Navajo. *Quarterly Journal of Studies on Alcohol* 30: 672–85.
Kurze, G.
    1887   Mikronesian und die mission daselbst. *Allgemeine Missions-Zeitschrift* 14: 64–80, 123–29.
La Barre, Weston
    1946   Some observations on character structure in the Orient. Pt. 2. The Chinese, parts I and II. *Psychiatry* 9: 215–37, 375–95.
    1971   Materials for a history of studies of crisis cults: a bibliographic essay. *Current Anthropology* 12: 3–44.
Laing, R. D.
    1962   *The self and others.* Chicago: Quadrangle Books.
Landis, C., and M. Bolles
    1950   *Textbook of abnormal psychology.* Rev. ed. New York: Macmillan.
Landman, Ruth H.
    1952   Studies of drinking in Jewish culture. Pt. 3. Drinking patterns of children and adolescents attending religious schools. *Quarterly Journal of Studies on Alcohol* 13: 87–94.
Larsen, D., and B. Abu-Laban
    1968   Norm qualities and deviant drinking. *Social Problems* 15: 441–50.

Laurie, Thomas
    n.d.   *The Spaniards and our mission in Micronesia.* Chicago: American Board of Commissioners for Foreign Missions.
Leach, Edmund R.
    1965   Two essays concerning the symbolic representation of time. In *Reader in comparative religion,* edited by William A. Lessa and Evon Z. Vogt. New York: Harper & Row.
Leacock, Eleanor
    1958   Status among the Montagnais-Naskapi of Labrador. *Ethnohistory* 5: 200–209.
LeBar, Frank, and A. Suddard
    1960   *Laos.* New Haven: Human Relations Area Files Press.
Leland, Joy
    1976   *Firewater myths. North American Indian drinking and alcohol addiction.* Rutgers Center of Alcohol Studies, monograph no. 11. New Brunswick, N.J.: Rutgers Center of Alcohol Studies.
Lemert, Edwin M.
    1954   *Alcohol and the Northwest Coast Indians.* University of California Publications in Culture and Society, no. 2: 303–406.
    1956   Alcoholism: theory, problems, and challenge. Pt. 3. Alcoholism and the sociocultural situation. *Quarterly Journal of Studies on Alcohol* 17: 306–17.
    1958   The use of alcohol in three Salish Indian tribes. *Quarterly Journal of Studies on Alcohol* 19: 90–107.
    1962   Alcohol, values and social control. In *Society, culture, and drinking patterns,* edited by David J. Pittman and Charles R. Snyder. New York: John Wiley & Sons.
    1976   Koni, kona, kava: orange-beer culture of the Cook Islands. *Journal of Studies on Alcohol* 37: 565–85.
Lerman, L. A.
    1958   Meditsinskie rabotniki i protivoalkogol'naia propaganda. *Sovetskoe Zdravookhranenie,* no. 11.
Leskov, N. S.
    1957   Nesmertel'nyi Golovan (Deathless Golovan). In *Complete Works.* Vol. 6, pp. 351–97. Moscow: Gos-izd-khudozh. lit. Originally published 1880.
Lessa, William, and Evon Z. Vogt
    1965   Dynamics in religion. In *Reader in comparative religion,* edited by William A. Lessa and Evon Z. Vogt. New York: Harper & Row.
Levin, I.
    1963   O vrede alkogolia. In *Za Kommunisticheskii Byt.* Leningrad.
Levy, Jerrold E., and Stephen J. Kunitz
    1969   Notes on some White Mountain Apache social pathologies. *Plateau* 42: 11–19.
    1971   Indian reservations, anomie, and social pathologies. *Southwestern Journal of Anthropology* 27: 97–128.
    1973   Indian drinking: problems of data collection and interpretation. In *Proceedings of the First Annual Alcoholism Conference of the National Institute on Alcohol Abuse and Alcoholism,* edited

by Morris E. Chafetz. Rockville, Md.: National Institute on Alcohol Abuse and Alcoholism.

1974   *Indian drinking: Navajo practices and Anglo-American theories.* New York: John Wiley & Sons.

Lewis, James L.
1967   *Kusaiean acculturation 1824–1948.* Saipan: Division of Land Management, Trust Territory of the Pacific Islands.

Lewis, Oscar
1961   *Children of Sanchez.* New York: Random House.

Lin, T. Y.
1953   A study of the incidence of mental disorder in Chinese and other cultures. *Psychiatry* 16: 313–36

Linton, Ralph
1936.   *The study of man.* New York: Appleton-Century.
1943   Nativistic movements. *American Anthropologist* 45: 230–40.

Literaturnaia gazeta
1967   13 December, p. 12.

Lolli, Giorgio
1961   Physiological, psychological, and social aspects of the cocktail hour. Unpublished paper.

Lolli, Giorgio; E. Serianni; G. Golder; and P. Luzzatto-Fegiz
1958   *Alcohol in Italian culture.* Glencoe, Ill.: The Free Press.

Longmate, Norman
1968   *The water drinkers: a history of temperance.* London: Hamilton.

Loomis, Albertine
1970   *To all people. A history of the Hawaii Conference of the United Church of Christ.* Honolulu: Hawaii Conference, United Church of Christ.

Lovett, Richard
1903   *James Chalmers, his autobiography and letters.* 6th ed. London: Religious Tract Society.

Lucas, A.
1948   *Ancient Egyptian materials and industries.* 3d ed. London: Arnold.

Lurie, Nancy Oestreich
1971   The world's oldest on-going protest demonstration: North American Indian drinking patterns. *Pacific Historical Review* 40: 311–32.

Lurie, Nancy Oestreich, ed.
1961   *Mountain Wolf Woman, sister of Crashing Thunder.* Ann Arbor: The University of Michigan Press.

Lutz, H. F.
1922   *Viticulture and brewing in the ancient Orient.* Leipzig: J. C. Hinrichs.

MacAndrew, Craig, and Robert B. Edgerton
1969   *Drunken comportment: a social explanation.* Chicago: Aldine.

MacCallum, Thomas M.
1934   *Adrift in the South Seas.* Los Angeles: Wetzel Publishing Co.

McCarthy, M. L.
1911   *Irish land and Irish liberty.* London.

McCarthy, Raymond G., ed.
  1959   *Drinking and intoxication. Selected readings in social attitudes and controls.* New Haven: College and University Press.
McClelland, David C.; William N. Davis; Rudolf Kalin; and Eric Wanner
  1972   *The drinking man.* New York: The Free Press.
McCord, William, and Joan McCord
  1960   *Origins of alcoholism.* Stanford: Stanford University Press.
McGrath, Thomas B.
  1973   Sakau in tomw. Sarawi in tomw. *Oceania* 44: 64–67.
McKinlay, Arthur P.
  1951   Attic temperance. *Quarterly Journal of Studies on Alcohol* 12: 61–102.
MacLysaght, E.
  1950   *Irish life in the seventeenth century.* Cork: Cork University Press.
Madsen, William
  1974a Alcoholics Anonymous as a crisis cult. *Alcohol Health and Research World,* spring. National Clearinghouse for Alcohol Information.
  1974b *The American alcoholic: the nature-nurture conflict in alcoholic research and therapy.* Springfield, Ill.: Charles C. Thomas.
Madsen, William, and Claudia Madsen
  1969   The cultural structure of Mexican drinking behavior. *Quarterly Journal of Studies on Alcohol* 30: 701–18
Mahlmann, John J.
  1918   *Reminiscences of an ancient mariner.* Yokohama: The *Japan Gazette* Printing and Publishing Co.
Mail, Patricia D.
  1967   The prevalence of problem drinking in the San Carlos Apache. M.P.H. thesis, Yale University School of Public Health.
Mail, Patricia D., and David R. McDonald
  1977   Native Americans and alcohol: a preliminary bibliography. *Behavior Science Research* 12: 169–96.
Mair, Lucy
  1934   *An African people in the twentieth century.* London: Routledge & Kegan Paul.
Malinowski, Bronislaw
  1948   *Magic, science and religion and other essays.* Boston: Beacon Press.
Mandelbaum, David G.
  1965   Alcohol and culture. *Current Anthropology* 6: 281–93.
Mangin, William
  1957   Drinking among Andean Indians. *Quarterly Journal of Studies on Alcohol* 18: 55–66.
Mann, M.
  1958   *New primer on alcoholism.* New York: Holt, Rinehart & Winston.
Marsack, C. C.
  1959   Provocation in trials for murder. *Criminal Law Review* (London), October, pp. 697–704.
Marshall, Mac
  1974a Report on working session on alcohol and kava use in Oceania.

Association for Social Anthropology in Oceania Newsletter 15: 3–4.
1974*b* Research bibliography of alcohol and kava studies in Oceania. *Micronesica* 10: 299–306.
1975   The politics of prohibition on Namoluk Atoll. *Journal of Studies on Alcohol* 36: 597–610.
1979   *Weekend warriors: alcohol in a Micronesian culture.* World Ethnology Series. Palo Alto, Calif.: Mayfield Publishing Co.
Marshall, Mac, and Leslie B. Marshall
1975   Opening Pandora's bottle: reconstructing Micronesians' early contacts with alcoholic beverages. *Journal of the Polynesian Society* 84: 441–65.
Maslow, A. H.
1961   Peak experience as acute identity experiences. *American Journal of Psychoanalysis* 21: 254–60.
1964   *Religions, values and peak experiences.* Columbus: Ohio State University Press.
1965   Lessons from peak experiences. In *Science and human affairs*, edited by R. Farson. Palo Alto, Calif.: Science and Behavior Books.
1971   *The farther reaches of human nature.* New York: The Viking Press.
Matsumoto, Yoshiharu S.
1960   Contemporary Japan: the individual and the group. *Transactions of the American Philosophical Society* 50, pt. 1, pp. 5–75.
Maude, H. E.
1968*a* Beachcombers and castaways. Appendix: the beachcomber books. In *Of islands and men*, by H. E. Maude. Melbourne: Oxford University Press.
1968*b* The coconut oil trade of the Gilbert Islands. In *Of islands and men*, by H. E. Maude. Melbourne: Oxford University Press.
1970   Baiteke and Binoka of Abemama, arbiters of change in the Gilbert Islands. In *Pacific Islands portraits*, edited by J. W. Davidson and Deryck Scarr. Canberra: Australian National University Press.
Maude, H. E., and Edwin Doran, Jr.
1966   The precedence of Tarawa Atoll. *Annals of the Association of American Geographers* 56: 269–89.
Mauss, Marcel
1967   *The gift.* New York: W. W. Norton & Co. First published in 1925.
Maxwell, Milton A.
1967   Alcoholics Anonymous: an interpretation. In *Alcoholism*, edited by David J. Pittman. New York: Harper & Row.
Mayer-Gross, W.
1932   Die Auslösung durch seelische und körperliche Schädigungen. In *Handbuch der Geisteskrankheiten*, edited by Oswald Bumke. Vol. 9, spec. pt. 5. Berlin: J. Springer.
Mayer-Gross, W.; E. Slater; and M. Roth
1969   *Clinical psychiatry.* 3d ed. London: Bailliere, Tindall & Cassell.
Mead, George H.
1934   *Mind, self and society.* Chicago: The University of Chicago Press.

Mead, Margaret
    1934   Kinship in the Admiralty Islands. *Anthropological Papers of the American Museum of Natural History* 34(2): 181–358.
Meditsinskaia gazeta
    1963   16 July, p. 2.
Meek, C. K.
    1931   *A Sudanese kingdom.* London: Kegan Paul.
Metzger, D.
    1963   Drinking in Aguacatenango. Unpublished paper.
Middleton, John
    1960   *Lugbara religion.* London: Oxford University Press.
    1962   Trade and markets among the Lugbara of Uganda. In *Markets in Africa*, edited by Paul Bohannon and George Dalton. Evanston: Northwestern University Press.
    1966   The resolution of conflict among the Lugbara of Uganda. In *Political anthropology*, edited by Marc Swartz, Victor Turner, and Arthur Tuden. Chicago: Aldine.
Midgley, J.
    1967   Conformity and control in the Cape Malay group. M.Soc.Sc. thesis, University of Cape Town.
Miller, Daniel R.
    1963   The study of social relationships: situation, identity, and social interaction. In *Psychology: a study of science*, edited by Sigmund Koch. New York: McGraw-Hill.
Minryoku, 1965 [National resources, 1965]
    1965   Tokyo: Asahi News.
Mironenko, Y.
    1967   The fight against alcoholism in the USSR. *Bulletin of the Institute for the Study of the USSR* (Munich) 14(9): 25–29.
Mischel, Walter, and Frances Mischel
    1958   Psychological aspects of spirit possession. *American Anthropologist* 60: 249–60.
Missionary Herald
    1853   "Voyage of exploration." By E. W. Clark. *MH* 49: 81–90.
    1854   Letters from Rev. Benjamin Snow, January–October 1853. *MH* 50: 50–54.
    1855   Journal of Dr. Gulick, April–September, 1854. *MH* 51: 225–29.
    1856   Letter from Mr. Doane, February 1856. *MH* 52: 376–78.
    1857a   Letter from Mr. Sturges, February–April 1856. *MH* 53: 105–7.
    1857b   "Micronesian mission." *MH* 53: 4.
    1860a   Journal of Mr. Sturges, October 24, 1859, to February 10, 1860. *MH* 56: 289–92.
    1860b   Letter from Mr. Sturges, January 4, and February 2, 1859, and extracts from his journal. *MH* 56: 34–37.
    1865   Letter from Mr. Sturges, January and February, 1865. *MH* 61: 293–96.
    1867   Intelligence from Captain of the *Pfiel* and Mr. Kanoa. *MH* 61: 122.
    1868   Letters from Mr. Sturges. *MH* 64: 252–54.
    1869a   Letters from Mr. Sturges, December 2, 1868 to January 18, 1869. *MH* 65: 235–36.

1869*b* Report from Mr. Bingham. *MH* 65: 130–32.
1870*a* Letters from Mr. Doane. *MH* 66: 280–85.
1870*b* Letters from Mr. Doane. *MH* 66: 365–70.
1876   Sturges—the work at Ponape—a fifteenth anniversary. *MH* 72: 308–11.
1881   "The Lagoon of Ruk." By E. T. Doane. *MH* 77: 208–10.
1882   Letter from Mr. Doane, February 12, 1882. *MH* 78: 272–74.
1886*a* Letters from Mr. Doane. *MH* 82: 451–52.
1886*b* Letters from Mr. Logan. *MH* 82: 15–18.
1888   Letter from Mr. Doane, May 4, 1888. *MH* 84: 442.
1889*a* Letter from Mr. Doane, July 25, 1889. *MH* 85: 544–45.
1889*b* The Morning Star's report to her stockholders for 1888–89. *MH* 85: 261–64.
1891   Account by Dr. Pease. *MH* 87: 418–21.
1893*a* Edited Summary from Messrs. Channon and Pease. *MH* 89: 231–34.
1893*b* Editorial paragraphs. *MH* 89: 215–21.
1898   Letter from Mr. Price. *MH* 94: 289–92.
1900   Letter from Mr. Nanpei. *MH* 96: 147–49.

Mooney, James
1896   Ghost dance religion and the Sioux outbreak of 1890. *Bureau of American Ethnology,* Annual Report 14 (1892–1893). Washington, D.C.

Moore, R. A.
1960   The conception of alcoholism as a mental illness: implications for treatment and research. *Quarterly Journal of Studies on Alcohol* 21: 172–75.
1964   Alcoholism in Japan. *Quarterly Journal of Studies on Alcohol* 25: 142–50.

Morley, Sylvanus G.
1956   *The ancient Maya.* 3d ed. Stanford: Stanford University Press.

Morrell, W. P.
1960   *Britain in the Pacific Islands.* Oxford: Clarendon Press.

Moryson, F.
1904   "The commonwealth of Ireland" and "The description of Ireland." In *Illustrations of Irish history,* edited by Caesar L. Falkiner. London.

Moss, Frederick J.
1889   *Through atolls and islands in the great South Sea.* London: Sampson Low, Marston, Searle & Rivington.

Mulford, Harold A., and D. W. Miller
1960   "Drinking in Iowa. Pt. 3. A scale of definitions of alcohol related to drinking behavior." *Quarterly Journal of Studies on Alcohol* 21: 267–78.

Mulford, Harold A., and R. W. Wilson
1966   Identifying problem drinkers in a household health survey. Public Health Service Publication no. 1000. Washington, D.C.: Government Printing Office.

Murdock, George P.
1965   Waging baseball in Truk. In *Culture and society,* by George P. Murdock. Pittsburgh: The University of Pittsburgh Press.

Murphy, William Barry
   1973   The great brandy caper and how it failed. *The Beacon, Magazine of Hawaii* 16: 56–57.
Myers, R. D., and W. L. Veale
   1971   The determinants of alcohol preference in animals. In *The biology of alcoholism*, edited by B. Bissin and H. Begleiter. Vol. 2. New York: Plenum.
Myerson, A.
   1940   Alcohol: a study of social ambivalence. *Quarterly Journal of Studies on Alcohol* 1: 13–20.
Nason, James D.
   1970   Clan and copra: modernization on Etal Island, Eastern Caroline Islands. Ph.D. dissertation, University of Washington.
Natal
   1909   *Blue Book on Native Affairs.*
National Institute of Mental Health
   1969   *Alcohol and alcoholism.* Washington, D.C.: Government Printing Office.
Nedelia
   1966   24–30 July, p. 2.
Netting, Robert McC.
   1964   Beer as a locus of value among the West African Kofyar. *American Anthropologist* 66: 375–84.
Nishinomiya City Office
   1962   *Kokusei Chōsa Kekka Gaiyō* (Summary of National Census Results). Nishinomiya.
Noguchi, S.
   1960   Current trends of alcoholism in Japan. *Psychiatria et Neurologia Japonica* 62: 1914–24.
Norbeck, Edward
   1954   *Takashima: a Japanese fishing community.* Salt Lake City: The University of Utah Press.
Norbeck, Edward, and M. Norbeck
   1956   Child training in a Japanese fishing community. In *Personal character and cultural milieu*, edited by D. Haring. Syracuse, N.Y.: Syracuse University Press.
Nozikov, N.
   1946   *Russian voyages around the world.* London: Hutchinson.
O'Brien, Ilma E.
   1971   Missionaries on Ponape: induced social and political change. *Australian National University Historical Journal* 8: 53–64.
Ogan, Eugene
   1966   Drinking behavior and race relations. *American Anthropologist* 68: 181–88.
O'Grady, H.
   1923   *Strafford in Ireland.* Dublin.
Opler, Morris K.
   1959   Anthropological aspects of psychiatry. In *Progress in psychotherapy*. vol. IV. *social psychotherapy*, edited by J. Masserman and J. L. Moreno. New York: Grune and Stratton.

Orley, J.
   1970   *Culture and mental illness*. Nairobi: East African Publishing
          House.
Orlovsky, L. V.
   1963   K metodike antialkogol'noi propagandy. In *Alkogolizm i alko-
          gol'nye psikhozy*, edited by I. I. Lukomsky. Moscow.
Parkman, F.
   1909   *The old regime in Canada*. London: Macmillan & Co.
Parsons, Elsie Clews
   1939   *Pueblo Indian religion*. 2 vols. Chicago: The University of Chi-
          cago Press.
Pelto, Pertti
   1970   *Anthropological research: the structure of inquiry*. New York:
          Harper & Row.
Petty, William
   1927   *The Petty papers*. London: Constable.
Pickthall, M. W., ed. and trans.
   1953   *The meaning of the glorious Koran*. New York: New American
          Library.
Pittman, David J., and Charles R. Snyder, eds.
   1962   *Society, culture and drinking patterns*. New York: John Wiley
          & Sons.
Pitts, J., and N. Ferris
   1969   The biochemistry of anxiety. *Scientific American* 220(2): 69–75.
Plath, David W.
   1964   *The after hours: modern Japan and the search for enjoyment*.
          Berkeley and Los Angeles: The University of California Press.
Platt, B. S.
   1955   Some traditional alcoholic beverages and their importance in
          indigenous African communities. *Proceedings of the Nutrition
          Society* 4: 132–40.
Platt, B. S., and R. A. Webb
   1946   Fermentation and human nutrition. *Proceedings of the Nutri-
          tion Society* 14: 115–24.
Popham, R. E., and W. Schmidt
   1958   *Statistics of alcohol use and alcoholism in Canada, 1871–1956*.
          Toronto: The University of Toronto Press.
Porot, A.
   1942   Le cannabisme (haschich—kif—chira—marihuana). *Annales
          Médico-Psychologiques* 100: 1–24.
Prakash, Om
   1961   *Food and drinks in ancient India*. Delhi: Munshi Ram Manohar
          Lal.
Pravda
   1969   6 April, p. 3.
Preston, Richard J.
   1967   Reticence and self-expression in a Cree community. Unpub-
          lished paper.
Purcell, David C., Jr.
   1971   Japanese entrepreneurs in the Mariana, Marshall and Caroline

Islands. In *East across the Pacific. Historical and sociological studies of Japanese immigration and assimilation*, edited by Hilary Conroy and T. Scott Miyakawa. Santa Barbara: American Bibliographical Center, Clio Press.

Ralston, Caroline
1970   The beach communities. In *Pacific Islands portraits*, edited by J. W. Davidson and Deryck Scarr. Canberra: Australian National University Press.

Ramos, S.
1938   El perfil del hombre y de la cultura en Mexico. Mexico City: Robredo.

Ravi Varma, L. A.
1950   Alcoholism in Ayurveda. *Quarterly Journal of Studies on Alcohol* 11: 484–91.

Redlich, F., and D. Freedman
1966   *The theory and practice of psychiatry*. New York: Basic Books.

Reichenbach, D. D.
1967   Autopsy incidence of diseases among southwestern American Indians. *Archives of Pathology* 84: 81–86.

Reiterer, K.
1915   *Altsteirisches*. Graz.

Renou, Louis
1954   *The civilization of ancient India*. Calcutta: Susil Gupta.

Republic of South Africa
1966   *Population census, 6 September 1960*. Vol. 2, no. 1. Report on the metropolitan area of Cape Town. Pretoria: Government Printer.

Resnick, H. L., and L. H. Dizmang
1971   Suicidal behavior among American Indians. *American Journal of Psychiatry* 127: 882–87.

Ridington, Robin
1968   The medicine fight: an instrument of political process among the Beaver Indians. *American Anthropologist* 70: 1152–60.

Riesenberg, Saul H.
1968a   *The native polity of Ponape*. Smithsonian Contributions to Anthropology no. 10. Washington, D.C.: Smithsonian Institution Press.
1968b   The tatooed Irishman. *Smithsonian Journal of History* 3: 1–18.

Riesman, David
1950   *The lonely crowd*. New Haven: Yale University Press.

Robbins, Michael, and R. Pollnac
1969   Drinking patterns and acculturation in rural Buganda. *American Anthropologist* 71: 276–84.

Rogers, Edward
1965   Leadership among the Indians of eastern subarctic Canada. *Anthropologica* 13: 263–84.

Romanucci-Ross, Lola
1966   Conflicts fanciers à Mokereng, village Matankor des Iles de L'Amiraute. *L'Homme* 6(2): 32–52.
1969   The hierarchy of resort in curative practices: the Admiralty Islands, Melanesia. *Journal of Health and Human Behavior* 10(3): 201–09.

Romney, Kimball, and Romaine Romney
1966   *The Mixtecans of Juxtlahuaca, Mexico.* Six Cultures Series, vol. 4. New York: John Wiley & Sons.
Rozhnov, V. E.
1969   *Po sledam zelenogo zmiia.* Moscow.
Sadoun, R.; G. Lolli; and M. Silverman
1965   *Drinking in French culture.* Rutgers Center of Alcohol Studies, monograph no. 5. New Brunswick, N.J.: Rutgers Center of Alcohol Studies, Publications Division.
Sahlins, Marshall D.
1965   On the sociology of primitive exchange. In *The relevance of models for social anthropology,* edited by Michael Banton. A.S.A. Monograph no. 1. London: Tavistock.
St. Johnston, Thomas R.
1922   *South Sea reminiscences.* London: T. Fisher Unwin.
Sakharov, A. B.
1961   *O lichnosti prestupnika i prichinakh prestupnosti v SSSR.* Moscow.
Salisbury, Richard
1962   *From stone to steel.* Melbourne: Melbourne University Press.
Salye, H.
1956   *The stress of life.* New York: McGraw-Hill.
Sangree, Walter H.
1962   The social functions of beer drinking in Bantu Tiriki. In *Society, culture, and drinking patterns,* edited by D. J. Pittman and C. R. Snyder. New York: John Wiley & Sons.
Savard, R. J.
1968   Effects of disulfiram therapy on relationships within the Navaho drinking group. *Quarterly Journal of Studies on Alcohol* 29: 909–16.
Sayres, William C.
1956   Ritual drinking, ethnic status, and inebriety in rural Colombia. *Quarterly Journal of Studies on Alcohol* 17: 53–62.
Scarr, Deryck
1970   Recruits and recruiters: a portrait of the labour trade. In *Pacific Islands portraits,* edited by J. W. Davidson and Deryck Scarr. Canberra: Australian National University Press.
Schaefer, Paul D.
1975   From "king" to pastor: the acquisition of Christianity on Kusaie. Paper read at the Fourth Annual Meeting of the Association for Social Anthropology in Oceania, 26–30 March 1975, Stuart, Florida.
Schwartz, Gary, and Don Merten
1968   Social identity and expressive symbols: the meaning of an initiation ritual. *American Anthropologist* 70: 1117–31.
Schwartz, Theodore
1962   The Paliau movement in the Admiralty Islands 1946–1954. *Anthropological Papers of the American Museum of Natural History* 49(2): 211–421.
1963   Systems of areal integration: some considerations based on the Admiralty Islands of northern Melanesia. *Anthropological Forum* 1(1): 56–97.

1973   Cult and context: the paranoid ethos in Melanesia. *Ethos* 1: 153–174.
Segal, B. M.
1967   *Alkogolizm: klinicheskie, sotsial'no-psikhologicheskie i biologicheskie problemy.* Moscow.
Severance, Craig J.
1974   Sanction and sakau: the accessibility and social control of alcohol on Pis-Losap. Paper read at the Third Annual Meeting of the Association for Social Anthropology in Oceania, 13–17 March 1974, Asilomar, Pacific Grove, California.
Shalloo, J. P.
1941   Some cultural factors in the etiology of alcoholism. *Quarterly Journal of Studies on Alcohol* 2: 464–78.
Sharp, Lauriston
1952   Steel axes for stone age Australians. In *Exploring human problems in technological change: a casebook,* edited by Edward Spicer. New York: Russell Sage Foundation.
Shineberg, Dorothy, ed.
1971   *The trading voyages of Andrew Cheyne 1841–1884.* Pacific History Series no. 3. Canberra and Honolulu: University of Hawaii Press.
Shore, J. H., and B. Von Fumetti
1972   Three alcohol programs for American Indians. *American Journal of Psychiatry* 128: 1450–54.
Shortt, A.
1914   The colony and its economic relations. In *Canada and its provinces,* edited by A. Shortt and A. G. Doughty, Vol. 2. Toronto and Glasgow: Brook & Co.
Sievers, M. L.
1968   Cigarette and alcohol usage by southwestern American Indians. *American Journal of Public Health* 58: 71–82.
Simmons, Ozzie G.
1959   Drinking patterns and interpersonal performance in a Peruvian mestizo community. *Quarterly Journal of Studies on Alcohol* 20: 103–11.
1960   Ambivalence and the learning of drinking behavior in a Peruvian community. *American Anthropologist* 62: 1018–27. Reprinted 1962. In *Society, culture and drinking patterns,* edited by David J. Pittman and Charles R. Snyder. New York: John Wiley & Sons.
Simpson, T. Beckford
1844   Pacific navigation and British seamen. *The Nautical Magazine and Naval Chronicle* 13: 99–103.
Smelser, N. J.
1963   Mechanisms of change and adjustment to change. In *Industrialization and society,* edited by B. F. Hoselitz and W. E. Moore. The Hague: UNESCO.
Snedecor, G. W., and Cochran, W. G.
1967   *Statistical methods.* 6th ed. Ames, Iowa: Iowa State University, Press.

Snyder, Charles R.
  1954   Culture and sobriety: a study of drinking patterns and sociocultural factors related to sobriety among Jews. Ph.D. dissertation, Yale University.
  1958   *Alcohol and the Jews: a cultural study of drinking and sobriety.* Rutgers Center of Alcohol Studies, monograph no. 1. New Brunswick, N.J.: Rutgers Center of Alcohol Studies Publications Division.
  1962   Culture and Jewish sobriety: the ingroup-outgroup factor. In *Society, culture and drinking patterns,* edited by David J. Pittman and Charles R. Snyder. New York: John Wiley & Sons.

Sobell, Linda C.; Mark B. Sobell; and William C. Christelman
  1972   The myth of one drink. *Behavior Research and Therapy* 10: 119–23.

Sokolov, I. S.
  1961   O protivoalkogol'noi propagande v SSSR i v kapitalisticheskikh stranakh. *Sovetskoe Zdravookhranenie,* no. 2.

Sovetskaia Rossiia
  1964   26 March, p. 4.

Sovetskaia torgovlia
  1959   12 May, 1959, p. 4.

Spaulding, P.
  1966   The social integration of a northern community: white mythology and métis reality." In *A northern dilemma: reference papers,* edited by A. K. Davis. 2 vols. Bellingham, Wash.: Western Washington State College.

Speck, Frank
  1931   Montagnais-Naskapi bands and early Eskimo distribution in the Labrador Peninsula. *American Anthropologist* 33: 557–600.

Speiser, Felix
  1913   *Two years with the natives in the western Pacific.* London: Mills & Boon.

Spindler, George D.
  1964   Alcohol symposium: editorial preview. *American Anthropologist* 66: 341–43.

Spoehr, Florence M.
  1963   *White Falcon. The house of Godeffroy and its commercial and scientific role in the Pacific.* Palo Alto: Pacific Books.

Spuhler, James N., and Clyde Kluckhohn
  1953   Inbreeding coefficients of the Ramah Navajo population. *Human Biology* 25: 295–317.

Srinivas, M. N.
  1955   The social system of a Mysore village. In *Village India,* edited by McKim Marriott. Chicago: The University of Chicago Press.

Srisavasi, B. C.
  1953   *Hill tribes of Siam.* Bangkok: Bamrung Nukoulit Press.

Stein, W. W.
  1961   *Hualcan: life in the highlands of Peru.* Ithaca: Cornell University Press.

Sterndale, H. B.
    1874   *Memoranda by Mr. Sterndale on some of the South Sea islands.*
            Wellington: George Didsbury, Government Printer.
Stevenson, Robert Louis
    1971   *In the South Seas.* Honolulu: University of Hawaii Press. Origi-
            nal edition 1900.
Stewart, Omer C.
    1964   Questions regarding Indian criminality. *Human Organization*
            23: 61–66.
Stoetzel, J.
    1955   *Without the chrysanthemum and the sword.* Paris: Heinemann.
    1958   Les caractéristiques de la consommation de l'alcool. Rapport à
            Presidence du conseil. Haut Comité d'étude et d'information
            sur l'alcoolisme.
Straus, R., and Selden D. Bacon
    1953   *Drinking in college.* New Haven: Yale University Press.
Strauss, W. Patrick
    1963   *Americans in Polynesia 1783–1842.* East Lansing: Michigan
            State University Press.
Suminoe, K.
    1962   *Nihon no sake.* (Japanese sake). Tokyo: Kawade shobō shinsha.
Szasz, T.
    1960   The myth of mental illness. *American Psychologist* 15: 113–18.
Szwed, John F.
    1966   Gossip, drinking and social control: consensus and communica-
            tion in a Newfoundland parish. *Ethnology* 5: 434–41.
Taylor, W. S.
    1948   Basic personality in orthodox Hindu culture patterns. *Journal of
            Abnormal and Social Psychology* 43: 3–12.
Thomas, Elizabeth
    1959   *The harmless people.* New York: Alfred A. Knopf.
Thompson, J. E. S.
    1940   *Mexico before Cortez.* New York: Scribner.
Thompson, Virginia, and Richard Adloff
    1971   *The French Pacific Islands. French Polynesia and New Caledo-
            nia.* Berkeley and Los Angeles: The University of California
            Press.
Thwaites, R. G., ed.
    1896   *The Jesuit Relations and allied documents.*73 vols. Cleveland:
            The Burrows Brothers.
Tkachevsky, I. M.
    1966   *Prestupnost' i alkogolizm.* Moscow.
Transkei
    1935   *Proceedings and reports.*
Transkeian Territories General Council
    1914   *Proceedings and reports.*
Transvaal Chamber of Mines
    1898   *Annual report.*
Transvaal, Liquor Commission
    1910   *Report of the Liquor Commission, 1910* (Annexure no. 10).

Transvaal, Mining Industry Commission
1897 *Minutes of evidence of the Mining Industry Commission.*
Turner, Lucien M.
1889–90 *Ethnology of the Ungava district, Hudson Bay Territory.* Eleventh Annual Report of the Bureau of American Ethnology. Washington, D.C.: Government Printing Office.
Turner, Victor W.
1957 *Schism and continuity in an African society.* Manchester: Manchester University Press.
Ullman, Albert D.
1958 Sociocultural backgrounds of alcoholism. *Annals of the American Academy of Political and Social Science* 315: 48–54.
1960 Ethnic differences in the first drinking experience. *Social Problems* 8: 45–56.
Union of South Africa
n.d. *Official Year Books.*
Union of South Africa, Commission of Assaults on Women
1913 *Report of the Commission of Assaults on Women* (U.G. 39–1913), pars. 57–58.
Union of South Africa, Economic Commission
1932 *Report of the Native Economic Commission* (U.G. 22–1932), par. 761.
Union of South Africa, Police Commission
1937 *Report of the Police Commission of Inquiry* (U.G. 50–1937), par. 276.
United Brethren, Church of the
1885 *Periodical accounts relating to the missions of the Church of the United Brethren* 33.
United States, Department of Health, Education and Welfare
1966 *Indian health highlights, 1966 edition.* Public Health Service, Bureau of Medical Services, Division of Indian Health. Washington, D.C.: Government Printing Office.
Uzzell, Douglas
1974 Susto revisited: illness as strategic role. *American Ethnologist* 1: 369–78.
Vaisberg, L., and S. Taibakova
1968 Alkogolizm i prestupnost' nesovershennoletnikh. In *Voprosy bor'by s prestupnost'iu nesovershennoletnikh,* edited by U. Dzhekebaev. Alma-Ata.
Veblen, Thorsten Bunde
1931 *The theory of the leisure class.* New York: Random House.
Viguera, Carmen, and Angel Palerm
1954 Alcoholismo brujeria, y homicidio en dos comunidades rurales de México. *América Indígena* 14: 7–36.
Vogel, E. F.
1963 *Japan's new middle class.* Berkeley and Los Angeles: University of California Press.
Waddell, Jack O.
1973 "Drink, friend!" Social contexts of convivial drinking and drunkenness among Papago Indians in an urban setting. In *Pro-*

ceedings of the First Annual Alcoholism Conference of the National Institute on Alcohol Abuse and Alcoholism, edited by Morris E. Chafetz. Rockville, Md.: National Institute on Alcohol Abuse and Alcoholism.

Walker, E. A.
1957   *A history of southern Africa.* 3d ed. London.

Wallace, Anthony F. C.
1956   Revitalization movements. *American Anthropologist* 58: 264–81.
1967   Identity processes in personality and in culture. In *Cognition, personality, and clinical psychology*, edited by Richard Jessor and Seymour Feshback. San Francisco: Jossey-Bass.
1970*a*   *The death and rebirth of the Seneca.* New York: Knopf.
1970*b*   Review of *New heaven, new earth*, by Kenelm Burridge. *American Anthropologist* 72: 1103–4.

Wallace, Anthony F. C., and Raymond D. Fogelson
1965   The identity struggle. In *Intensive family therapy*, edited by Ivan Boszormenyi-Nagy and James F. Framo. New York: Harper & Row.

Wallace, G. B.
1944   The marihuana problem in the city of New York: sociological, medical, psychological and pharmacological studies. New York: Cattell.

Walsh, B. M., and D. J. Walsh
1970   Economic aspects of alcohol consumption in the Republic of Ireland. *Economic and Social Review* 2: 115–38.

Ward, Roger L.
1974   Ponapean apology rituals: elaborations of the apology pattern in modern Ponape. Paper read at the Third Annual Meeting of the Association for Social Anthropology in Oceania, 13–17 March 1974, Asilomar, Pacific Grove, California.

Washburne, Chandler
1961   *Primitive drinking.* New York and New Haven: The College and University Press.

Watson, George
1972   *Nutrition and your mind: the psychochemical response.* New York: Harper & Row.

Wawn, William T.
1973   *The South Sea islanders and the Queensland labour trade*, edited by Peter Corris. Canberra and Honolulu: The University Press of Hawaii.

Wax, Rosalie, and Robert Thomas
1961   American Indians and white people. *Phylon* 22: 305–17.

Wedge, B. M., and S. Abe
1949   Racial incidence of mental diseases in Hawaii. *Hawaii Medical Journal* 8: 337–38.

Weld, I., Jr.
1800   *Travels through the states of North America and the provinces of upper and lower Canada during the years 1795, 1796, 1797.* London: John Stockdale.

Westermeyer, Joseph
    1968   The use of alcohol and opium by two ethnic groups in Laos. M.A. thesis, University of Minnesota.
    1972a Chippewa and majority alcoholism in the Twin Cities: a comparison. *Journal of Nervous and Mental Diseases* 155: 322–27.
    1972b Options regarding alcohol use among the Chippewa. *American Journal of Orthopsychiatry* 42: 398–403.
Westermeyer, Joseph, and J. Brantner
    1972   Violent death and alcohol use among the Chippewa in Minnesota. *Minnesota Medicine* 55: 749–52.
Westermeyer, Joseph, and G. Lange
    n.d.   Ethnic differences in use of alcoholism facilities. Unpublished paper.
Westwood, John
    1905   *Island stories.* Shanghai: *North China Herald* Office.
Wetmore, Charles H.
    1886   Report of visit to the mission of the Marshall and Caroline Islands. Unpublished paper.
Whittaker, James O.
    1963   Alcohol and the Standing Rock Sioux tribe. Pt. 2. Psychodynamic and cultural factors in drinking. *Quarterly Journal of Studies on Alcohol* 24: 80–90.
Wikler, Abraham
    1952   Mechanisms of actions of drugs that modify personality function. *American Journal of Psychiatry* 108: 590–99.
Wikler, Abraham, and Robert W. Rasor
    1953   Psychiatric aspects of drug addiction. *American Journal of Medicine* 14: 566–70.
Wilkes, Charles
    1845   *Narrative of the United States exploring expedition during the years 1838, 1839, 1840, 1841, 1842.* Vol. 5. Philadelphia: Lea & Blanchard.
Willems, E.
    1955   Protestantism as a factor of culture change in Brazil. *Economic Development and Culture Change* 3: 327–33.
Wolcott, Harry F.
    1974   *The African beer gardens of Bulawayo.* Rutgers Center of Alcohol Studies, monograph no. 10. New Brunswick, N.J.: Rutgers Center of Alcohol Studies.
Wolf, Eric R.
    1959   *Sons of the shaking earth.* Chicago: The University of Chicago Press.
    1966   *Peasants.* Englewood Cliffs, N.J.: Prentice-Hall.
Wolff, P. H.
    1973   Vasomotor sensitivity to alcohol in diverse Mongoloid populations. *American Journal of Human Genetics* 25: 193–99.
Wolff, P. O.
    1949   Problems of drug addiction in South America. *British Journal of Addiction* 46: 66–78.

Wood, C. F.
  1875   *A yachting cruise in the South Seas.* London: Henry S. King & Co.
Woolf, C. M., and F. C. Dukepoo
  1969   Hopi Indians: inbreeding and albinism. *Science* 164: 30–37.
Woolf, C. M., and R. B. Grant
  1962   Albinism among the Hopi Indians in Arizona. *American Journal of Human Genetics* 14: 391–400.
Worsley, Peter
  1957   *The trumpet shall sound: a study of "cargo" cults in Melanesia.* London: Macgibbon & Kee.
Wright, Louis B., and Mary Isabel Fry
  1936   *Puritans in the South Seas.* New York: Henry Holt & Co.
Yamamuro, Bufo
  1958   Japanese drinking patterns: alcoholic beverages in legend, history and contemporary religions. *Quarterly Journal of Studies on Alcohol* 19: 482–90.
Yanagida, K., ed.
  1957   *Japanese manners and customs in the Meiji era,* translated by C. S. Terry. Tokyo Ōbunsha.
Yanaihara, Tadao
  1940   *Pacific islands under Japanese mandate.* London: Oxford University Press.
Yih-fu, R.
  1962   The Miao: their origin and southward migration. Mimeographed. Proceedings of the Second Biennial Conference of the International Association of Historians of Asia, Taipei, Taiwan.
Young, A. C.
  1892   *A tour in Ireland in the years 1776, 1777, and 1778.* London: A. W. Hutton.
Young, G.
  1961   *Hill tribes of northern Thailand.* Bangkok: Siam Society.
Zeiner, Arthur R.
  1978   Are differences in the disulfiram-alcohol reaction the basis of racial differences in biological sensitivity to ethanol? Paper read at the National Drug Abuse Conference, April 1978, Seattle, Washington.

The University of Mi
Imprint Series in Ant

Vern Carroll, Series Editor

David M. Schneider and Raymond T. Smith
Class Differences in American Kinship

Mac Marshall, ASAO Monograph Series Editor

James Boutilier, Daniel Hughes, and Sharon Tiffany, editors
Mission, Church, and Sect in Oceania
(ASAO Monograph no. 6)

Margaret Rodman and Matthew Cooper, editors
The Pacification of Melanesia
(ASAO Monograph no. 7)

Available from University Microfilms International,
300 North Zeeb Road, Ann Arbor, Michigan 48106.